Fundamentals of
Body CT

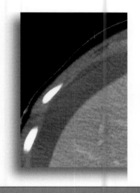

FUNDAMENTALS OF BODY CT

Third Edition

W. Richard Webb, M.D.
Chief, Thoracic Imaging, Professor of Radiology,
University of California San Francisco Medical School,
Department of Radiology, San Francisco, California, USA

William E. Brant, M.D.
Professor of Radiology, Director, ThoracoAbdominal
Imaging Division, University of Virginia Health System,
Department of Radiology, Charlottesville,
Virginia, USA

Nancy M. Major, M.D.
Associate Professor of Radiology and Surgery,
Duke University Medical Center, Division of
Musculoskeletal Imaging, Durham, North Carolina, USA

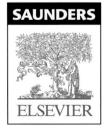

SAUNDERS

ELSEVIER

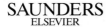

SAUNDERS
ELSEVIER

1600 John F. Kennedy Blvd.
Ste 1800
Philadephia, PA 19103-2899

FUNDAMENTALS OF BODY CT   ISBN 13: 978-1-4160-0030-3
Copyright 2006, 1998, 1991, Elsevier Inc. All rights reserved.   ISBN 10: 1-4160-0030-5

Notice

Knowledge and best practice in this field are constantly changing. As new research and experience
broaden our knowledge, changes in practice, treatment and drug therapy may become necessary or
appropriate. Readers are advised to check the most current information provided (i) on procedures
featured or (ii) by the manufacturer of each product to be administered, to verify the recommended dose
or formula, the method and duration of administration, and contraindications. It is the responsibility of
the practitioner, relying on their own experience and knowledge of the patient, to make diagnoses, to
determine dosages and the best treatment for each individual patient, and to take all appropriate safety
precautions. To the fullest extent of the law, neither the Publisher nor the Authors assume any liability
for any injury and/or damage to persons or property arising out of or related to any use of the material
contained in this book.

The Publisher

First Edition 1991.
Second Edition 1998.

Library of Congress Cataloging-in-Publication Data
  Webb, W. Richard (Wayne Richard), Fundamentals of body CT / W. Richard Webb,
William E. Brant, Nancy M. Major.—3rd ed.
    p.; cm.
  Includes bibliographical references and index.
  ISBN-13: 978-1-4160-0030-3   ISBN-10: 1-4160-0030-5
  1. Tomography. I. Brant, William E. II. Major, Nancy M. III. Title.
  [DNLM: 1. Tomography, X-Ray Computed. WN 206 W368f2006]
  RC78.7.T6W433 2006
  616.07'572–dc22   2005050437

Acquisitions Editor: *Meghan McAteer*
Editorial Assistant: *Ryan Creed*
Design Direction: *Steven Stave*

Printed in the United States of America

Last digit is the print number: 9 8 7 6 5 4

Working together to grow
libraries in developing countries

www.elsevier.com | www.bookaid.org | www.sabre.org

ELSEVIER   BOOK AID
               International   Sabre Foundatior

Preface

Writing the preface to a third edition is a pleasure for three reasons. First, it means the first two editions were successful, and the publishers are willing to go through the whole process again; second, it means that you are finally finished with the writing; and lastly, and most important, a new edition gives you the chance to add new material, correct mistakes, and bring things up to date.

The half dozen or so years since the second edition was published have seen a number of innovations and advances in CT techniques, most notably the development and maturation of multidetector spiral/helical CT. In this edition, we have updated our descriptions of CT techniques to include the various spiral/helical CT protocols now accepted in clinical practice for the diagnosis of chest, abdominal, and musculoskeletal abnormalities and have included some discussion of the role of spiral CT, three-dimensional CT, and CT angiography. Other recent CT developments are also included in this edition, and new topics and illustrations have been added to all chapters.

For example, in the chest section, discussions of high-resolution lung CT, CT diagnosis of pulmonary embolism, and aortic abnormalities have been expanded, in a fashion paralleling the expanded clinical use of these techniques. Also added in this edition is a chapter on abdominal trauma and discussions of CT for renal stone diagnosis. The musculoskeletal section has been revised and expanded to include three chapters dealing with traumatic and nontraumatic abnormalities and problematic bone findings detected incidentally on body CT exams.

At the same time, we have tried keep things simple, and have condensed some of the text in favor of lists and tables. We hope you enjoy and profit from our efforts.

W. Richard Webb
William E. Brant
Nancy M. Major

Preface to the First Edition

Instead of writing a text intended to record everything that is known about body CT or even everything that we know about body CT, we have attempted to write one that teaches how to perform and read body CT scans. In doing this, we have tried to limit ourselves to discussing what is key to understanding body CT from a practical clinical standpoint—the key anatomy, the key concepts, the key diseases, and the key controversies. We have done this at the risk of leaving a few things out, but it isn't necessary to read about everything when you are first learning a subject. In other words, *Fundamentals of Body CT* is not intended to provide more than the best CT texts on the market do, but rather less, with a different emphasis, and in a more manageable package.

Each of us has written a different part of this book, obviously depending on our areas of expertise. Since each of us teaches in a slightly different way, each of the three sections of the book—the thorax, the abdomen, and the musculoskeletal system—is somewhat different in approach. We hope that by preserving our individual styles we have made the book more interesting to read, and for us, it certainly made this book easier to write.

Contents

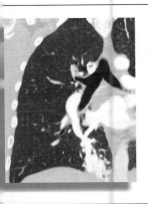

PART ONE

THE THORAX

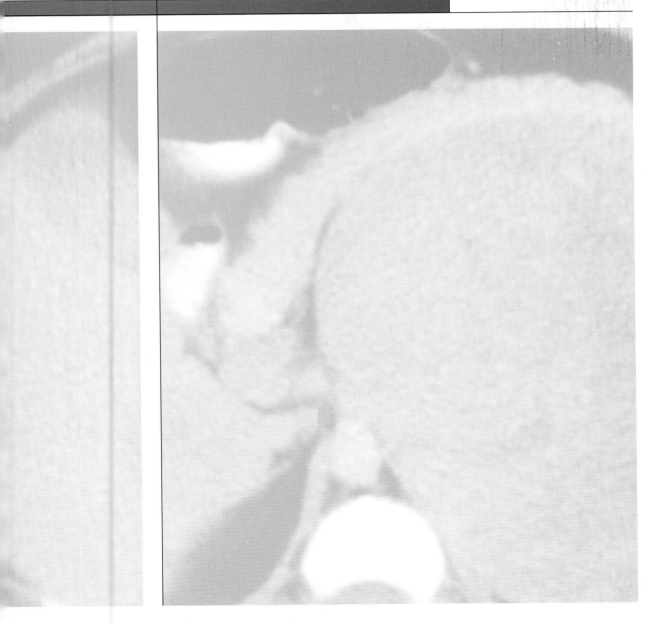

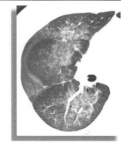

Introduction to CT of the
Thorax: Chest CT Techniques

W. Richard Webb, M.D.

Spiral computed tomography (CT) allows the entire chest to be imaged during a single breath hold in cooperative patients, with volumetric acquisition and exact registration or overlapping of slices. Three-dimensional reformations may be performed. Because scanning is rapid, contrast agents can be injected quickly, and excellent vascular opacification can be achieved.

☐ SPIRAL CT: TYPES OF SCANNERS

Spiral CT scanners are of two types: single-detector CT (SDCT) and multidetector CT (MDCT) scanners. The techniques used for chest CT vary significantly depending on whether an SDCT or MDCT scanner is used. The next section briefly reviews these techniques.

Single-Detector Spiral CT

Single-detector scanners have a single row of x-ray detectors that are used to record data as the gantry rotates around the patient and the patient moves through the gantry. A single continuous spiral acquisition is obtained. The thickness of the slice is determined primarily by the thickness of the x-ray beam (collimation).

With SDCT, five scan parameters must be chosen prospectively. These are (1) gantry rotation time (time for a complete rotation of the scanner gantry), (2) total scan duration, (3) the scan volume, (4) collimation (the thickness of the x-ray beam used), and (5) pitch (table excursion during a complete gantry rotation divided by collimation). The relation of these factors is governed by a simple formula (Fig. 1-1).

Values for gantry rotation time, scan volume, and scan duration are described later in this chapter and are usually determined by the patient's ability to suspend respiration. Of the remaining two variables, collimation and pitch, only one can be controlled independently. Pitch varies at intervals between 1 and 2, depending on the scanner (e.g., 1, 1.3, 1.7, 2). Collimation varies at intervals from 1 to 10 mm (e.g., 1, 3, 5, 7, 10 mm).

Multidetector Spiral CT

MDCT scanners, also known as multidetector row CT, have multiple parallel rows of x-ray detectors (currently, 4, 8, 16, or 64 for different machines). Each of the rows records data independently as the gantry rotates; consequently, a much larger patient volume is imaged with each rotation. Having a 16-detector MDCT

Parameters for SDCT

$$\text{Scan duration (sec)} = \frac{\text{rotation time (sec)} \times \text{scan volume (mm)}}{\text{collimation (mm)} \times \text{pitch}}$$

FIGURE 1-1 Parameters for single-detector computed tomography (SDCT).

scanner is like having 16 SDCT scanners working together.

An MDCT scanner has the advantages of being much faster than an SDCT and allows images to be reconstructed with different thicknesses after the study is done. In clinical practice, SDCT scanners are gradually being replaced by MDCT, and MDCT with 16 or 64 rows are gradually upgrading those with fewer rows.

With MDCT, pitch is determined by the table excursion during a complete gantry rotation divided by the width of all the detectors used (e.g., detector width × number of detector rows). As with SDCT, pitch usually ranges from 1 to 2. Although it varies with the scanner and manufacturer, the thinnest detector rows are about 0.5 to 1 mm in width, and the multiple scanner rows add up to about 20 mm for 16 detector scanners and 40 mm for 64 detector scanners. For MDCT, the formula relating scan parameters is shown in Fig. 1-2.

☐ SPIRAL CHEST CT: GENERAL PRINCIPLES

The specific protocols used for chest CT depend on the type of scanner used, the scanner manufacturer, and the reason for the study. However, several general principles apply to all chest scans (Table 1-1).

Scan Levels

Chest CT is usually obtained from a level just above the lung apices (near the suprasternal notch) to the level of the posterior costophrenic angles; these scans also encompass the diaphragm and the upper abdomen. The distance (or volume) needed to cover the thorax is determined by a preliminary projection scan (e.g., "scout view"), and usually it is about 25 cm.

Patient Position

Routinely, patients are scanned supine. Prone scans may be obtained for high-resolution CT (HRCT) or to assess movement of pleural fluid collections. The patient may also be positioned prone for biopsy of posterior lung lesions.

Lung Volume

Scans are routinely obtained after a full inspiration (i.e., at total lung capacity) and during suspended respiration. Expiratory scans may be performed in some cases (particularly on HRCT) to assess air trapping.

Gantry Rotation Time

A rapid gantry rotation time is used to reduce scan time. Times are usually less than 1 second (e.g., 0.6 to 0.8 second).

TABLE 1-1

Chest CT: General Principles

Scan levels: lung apices to the posterior costophrenic angles

Patient position: supine

Lung volume: full inspiration; single breath hold if possible

Gantry rotation time: rapid

Scan duration: total scan duration determined by breath hold; trade-off between scan duration and resolution

Slice thickness and pitch: increase pitch (up to 2) rather than collimation or detector thickness

Reconstruction algorithm: high-resolution algorithm used for most studies; standard or soft-tissue algorithm for vascular studies

Three-dimensional reconstructions: occasionally useful for lung, airway, or vascular studies

Contrast agents: intravenous contrast injection in some cases; oral contrast agents only for gastrointestinal abnormalities

Window settings: viewed using lung and soft-tissue (mediastinal) windows

Parameters for MDCT

$$\text{Scan duration (sec)} = \frac{\text{rotation time (sec)} \times \text{scan volume (mm)}}{\text{detector row width (mm)} \times \text{number of detectors} \times \text{pitch}}$$

FIGURE 1-2 Parameters for multidetector computed tomography (MDCT).

Slice Thickness and Pitch

The collimation (SDCT) or detector row width (MDCT) chosen for a CT examination depends on the reason for the study. Thinner slices are required for some specific indications, whereas thicker slices are appropriate for routine studies.

Keep in mind that with spiral technique, the actual thickness of the slice you view (i.e., "effective slice thickness") may be greater than the collimation or detectors used, depending on the pitch; the greater the pitch is, the greater the effective slice thickness is. With a pitch of 1, the effective slice thickness is approximately equal to collimation; with a pitch of 2, the effective slice thickness is about 30% greater than the collimation.

A general rule with spiral CT of the chest is that it is better to increase the pitch to cover a given area during the patient's breath hold than it is to increase the collimation or detector width; increasing the pitch generally results in better resolution. For example, doubling the pitch (i.e., from 1 to 2) results in an increase in effective slice thickness of only about 30%; doubling the collimation or detector width results in a doubling of the effective slice thickness.

Scan Duration

The total scan duration or imaging time is generally determined by the patient's ability to suspend respiration; most patients can hold their breath for 20 to 25 seconds, and these values are often assumed for routine scanning. If the patient is uncooperative (i.e., cannot hold his or her breath) or a longer scan duration is needed, then image degradation resulting from respiratory motion is likely to occur.

There is a fundamental trade-off in chest CT between the duration of the scan and the resolution obtainable. If thin scans and high resolution are desired, the scan takes longer to obtain and artifacts resulting from respiratory motion are more likely to occur. If thicker scans are obtained, then the scan may be obtained quickly without a risk of respiratory motion, but spatial resolution is reduced. This trade-off must be kept in mind when deciding on a scan protocol.

Reconstruction Algorithm

Once the scans have been performed, the scan data are reconstructed using an algorithm that determines some characteristics of the resul-

ting image. For routine chest imaging, a high-resolution algorithm is often used to optimize detail, but this makes the image somewhat grainy in appearance.

A standard or soft-tissue algorithm, which produces a smoother image, is better for assessing thoracic vascular structures (e.g., studies performed for diagnosis of pulmonary embolism, aneurysm, or aortic dissection) but is not optimal for other chest imaging. This algorithm is often used for abdominal imaging.

Three-Dimensional Reconstruction

Because the scan data are acquired continuously and volumetrically using spiral CT, scans may be reconstructed in any plane desired, if appropriate workstations are available. However, these techniques may be time-consuming to perform, and depending on the collimation or detector row width selected, reconstructed images may have reduced spatial resolution. A variety of display techniques have been used for imaging the thorax. These include multiplanar reconstructions, three-dimensional shaded surface or volume rendering from an external perspective, or shaded surface or volume rendering from an internal (endoluminal) perspective, also known as virtual bronchoscopy.

Multiplanar, two-dimensional reconstructions offer the advantage of being quickly performed and are sufficient for diagnosis in most cases in which a reformation is considered desirable. Subsequent chapters provide a number of examples of two-dimensional reconstructions. Three-dimensional techniques, such as shaded surface display and volume rendering, can be valuable in selected cases, but they are time-consuming and require considerable operator experience. These techniques are not commonly used in clinical chest imaging, with exception of virtual bronchoscopy or airway imaging and specialized vascular imaging.

Maximum- or minimum-intensity projection images representing a slab of three-dimensional data reconstructed from a volumetric data set may sometimes be useful in imaging pulmonary, airway, or vascular abnormalities.

Contrast Agents

Chest CT can be performed with or without the administration of an intravenous contrast agent, depending on the indication for the study. Scans obtained to rule out pulmonary metastases or to assess lung disease generally do not require contrast. Contrast should be used in patients with suspected hilar, mediastinal, or pleural abnormalities and in patients with possible vascular abnormalities.

With a spiral scanner, injecting contrast at 2.5 to 4 mL/second, 10 to 30 seconds before scanning begins and for the duration of the scan series, provides excellent opacification of vascular structures. The rate of contrast injection and the scan delay (the time between the start of contrast injection and the start of scanning) vary depending on the reason for the study.

Scanning is begun when the vessels of interest are opacified. For pulmonary embolism diagnosis, the pulmonary arteries need to be opacified; this usually requires a 15- to 20-second delay. For diagnosis of aortic abnormalities, a longer delay of usually 20 to 30 seconds is needed. The delay varies in individual patients according to a number of factors. Timing the scan delay is usually done using software available on the scanner, which shows vascular opacification during the injection. The use of an oral contrast agent for opacification of the esophagus and gastrointestinal tract is not necessary unless a specific gastrointestinal (i.e., esophageal) abnormality is suspected.

Window Settings

For chest CT, scans must be viewed using at least two different window settings. These two windows are appropriately named "lung" and "soft-tissue" (or "mediastinal") windows, which also describe their primary use.

Lung windows typically have a window mean of approximately −600 to −700 H and a window width of 1000 to 1500 H. Lung windows best demonstrate lung anatomy and pathology, contrasting soft-tissue structures with surrounding air-filled lung parenchyma.

Mediastinal or *soft-tissue windows* (window mean, 20 to 40 H; width, 450 to 500 H) demonstrate soft-tissue anatomy in the mediastinum and in other areas of the thorax, allowing the differentiation of fat, fluid, tissue, calcium, and contrast-opacified vessels. This window is also of value in providing information about consolidated lung, the hila, pleural disease, and structures of the chest wall. Subsequent chapters discuss more specific uses of these two windows.

☐ SPIRAL CHEST CT: PROTOCOLS

In most patients, chest CT is performed using a routine protocol. This technique is designed to provide useful (although not necessarily optimal) information about the lung, mediastinum, hila, pleura, and chest wall. It is valuable in the diagnosis of a variety of diseases and types of abnormalities.

Modified CT techniques are used in specific clinical settings or to look for specific abnormalities (e.g., pulmonary embolism, aortic dissection, and diffuse lung disease). Subsequent chapters provide detailed reviews of some specific protocols.

Routine Chest CT

A useful routine technique is to obtain scans with 5-mm collimation when using SDCT. With a gantry rotation time of 0.8 second and assuming a volume of 25 cm for the entire thorax, a breath hold of less than 25 seconds requires a pitch of 1.7 and results in an effective slice thickness of about 6 mm (Table 1-2). Other scan techniques may be used (see Table 1-2), but they result in differences in effective slice thickness, breath hold duration, scan volume, and the volume of contrast used (if contrast is injected). Scans may be reconstructed at contiguous levels (i.e., 5-mm collimation scans reconstructed every 5 mm), or they may be reconstructed at overlapping levels (i.e., 5-mm collimation scans reconstructed every 3 mm). Overlapping of reconstructions has been shown to improve the detection of small lesions (e.g., small nodules). With SDCT, resolution can be optimized by decreasing collimation and pitch and scanning a limited volume (e.g., 2 cm; see Table 1-2).

With a 16-row detector MDCT scanner, I routinely scan the chest using 1.25-mm detector width, with a pitch of 1.6 and a gantry rotation time of 0.6 second. This allows the entire thorax to be scanned in less than 5 seconds. The scan data can be reconstructed with a thickness of 5 mm (effective slice thickness, 6 mm) for routine reading or 1.25 mm (effective slice thickness, 1.5 mm) for high-resolution imaging (see Table 1-2). If MDCT is available, this is the preferred technique for routine chest imaging. As indicated earlier, the use of intravenous or oral

TABLE 1-2
Possible Variations in Routine Spiral CT Protocol

Scanner Type	Collimation Detectors and Pitch	Effective Slice Thickness (mm)	Gantry Rotation Time (seconds)	Breath Hold (seconds)	Scan Volume (cm)	Contrast Injection Rate (mL/second)	Contrast Volume (15-second delay) (mL)
SDCT	7-mm collimation; pitch of 1	7	0.8	28	25	2.5	107.5
	5-mm collimation; pitch of 1.7	6	0.8	24	25	2.5	97.5
	5-mm collimation; pitch of 1.5	5.5	0.8	27	25	2.5	105
	3-mm collimation; pitch of 2	4	0.8	33	25	2.5	120
	1-mm collimation; pitch of 1	1	0.8	16	2		
MDCT	16 × 1.25-mm detectors; pitch of 1.6	1.5 or 6	0.6	4.7	25	3.5	70

contrast agents depends on the indication for the study.

Vascular Imaging Protocols

In some patients, chest CT is performed primarily for the diagnosis of a vascular abnormality suspected on the basis of clinical symptoms or radiographic findings. Common thoracic vascular abnormalities assessed using CT include pulmonary embolism, aortic dissection or aneurysm, and traumatic aortic rupture (Table 1-3). Examples of protocols are listed in Table 1-3, although these vary among scanners and institutions. Vascular protocols attempt to optimize the degree of contrast enhancement and image resolution while keeping the length of breath hold and the amount of contrast injected at a reasonable value.

Pulmonary Embolism

For diagnosis of pulmonary embolism with a single-detector spiral CT, one obtains scans with 3-mm collimation and a pitch of 2 through the central pulmonary arteries only, a volume measuring approximately 12 cm (see Table 1-3). This requires a 16-second breath hold and yields scans with an effective slice thickness of approximately 4 mm. Reconstruction of scans at 2-mm intervals (i.e., overlapping of images) is typical and improves accuracy.

With MDCT, scanning with 1.25-mm detectors requires a breath hold of less than 5 seconds and provides scans with an effective slice thickness of 1.5 mm through the entire thorax. Overlapping of scan reconstruction is not necessary. The advantages of using MDCT are obvious.

Intravenous contrast is injected rapidly (e.g., 4 mL/second). Scanning is begun when the scanner shows the pulmonary arteries or left atrium to be opacified. This delay varies, but it averages about 15 seconds. Because of its more rapid scan time, less contrast is injected when MDCT is used (see Table 1-3).

Aortic Disease

Aortic abnormalities assessed using CT include dissection, aneurysm, and traumatic aortic rupture. With SDCT, scans may be obtained from just above the aortic arch to the diaphragm, a distance of about 20 cm. With MDCT, scans through the entire thorax may be obtained with the same protocol used for pulmonary embolism diagnosis, if only the thoracic aorta is being examined (see Table 1-3).

If imaging of the abdominal aorta is also required (e.g., for aortic dissection), scans are usually obtained using a thicker collimation or detector width (e.g., 5 mm for SDCT and 2.5 mm for MDCT). This enables scanning of the much larger volume during the continuous injection of contrast. Breath holding is required only for scans through the thorax. Quiet breathing during the abdominal portion of the scan is usually allowed.

Intravenous contrast is injected rapidly (e.g., 4 mL/second) for imaging of the thoracic aorta. If scanning of the abdominal aorta is also necessary, the rate of injection is usually reduced (e.g., 2.5 mL/second) to keep the total contrast volume at a reasonable level. Scanning is begun when the scanner shows the aorta to be opacified. The delay may range from 20 to 30 seconds.

High-Resolution CT

HRCT is used to diagnose diffuse lung diseases, emphysema, bronchiectasis, and focal lung lesions (i.e., a solitary nodule). HRCT requires thin collimation or detector width (1 to 2 mm) and image reconstruction using a sharp (high-resolution) algorithm. Injection of contrast is not necessary for HRCT.

With 7-, 5-, or even 3-mm collimation or detector width, volume averaging in the plane of scan significantly reduces the ability of CT to resolve small structures. Volume averaging means that various different densities and structures present in the same volume element (voxel) are averaged together in the final image or picture element (pixel) representing that voxel, thus obscuring details or edges that may be important in diagnosis. Thin collimation allows anatomic detail to be seen more clearly.

Reconstruction of the scan data using a sharp or high-resolution algorithm (e.g., the "bone" algorithm available on some machines) reduces image smoothing and increases spatial resolution, making structures appear sharper. Although using a sharp algorithm also increases image noise, only rarely does this create a problem in interpretation.

HRCT protocols are described further in Chapter 6. Basically, HRCT may be performed in two different ways:

TABLE 1-3

Spiral CT Protocols for Vascular Diseases

Scanner Type	Indication	Collimation, Detectors, and Pitch	Effective Slice Thickness (mm)	Gantry Rotation Time (seconds)	Breath Hold (seconds)	Scan Volume	Contrast Injection Rate (mL/second)	Contrast Volume (15-second delay) (mL)
SDCT	PE	3-mm collimation; pitch of 2	4	0.8	16	12 cm	4	124
MDCT	PE	16 × 1.25-mm detectors; pitch of 1.6	1.5	0.6	4.7	25 cm	4	79
SDCT	Thoracic aorta	5-mm collimation; pitch of 2	6.5	0.8	16	Aortic arch to diaphragm (20 cm)	4	124
MDCT	Thoracic aorta	16 × 1.25-mm detectors; pitch 1.6	1.5	0.6	4.7	25 cm	4	79
MDCT	Dissection	8 × 2.5-mm detectors; pitch 1.6	3	0.6	4.7 (for thorax)	Aortic arch to aortic bifurcation	2.5	79 (for thorax)

MDCT, multidetector spiral computed tomography; PE, pulmonary embolism; SDCT, single-detector spiral computed tomography.

1. HRCT is often obtained without spiral technique, even if a spiral scanner is used. Thin slices are performed individually (or in clusters) at spaced intervals (i.e., 1 to 2 cm) without table movement to optimize spatial resolution.
2. Volumetric HRCT may be performed using the spiral technique. MDCT and 1- to 1.25-mm detector rows are required to image the entire thorax during a single breath hold. However, volumetric imaging usually is not necessary for diagnosis and results in an increased radiation dose.

Dynamic CT

The term *dynamic CT* means that a number of scans are performed in sequence. Because spiral scanning is continuous, it is a dynamic technique, but dynamic scanning can also be performed without a spiral technique (i.e., without table and patient motion during the acquisition of scans). Dynamic scanning may be performed at a single level during expiration to detect air trapping or to assess tracheal or bronchial collapse in patients with tracheomalacia or airways disease. Dynamic scanning may also be performed to assess some vascular abnormalities.

Low-Dose CT

Reducing radiation dose is desirable when possible, but it generally results in a decrease in image quality because of increased noise. CT radiation dose may be reduced to some degree by increasing gantry rotation time, pitch, or slice thickness; by spacing scans (as in HRCT); or by using other more complicated techniques. However, the term *low-dose CT* usually implies the use of a reduced tube current (milliamperage, mA) or sometimes the kilovolt peak (kVp) during the scan. Reducing milliamperage to one-fourth of routine milliamperage still results in readable images in most patients. In large patients, however, low-dose CT may not be possible. Low-dose chest CT is usually used in children, for screening patients (i.e., for lung cancer screening), or if multiple follow-up examinations are necessary.

▨ SUGGESTED READING

ARAKAWA H, WEBB WR: Expiratory high-resolution CT scan. Radiol Clin N Am 36:189–209, 1998.

COSTELLO P, DUPUY DE, ECKER CP, TELLO R: Spiral CT of the thorax with reduced volume of contrast material: A comparative study. Radiology 185:663–666, 1992.

DILLON EH, VAN LEEUWEN MS, FERNANDEZ MA, MALI WP: Spiral CT angiography. AJR Am J Roentgenol 160:1273–1278, 1993.

HEIKEN JP, BRINK JA, VANNIER MW: Spiral (helical) CT. Radiology 189:647–656, 1993.

KALENDER WA, SEISSLER W, KLOTZ E, VOCK P: Spiral volumetric CT with single-breath-hold technique, continuous transport, and continuous scanner rotation. Radiology 176:181–183, 1990.

LAWLER LP, FISHMAN EK: Multi-detector row CT of thoracic disease with emphasis on 3D volume rendering and CT angiography. Radiographics 21:1257–1273, 2001.

MAHESH M: Search for isotropic resolution in CT from conventional through multiple-row detector. Radiographics 22:949–962, 2001.

MAYO JR: The high-resolution computed tomography technique. Semin Roentgenol 26:104–109, 1991.

MAYO JR, WEBB WR, GOULD R, et al: High-resolution CT of the lungs: An optimal approach. Radiology 163:507–510, 1987.

PARANJPE DV, BERGIN CJ: Spiral CT of the lungs: Optimal technique and resolution compared with conventional CT. AJR Am J Roentgenol 162:561–567, 1994.

RUBIN GD, NAPEL S, LEUNG AN: Volumetric analysis of volumetric data: Achieving a paradigm shift. Radiology 200:312–317, 1996.

ZWIREWICH CV, MAYO JR, MÜLLER NL: Low-dose high-resolution CT of lung parenchyma. Radiology 180:413–417, 1991.

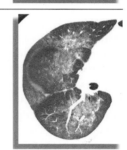

Mediastinum: Introduction and Normal Anatomy

W. Richard Webb, M.D.

Computed tomography (CT) is commonly used in patients suspected of having a mediastinal mass or vascular abnormality (e.g., an aortic aneurysm), because its ability to image mediastinal anatomy is far superior to that of conventional radiographic techniques. In general, CT of the mediastinum is obtained in two situations.

First, CT is almost always performed in patients who have an abnormality visible on plain radiographs that is suggestive or indicative of mediastinal pathology. In patients with a visible mass, CT can be helpful in confirming the presence of a significant lesion (mediastinal contour abnormalities seen, or imagined, on plain films do not always reflect a real abnormality); defining its location; determining the relation of the lesion to vascular or nonvascular structures from which it may be arising or is involving; showing other, unrecognized mediastinal lesions; and characterizing the mass as solid, cystic, vascular, enhancing, calcified, inhomogeneous, fatty, and so on. Although CT may not be able to diagnose a lesion with certainty, it may be possible to limit the differential diagnosis to a few entities, and this may determine the most appropriate next step, be it percutaneous biopsy, mediastinoscopy, surgery, arteriography, or no further testing.

Second, CT is often used to evaluate the mediastinum in patients who have normal chest radiographs but who also have a clinical reason that makes one suspect mediastinal disease. Chest films are relatively insensitive to mediastinal abnormalities. One example is a patient with lung cancer in whom enlarged mediastinal nodes might be detected using CT despite a normal chest radiograph. Another example is a patient with myasthenia gravis who, therefore, has a significant chance of having a thymoma (approximately 15%) that may be detected on CT.

☐ NORMAL MEDIASTINAL ANATOMY

The mediastinum is the tissue compartment situated between the lungs, marginated on each side by the mediastinal pleura, anteriorly by the sternum and chest wall, and posteriorly by the spine and chest wall. It contains the heart, great vessels, trachea, esophagus, thymus, considerable fat, and a number of lymph nodes, which are grouped together in specific regions. Many of these structures can be reliably identified on CT by their location, appearance, and attenuation.

11

In general, the mediastinum can be thought of as consisting of three almost equal divisions, the first beginning at the thoracic inlet and the third ending at the diaphragm. In adults, each of these divisions is made up of about 15 contiguous 5-mm slices. For lack of official anatomic names, these can be remembered as follows:

1. The *supra-aortic mediastinum*: from the thoracic inlet to the top of the aortic arch.
2. The *subaortic mediastinum*: from the aortic arch to the superior aspect of the heart.
3. The *paracardiac mediastinum*: from the heart to the diaphragm.

In each of these compartments, specific structures are consistently seen, and these need to be evaluated in every patient. Although very detailed mediastinal anatomy can be seen using CT, this description of normal anatomy is limited to the most significant structures. If a more detailed knowledge of mediastinal anatomy is desired, there are a number of excellent atlases of cross-sectional anatomy. My main goal here is to provide an approach to viewing the mediastinum.

Supra-Aortic Mediastinum

In evaluating a CT scan of this part of the mediastinum, it is a good idea to localize the trachea before doing anything else (Fig. 2-1*A*). The trachea is easy to recognize because it contains air, is seen in cross section, and has a reasonably consistent round or oval shape. It is relatively central in the mediastinum, from front to back and from right to left, and it serves as an excellent reference point. Many other mediastinal structures maintain a consistent relation to it. If you are unable to find the trachea on a scan of this part of the mediastinum, I would suggest giving up right now.

At or near the thoracic inlet, the mediastinum is relatively narrow from front to back. The esophagus lies posterior to the trachea at this level (see Fig. 2-1), but depending on the position of the trachea relative to the spine, the esophagus can be displaced to one side or the other, usually the left side. It is usually collapsed and appears as a flattened structure of soft-tissue attenuation, but small amounts of air or air and fluid are often seen in its lumen.

In the supra-aortic mediastinum, the great arterial branches of the aortic arch and the great veins are the most important structures to recognize. At or near the thoracic inlet, the brachiocephalic veins are the most anterior and lateral vascular branches visible, lying immediately behind the clavicular heads (see Fig. 2-1*A* and *B*). Although they vary in size, their positions are relatively constant. The great arterial branches (innominate, left carotid, and left subclavian arteries) are posterior to the veins and lie adjacent to the anterior and lateral walls of the trachea. They can be reliably identified by their relative positions.

Below the thoracic inlet, anterior to the arterial branches of the aorta, the left brachiocephalic vein crosses the mediastinum from left to right (see Fig. 2-1*C*), to join the right brachiocephalic vein, thus forming the superior vena cava (see Fig. 2-1*C* and *D*). The left subclavian artery is most posterior and is situated adjacent to the left side of the trachea, at the 3 or 4 o'clock position relative to the tracheal lumen. The left carotid artery is anterior to the left subclavian artery, at 1 or 2 o'clock, and is somewhat variable in position. The innominate artery is usually anterior and somewhat to the right of the tracheal midline (11 o'clock), but it is the most variable of all the great vessels and can have a number of different appearances in different patients or in the same patient at different levels (see Fig. 2-1*D*).

Near its origin from the aortic arch, the innominate artery is usually oval, being somewhat larger than the other aortic branches. As it ascends toward the thoracic outlet, it may appear oval or elliptical, because of its orientation or because of its bifurcation into the right subclavian and carotid arteries. Also, this vessel can be quite tortuous and can appear double if both limbs of a U-shaped part of the vessel are imaged in the same slice. Usually, these vessels can be traced from their origin at the aortic arch to the point they leave the chest, if there is any doubt as to what they represent.

Other than the great vessels, trachea, and esophagus, little is usually seen in the supra-aortic mediastinum. Some lymph nodes are sometimes visible. Small vascular branches, particularly the internal mammary veins, can be seen in this part of the mediastinum. In some patients, the thyroid gland may extend into this portion of the mediastinum, and the right and left thyroid lobes may be visible on each side of the trachea. This appearance is not abnormal and does not imply thyroid enlargement or "sub-

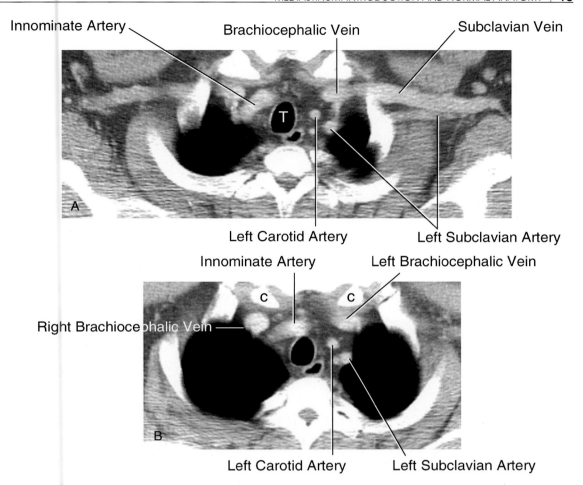

FIGURE 2-1 **Supra-aortic mediastinum.** *A,* At the thoracic inlet, the trachea (T) is clearly seen, with the air-filled esophagus posterior and to the left of it. The right and left brachiocephalic veins are anterior and lateral, being seen behind the clavicular heads. At this level, the axillary veins are also visible (within the axilla). The great arterial branches (innominate, left carotid, and left subclavian arteries) are posterior to the veins, lying adjacent to the anterior and lateral walls of the trachea. The innominate artery appears elliptical because of its orientation in the plane of scan. *B,* Just below *A,* the brachiocephalic veins are visible posterior to the clavicular heads (C). The left subclavian artery is most posterior and is situated lateral to the left tracheal wall, at the 3 or 4 o'clock position relative to the tracheal lumen, and contacting the mediastinal pleura. The left carotid artery is anterior to the left subclavian artery, at about the 2 o'clock position, and is somewhat variable in position. The innominate artery is usually anterior and to the right of the tracheal midline.

Continued

sternal thyroid." On CT, the thyroid can be distinguished from other tissues or masses because its attenuation is greater than that of soft tissue (because of its iodine content).

Subaortic Mediastinum

Like the supra-aortic region, in adults, the subaortic mediastinum consists of approximately fifteen 5-mm scans, extending from the aortic arch to the upper heart (Fig. 2-2). Whereas the supra-aortic region largely contains arterial and venous branches of the aorta and vena cava, this compartment contains many of the undivided mediastinal great vessels, such as the aorta, superior vena cava, and pulmonary arteries. This compartment also contains most of the important lymph nodes groups, which may be abnormal in patients with lung cancer, infectious diseases, sarcoidosis, or lymphoma. In other words, on most CT studies of the mediastinum, this is where the action is. A few key levels in this part of the mediastinum need to be discussed in detail.

Aortic Arch Level

In the upper portion of the subaortic mediastinum compartment, the aortic arch is seen easily

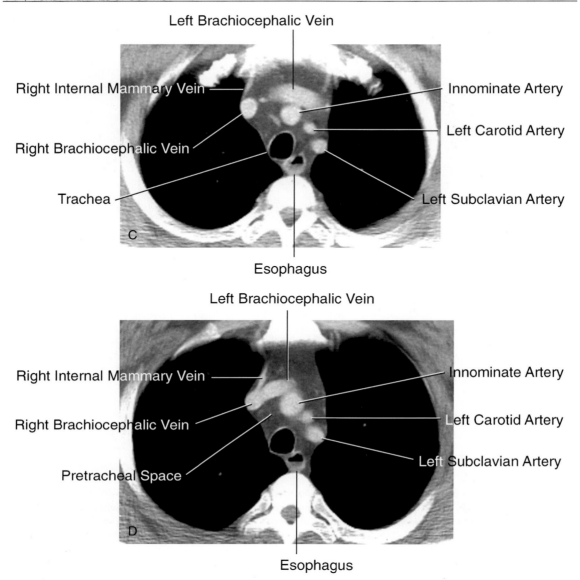

FIGURE 2-1 Cont'd C, At a level below B, the left brachiocephalic vein is visible crossing the mediastinum from left to right. The subclavian, carotid, and innominate arteries maintain the same relative positions as in B. The right internal mammary vein is visible arising from the right brachiocephalic vein. The esophagus contains a small amount of fluid in its lumen, with an air–fluid level visible. D, At a level below C, the left brachiocephalic vein joins the right brachiocephalic vein, forming the superior vena cava. The major aortic branches are again clearly seen. The pretracheal space is anterior to the trachea and posterior to the arteries and veins.

Continued

and has a characteristic but somewhat variable appearance (see Fig. 2-2*A* and *B*). The anterior aspect of the arch is seen anterior to the trachea, with the arch itself passing to the left of the trachea, and the posterior arch is usually lying anterior and lateral to the spine. Usually, the aortic arch is about the same diameter in its anterior and midportion, although the posterior arch is typically a little smaller. The position of the anterior and posterior aspects of the arch can vary in the presence of atherosclerosis and aortic tortuosity; in patients with a tortuous aorta, the anterior arch is displaced anteriorly and to the right, whereas the posterior aorta is displaced more laterally and posteriorly, to a position to the left of the spine.

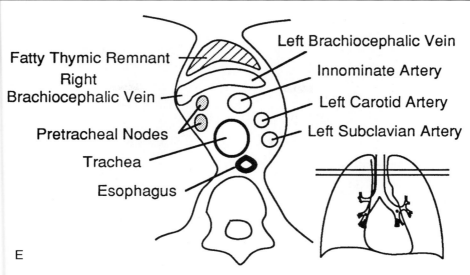

E

FIGURE 2-1 **Cont'd** *E,* Diagram of supra-aortic anatomy at the level of *D.* The location of pretracheal lymph nodes is shown, although these are not visible in the scan. Also, although not seen well in *D,* the location of the thymic remnant is marked. The approximate level of the scan in *D* is indicated by *horizontal lines.* Some structures indicated here are not visible in the scans.

At this level, the superior vena cava is visible anterior and to the right of the trachea, usually being oval in shape (see Fig. 2-2*A* to *D*). The esophagus appears the same as at higher levels and is variable in position. Often, it lies somewhat to the left of the midline of the trachea (and, of course, is behind the trachea).

The aortic arch on the left, the superior vena cava and mediastinal pleura on the right, and the trachea posteriorly serve to define a

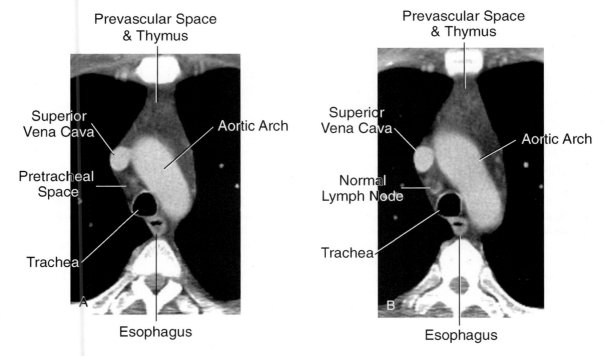

FIGURE 2-2 **Subaortic mediastinum.** *A,* Aortic arch level. The aortic arch extends from a position anterior to the trachea, to the left, with the posterior part of the arch usually lying anterior and lateral to the spine. The superior vena cava contacts the right mediastinal pleura and together with the aortic arch delineates the anterior aspect of the pretracheal space. The prevascular space is anterior to the great vessels and contains the thymus, which is largely replaced by fat in this patient. *B,* The locations of the pretracheal node-bearing space and prevascular space, containing the thymic remnant, are indicated. A normal pretracheal node is visible.

Continued

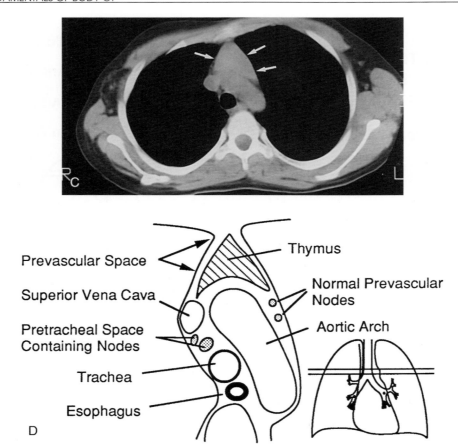

FIGURE 2-2 Cont'd *C,* A large normal thymus *(arrows)* in a young patient occupies most of the prevascular space. *D,* Diagram of the anatomy at the aortic arch level.

Continued

roughly triangular space (with the apex of the triangle directed anteriorly), which has been named the *pretracheal* or *anterior paratracheal* space (see Fig. 2-2*A, B,* and *D*). This fat-filled space is important because it contains middle mediastinal lymph nodes in the paratracheal chain, which are commonly involved in various lymph node diseases. Whenever the mediastinum is being viewed for the diagnosis of lymphadenopathy, one should look here first. Other mediastinal node groups are closely related to this group both spatially and in regard to lymphatic drainage. It is not uncommon to see a few normal-sized lymph nodes (short axis diameter, <1 cm) in the pretracheal space (see review of mediastinal lymphadenopathy in Chapter 4 for a detailed discussion of this topic).

Anterior to the great vessels (aorta and superior vena cava) is another roughly (very roughly) triangular space called the *prevascular* space (see Fig. 2-2*A, B,* and *D*). This compart-ment represents the anterior mediastinum and primarily contains the thymus, lymph nodes, and fat. The apex of this triangular space represents the anterior junction line, which is sometimes visible on chest radiographs.

In young patients, usually teenagers or adults in their early 20s, CT shows the thymus to be of soft-tissue attenuation and bilobed or arrowhead shaped, with each of the two lobes (right and left) contacting the mediastinal pleura. Each lobe usually measures 1 to 2 cm in thickness (measured perpendicular to the pleura), but this varies (see Fig. 2-2*C*). In adulthood, the thymus involutes, with soft tissue being replaced by fat. In patients older than 30 years, the prevascular space appears primarily fat filled, with thin wisps of tissue passing through the fat. Most of this, including the fat, actually represents the thymus. At higher levels, the thymus is sometimes visible anterior to the

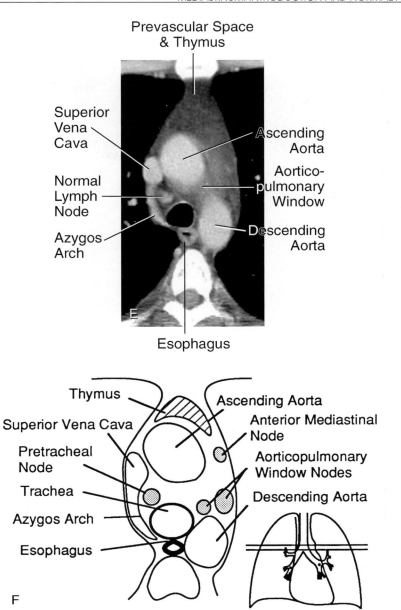

FIGURE 2-2 **Cont'd** *E,* Azygos arch and aortopulmonary window level. The azygos arch is visible arising from the posterior aspect of the superior vena cava, contacting the right mediastinal pleura, and forming the lateral margin of the pretracheal space. Fat visible under the aortic arch is in the aortopulmonary window. *F,* Locations of lymph nodes in the pretracheal space, aortopulmonary window, and anterior mediastinum at this level are shown, although they are not visible in *E.*

Continued

brachiocephalic arteries and veins, also within the prevascular space.

Azygos Arch and Aortopulmonary Window Level

At a level slightly below the aortic arch, the ascending aorta and descending aorta are visible as separate structures. Characteristically, the ascending aorta (25 to 35 mm in diameter) is slightly larger than the descending aorta (20 to 30 mm).

At or near this level, the trachea bifurcates into the right and left main bronchi. Near the carina, the trachea commonly assumes a somewhat oval or triangular shape (see Fig. 2-2*G*). The carina itself is usually visible on CT. On the right side, the arch of the azygos vein (*azygos,*

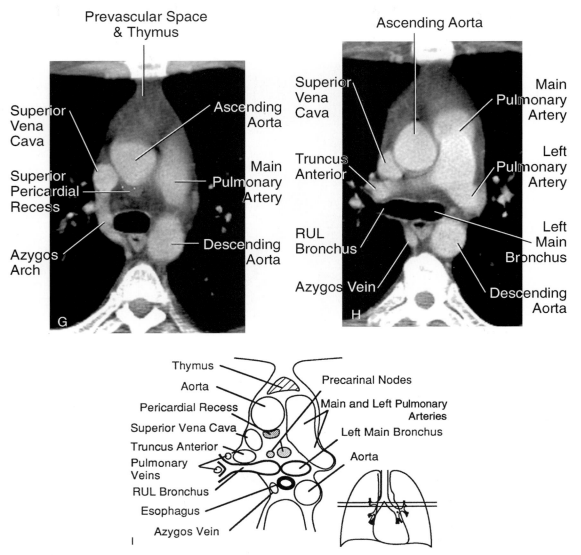

FIGURE 2-2 Cont'd *G,* At the tracheal carina, the trachea assumes an oval shape. The azygos arch remains visible. The upper aspect of the main pulmonary artery, which marginates the caudal aspect of the aortopulmonary window, should not be confused with a mass lesion. *H* and *I,* Scan and diagram at the level of the left pulmonary artery and right upper lobe (RUL) bronchus. The superior pericardial recess posterior to the aorta appears larger in *I* than in *H.*

Continued

incidentally, means "unpaired") arises from the posterior wall of the superior vena cava, passes over the right main bronchus (thus it is seen at a higher level than the bronchus itself), and continues posteriorly along the mediastinum, to lie to the right and anterior of the spine (see Fig. 2-2*E* to *G*). (Below the level of the azygos arch, the azygos vein remains visible in this position.) The azygos arch is often visible on one or two adjacent slices and sometimes appears "nodular." However, its characteristic location is usually sufficient to correctly identify this structure.

When the azygos arch is visible, it marginates the right border of the pretracheal space.

On the left side of the mediastinum, under the aortic arch but above the main pulmonary artery, is the region termed the *aortopulmonary* (or *aorticopulmonary*) *window.* The aortopulmonary window contains fat, lymph nodes (middle mediastinal), the recurrent laryngeal nerve, and the ligamentum arteriosum (the latter two are usually invisible; see Fig. 2-2*E* and *F*). Aortopulmonary window lymph nodes freely communicate with those in the pretracheal space, and,

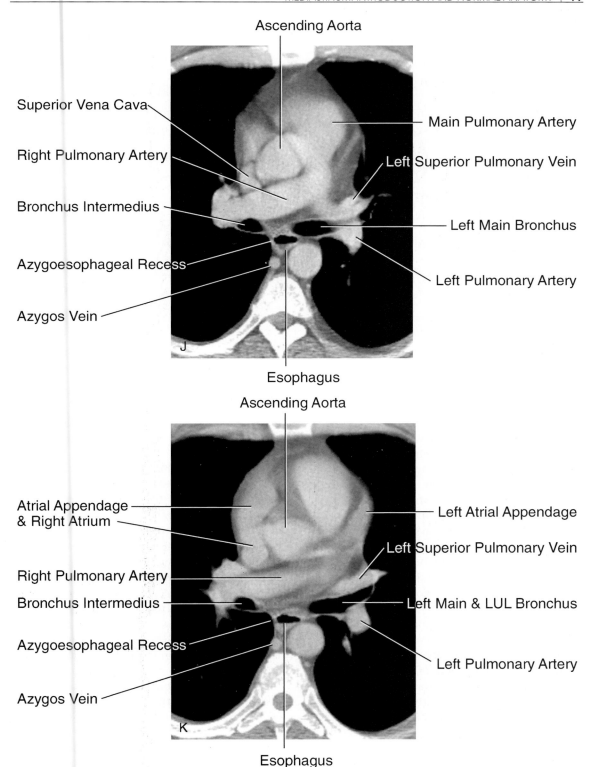

Ascending Aorta

Superior Vena Cava

Right Pulmonary Artery

Bronchus Intermedius

Azygoesophageal Recess

Azygos Vein

Main Pulmonary Artery

Left Superior Pulmonary Vein

Left Main Bronchus

Left Pulmonary Artery

J

Esophagus

Ascending Aorta

Atrial Appendage
& Right Atrium

Right Pulmonary Artery

Bronchus Intermedius

Azygoesophageal Recess

Azygos Vein

Left Atrial Appendage

Left Superior Pulmonary Vein

Left Main & LUL Bronchus

Left Pulmonary Artery

K

Esophagus

FIGURE 2-2 **Cont'd** *J,* Main pulmonary arteries, subcarinal space, and azygoesophageal recess level. Slightly below the tracheal carina, the right pulmonary artery is visible crossing the mediastinum, filling the pretracheal and precarinal space. A small amount of fat is visible in the subcarinal space, slightly anterior to the esophagus, azygos vein, and azygoesophageal recess. *K* and *L,* Scan and diagram at the level of the azygoesophageal recess. The recess appears concave laterally, with the mediastinal pleura closely related to the azygos vein and esophagus. Some structures indicated here are not visible in the scans. LUL, left upper lobe.

Continued

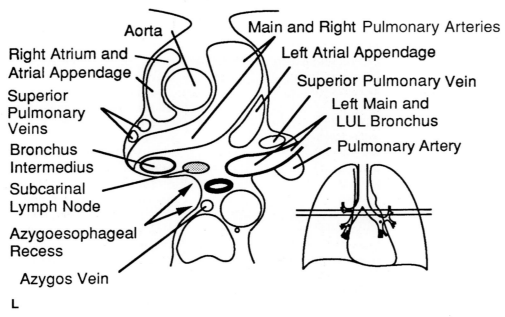

Aorta

Right Atrium and Atrial Appendage

Superior Pulmonary Veins

Bronchus Intermedius

Subcarinal Lymph Node

Azygoesophageal Recess

Azygos Vein

Main and Right Pulmonary Arteries

Left Atrial Appendage

Superior Pulmonary Vein

Left Main and LUL Bronchus

Pulmonary Artery

L

FIGURE 2-2 Cont'd

in fact, it may be difficult to distinguish nodes in the medial aortopulmonary window from those in the left part of the pretracheal space. In some patients, the aortopulmonary window is not well seen, with the main pulmonary artery lying immediately below the aortic arch. In such patients, it is usually difficult to distinguish lymph nodes from volume averaging of the adjacent aorta and pulmonary artery (see Fig. 2-2*G*); therefore, caution should be exercised. However, sometimes scans with thin collimation are helpful in distinguishing nodes from volume averaging.

At or slightly below the aortopulmonary window, at the level the ascending aorta is first clearly seen in cross section (i.e., it is round or nearly round), a portion of the pericardium, usually containing a small amount of pericardial fluid, extends up from below into the pretracheal space and immediately behind the ascending aorta. This part of the pericardium is called the *superior pericardial recess* (see Fig. 2-2*G* to *I*). Although it can sometimes be confused with a lymph node, its typical location, immediately behind and hugging the aortic wall, its oval or crescentic shape, and its relatively low (water) attenuation allow it to be distinguished from a significant abnormality. Another part of the peri-

cardial recess can sometimes be seen anterior to the ascending aorta and pulmonary artery.

Main Pulmonary Arteries, Subcarinal Space, and Azygoesophageal Recess

Below the level of the carina and azygos arch (see Fig. 2-2*H* to *L*), the medial aspect of the right lung tucks into the posterior portion of the middle mediastinum, in close association with the azygos vein and esophagus. This part of the mediastinum, reasonably called the *azygoesophageal recess,* is important because of the adjacent subcarinal lymph nodes and its close relation to the esophagus and main bronchi. The contour of the azygoesophageal recess is concave laterally in most normal subjects, and a convexity in this region indicates the possibility of an underlying pathologic process. However, a convexity in this region may be produced by a normal esophagus or azygos vein. Of course, the great value of CT is that we do not need to rely on contours, as we do on plain radiographs, to make a diagnosis of mediastinal disease. If a contour abnormality is detected (usually on lung window scans, which best show mediastinal contours), a close look at the mediastinal windows should be sufficient to delineate the cause of the abnormal contour. If the contour abnormality does not reflect the esophagus or azygos vein, then it is abnormal and subcarinal node enlargement is the usual culprit.

In many subjects, the azygoesophageal recess is somewhat posterior to the node-bearing subcarinal space, which lies between the main bronchi. Normal nodes are commonly visible in this space, because they are larger than normal nodes in other parts of the mediastinum and up to 1.5 cm in short-axis diameter. The esophagus is usually seen immediately behind the subcarinal space, and distinguishing nodes and esophagus may be difficult, unless the esophagus contains air or contrast material. At levels below the subcarinal space, the appearance of the azygoesophageal recess is relatively constant, although it narrows somewhat in a retrocardiac region.

Also at or near this level, the main pulmonary artery divides into its right and left branches. The left pulmonary artery (see Fig. 2-2*G* to *I*) is somewhat higher than the right, usually being seen 1 cm above it, and appears to be the continuation of the main pulmonary artery, directed posterolaterally and to the left. The right pulmonary artery arises at an angle of nearly 90 degrees to the main and left pulmonary artery and crosses the mediastinum, anterior to the carina or main bronchi. In this location, the right pulmonary artery effectively fills in the pretracheal space. At the point the main bronchi and pulmonary arteries exit the mediastinum, the pulmonary hila are entered (see Chapter 5).

Paracardiac Mediastinum

As one progresses caudad through the mediastinum, the origins of the great vessels from the cardiac chambers can be seen to a variable degree. Although CT is not commonly used to diagnose cardiac abnormalities (echocardiography or magnetic resonance imaging is usually preferred), some simple understanding of cardiac anatomy on CT can be helpful in diagnosis.

The main pulmonary artery is most anterior, arising from the right ventricle, which can be seen at lower levels to be anterior and to the right of the left ventricle (Fig. 2-3*A* and *B*). The superior vena cava enters the right atrium, which is elliptical or crescentic. The right atrial appendage extends anteriorly from the upper atrium, bordering the right mediastinal pleura.

Between the right atrium and the main pulmonary artery or pulmonary outflow tract, the aortic root enters the left ventricle. At this level, it is common in adults to see some coronary artery calcification (see Fig. 2-3*C*), and, often, uncalcified coronary arteries are visible surrounded by mediastinal fat. Calcification of the left coronary artery, left anterior descending coronary artery, circumflex coronary artery, and right coronary artery can be identified. The left atrium is posteriorly located, appearing larger than the right. The left atrial appendage extends anteriorly and to the left and is visible below the left pulmonary artery, bordering the pleura. On each side, superior and inferior pulmonary veins can be seen entering the left atrium (see Fig. 2-3*A, B, D,* and *E*; see Chapter 5 for further discussion).

Near the level of the diaphragm, the inferior vena cava is visible as an oval structure extending caudad from the posterior right atrium; it is easy to identify.

The only other structures of consequence at this level that need to be mentioned are the esophagus, which lies in a retrocardiac location; the azygos vein, which is often still visible in the same relative position as at higher levels; and the hemiazygos vein, which is usually smaller than the azygos and on the opposite side, behind the descending aorta. Paravertebral nodes lie in association with the azygos and hemiazygos veins but are not normally visible.

☐ NORMAL CARDIAC ANATOMY

Without the injection of contrast medium, little cardiac anatomy is discernible on CT, but some differentiation of cardiac chambers is possible because of the presence of epicardial fat collections. When contrast medium is used, additional features of cardiac anatomy are visible, depending on the amount and rapidity of contrast medium injection; the myocardium opacifies less than the intracardiac blood and is often visible as a relatively low-attenuation band after rapid infusion of a large-contrast medium bolus. The interventricular septum is usually visible if contrast medium has been infused; it is typically oriented at an angle at about 2 o'clock to the vertical and is convex anteriorly because of the greater left ventricular pressure (see Fig. 2-3). However, other segments of the myocardium may be difficult to appreciate as distinct from

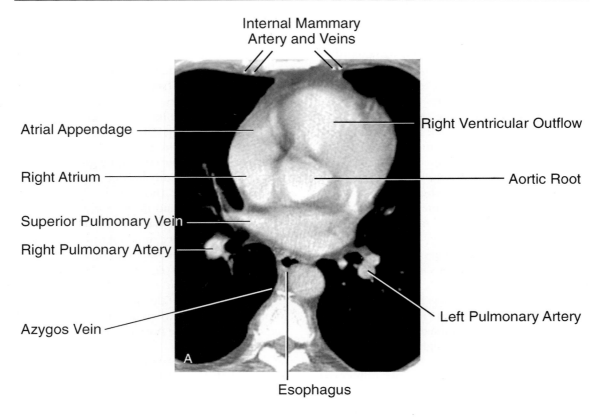

Internal Mammary
Artery and Veins

Atrial Appendage

Right Atrium

Superior Pulmonary Vein

Right Pulmonary Artery

Azygos Vein

Right Ventricular Outflow

Aortic Root

Left Pulmonary Artery

Esophagus

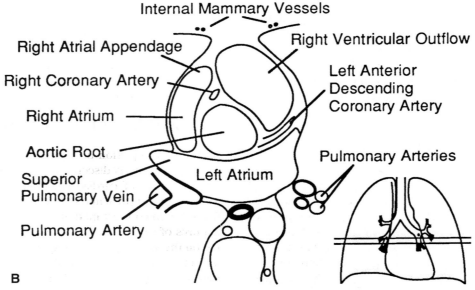

Internal Mammary Vessels

Right Atrial Appendage

Right Coronary Artery

Right Atrium

Aortic Root

Superior
Pulmonary Vein

Pulmonary Artery

Right Ventricular Outflow

Left Anterior
Descending
Coronary Artery

Left Atrium

Pulmonary Arteries

FIGURE 2-3 **Paracardiac mediastinum.** *A,* Most cephalad, the origins of the aorta and pulmonary artery are visible, with the aortic root being central. The right ventricular (pulmonary) outflow tract or main pulmonary artery are anterior and to the left of the aortic root at this level. The right atrium, with its appendage extending anteriorly, borders the right mediastinal pleura. The superior pulmonary veins enter the upper aspect of the left atrium at this level or slightly above. Anteriorly, the right internal mammary vessels are visible *(arrow). B,* Diagram at the level of *A.* The positions of left and right coronary arteries are shown.

Continued

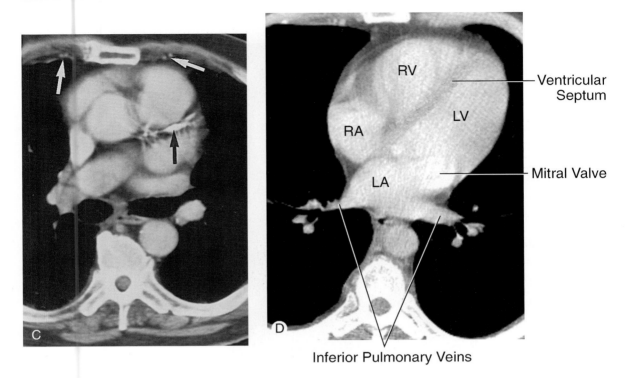

RV

RA

LV

LA

Ventricular Septum

Mitral Valve

Inferior Pulmonary Veins

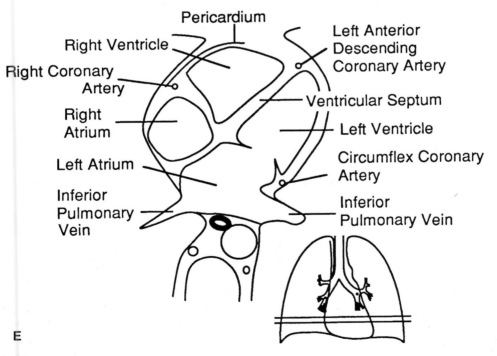

Pericardium

Right Ventricle

Right Coronary Artery

Right Atrium

Left Atrium

Inferior Pulmonary Vein

Left Anterior Descending Coronary Artery

Ventricular Septum

Left Ventricle

Circumflex Coronary Artery

Inferior Pulmonary Vein

E

FIGURE 2-3 Cont'd C, In another subject, calcification of the left anterior descending coronary artery *(black arrow)* is easily seen. The left coronary artery arises from the posterolateral aortic root. The internal mammary vessels *(white arrows)* are also visible. *D* and *E,* At a lower level, the right and left atria and ventricles are visible. The right ventricle (RV) is located anterior and to the right of the left ventricle (LV). At this level, the inferior pulmonary veins enter the left atrium (LA).

Continued

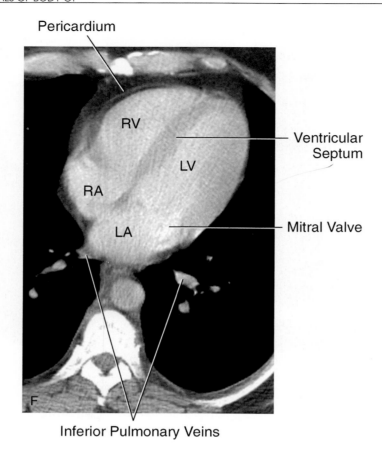

Pericardium

RV

Ventricular
Septum

LV

RA

Mitral Valve

LA

F

Inferior Pulmonary Veins

FIGURE 2-3 Cont'd *F,* At this level, both atria and ventricles are visible. The ventricular septal and left ventricular walls are thicker than the right ventricular wall, and the septum is convex toward the RV.

Continued

the opacified cardiac chambers on clinical scans unless contrast medium is infused rapidly. The lateral or "free" left ventricular wall is about three times thicker (it is about 1 cm in thickness) than the right ventricular wall.

Cardiac anatomy is easiest to understand if we start with a scan near the cardiac apex (and diaphragm). At this level, the left ventricle is elliptical, with its long axis directed laterally and anteriorly (see Fig. 2-3F to H). Being the highest pressure chamber, it dominates cardiac anatomy, and the other cardiac chambers mold themselves to its shape. The right ventricle, which is anterior and to the right, is triangular. On scans at this level or slightly above, the line of the interventricular septum, if continued posteriorly and to the right, separates the lower right atrium anteriorly (and in contiguity with the right ventricle), from the lower left atrium

posteriorly. The mitral and tricuspid valves are located at or near this level and can be seen if there is good contrast opacification of the cardiac chambers.

At higher levels (see Fig. 2-3A and B), the left ventricular outflow tract and aortic valve are centrally located within the heart. The right ventricular outflow tract is directed toward the left and is visible anterior or to the left of the left ventricular outflow tract. That is, because of twisting of the heart during development, the left ventricular outflow tract is directed rightward and the right ventricular outflow tract is directed leftward. This accounts for the location of the aorta on the right and the pulmonary artery on the left. The aortic and pulmonic valves are located near this level and are sometimes visible in normal subjects.

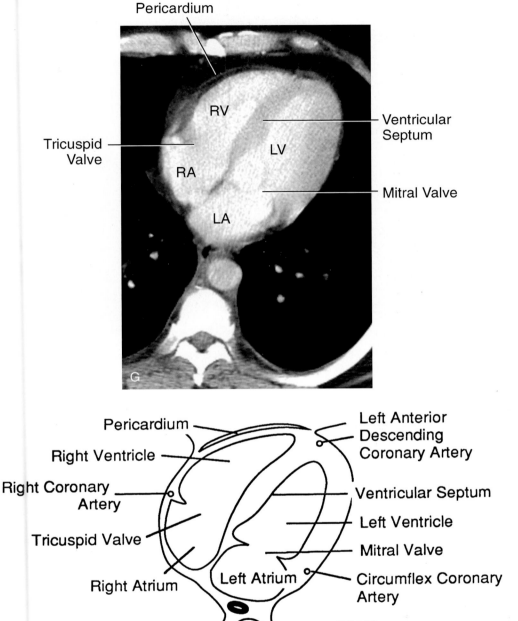

FIGURE 2-3 Cont'd *G* and *H,* All four chambers are visible, and the location of both tricuspid and mitral valves can be identified. The interventricular septum and free wall of the LV are considerably thicker than the wall of the RV. The pericardium is visible as a thin white line surrounded by mediastinal fat. It should appear 1 to 2 mm in thickness.

Continued

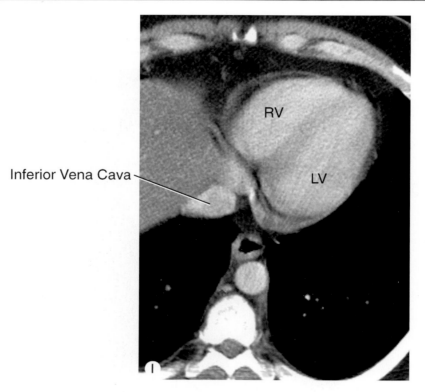

FIGURE 2-3 **Cont'd** *I*, Near the diaphragm, the inferior vena cava is visible as a separate structure, below the level of the right atrium. Some structures indicated here are not visible in the scans. RA, right atrium.

The Normal Pericardium

The normal pericardium (the visceral and parietal pericardium and pericardial contents) is visible as a 1- to 2-mm stripe of soft-tissue attenuation parallel to the heart and outlined by mediastinal fat (outside the pericardial sac) and epicardial fat. It is best seen near the diaphragm, along the anterior and lateral aspects of the heart, where the fat layers are thickest (Fig. 2-3*F* to *H*). As stated earlier, extensions of the pericardium into the upper mediastinum can also be seen in healthy persons.

☐ **THE RETROSTERNAL SPACE**

In a retrosternal location, the internal mammary arteries and veins are normally visible 1 or 2 cm lateral to the edge of the sternum on good CT scans (see Fig. 2-3*A* to *C*); up to three vessels can be seen on each side (one artery, two veins). These vessels are not of much diagnostic significance, although the veins commonly enlarge in patients with superior vena caval obstruction, but they are important because they serve to localize the internal mammary chain of lymph nodes. Although normal nodes can be seen in several areas of the mediastinum (most notably the pretracheal space, aortopulmonary window, and subcarinal space), normal internal mammary nodes are not large enough to be recognized. A lymph node in this region that is large enough to be visible should be regarded as abnormal. Internal mammary node enlargement is most common in patients with breast cancer or lymphoma.

▣ **SUGGESTED READING**

Aronberg DJ, Peterson RR, Glazer HS, Sagel SS: The superior sinus of the pericardium: CT appearance. Radiology 153:489–492, 1984.

Francis I, Glazer GM, Bookstein FL, Gross BH: The thymus: Reexamination of age-related changes in size and shape. AJR Am J Roentgenol 145: 249–254, 1985.

GLAZER HS, ARONBERG DJ, SAGEL SS: Pitfalls in CT recognition of mediastinal lymphadenopathy. AJR Am J Roentgenol 144:267–274, 1985.

KIYONO K, SONE S, SAKAI F, et al: The number and size of normal mediastinal lymph nodes: A post-mortem study. AJR Am J Roentgenol 150:771–776, 1988.

MÜLLER NL, WEBB WR, GAMSU G: Paratracheal lymph-adenopathy: Radiographic findings and correlation with CT. Radiology 156:761–765, 1985.

MÜLLER NL, WEBB WR, GAMSU G: Subcarinal lymph node enlargement: Radiographic findings and CT correlation. AJR Am J Roentgenol 145:15–19, 1985.

ZYLAK CJ, PALLIE W, PIRANI M, et al: Anatomy and computed tomography: A correlative module on the cervicothoracic junction. Radiographics 3:478–530, 1983.

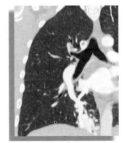

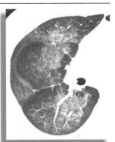

Mediastinum: Vascular Abnormalities

W. Richard Webb, M.D.

3

On any thoracic CT in a patient with a mediastinal mass, the first objective is often to prove that the mass is or is not vascular in origin.

☐ AORTIC ABNORMALITIES

A variety of aortic arch and great arterial abnormalities are visible on CT scans, and CT is commonly used to diagnose aortic disease when it is suspected clinically or when chest radiographs are abnormal.

Congenital Anomalies

Congenital abnormalities of the aorta and its mediastinal branches are diagnosed easily using CT, and no other study is usually needed unless the anomaly is complex or is associated with congenital heart disease. Magnetic resonance imaging is often used to study coarctation.

Aberrant Right Subclavian Artery

An aberrant right subclavian artery is a relatively common anomaly (1/100 patients) that does not usually produce a recognizable mediastinal abnormality on chest radiographs, and thus is usually detected incidentally on CT scans obtained

for another reason. Its main significance is that it should not be misinterpreted as something else. In patients with this anomaly, the aortic arch is often somewhat higher than normal. The aberrant artery arises from the medial wall of the aorta, as its last branch (Fig. 3-1). It passes to the right, behind the esophagus, and then ascends on the right toward the thoracic inlet. It lies much more posterior than is normal for the subclavian artery, often anterolateral to the spine. At its point of origin, the artery may be dilated, or if you wish to think of it in a more complicated way, the artery may arise from an aortic diverticulum *(diverticulum of Kommerell)*. This may cause compression of the esophagus and symptoms of dysphagia. In some patients, the diverticulum or the anomalous artery becomes aneurysmal (Fig. 3-2).

Right Aortic Arch

There are two main types of right aortic arch: *right arch associated with aberrant left subclavian artery* and *mirror image right arch*. Right arch with an aberrant left subclavian artery is most common, being present in about 1 in 1000 people. It is the reverse of a left arch with an aberrant right subclavian artery (Fig. 3-3). An aortic diverticulum is more common in the presence of a right arch. With this anomaly,

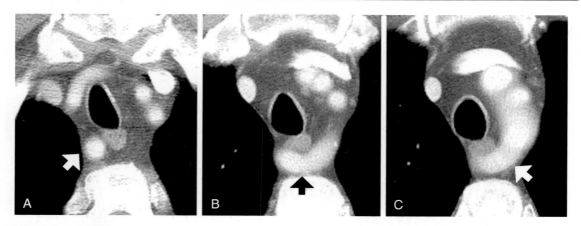

FIGURE 3-1 **Aberrant right subclavian artery.** *A,* An aberrant right subclavian artery *(arrow)* is located posteriorly in the right superior mediastinum. *B,* At a level 7 mm below *A,* the anomalous artery *(arrow)* passes posterior to the esophagus. *C,* At 7 mm below *B,* the origin *(arrow)* of the anomalous artery from the posterior superior aortic arch is visible.

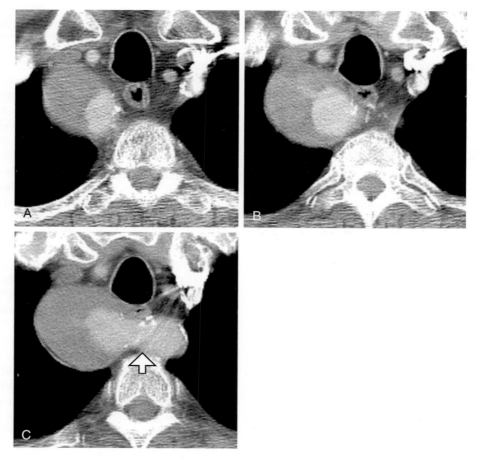

FIGURE 3-2 **Aneurysm of aberrant right subclavian artery.** *A,* As in Figure 3-1*A,* an aberrant right subclavian artery is situated in the right mediastinum. It is dilated, and its lumen is partially filled with clot. *B* and *C,* At lower levels, the aberrant artery is located posterior to the esophagus, and its origin *(arrow)* from the posterior superior aortic arch is visible.

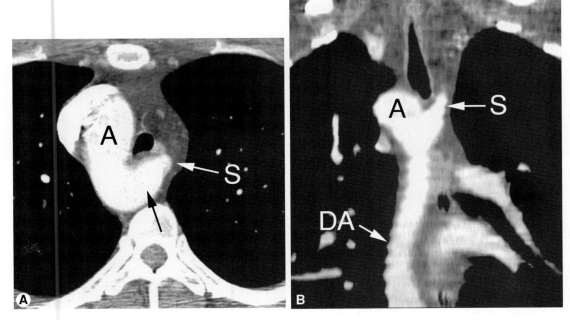

FIGURE 3-3 **Right aortic arch with aberrant left subclavian artery.** *A,* In a patient with no evidence of congenital heart disease and with a right aortic arch (A), an aberrant left subclavian artery (S) arises from a retroesophageal aortic diverticulum *(black arrow)*. The esophagus is compressed by the diverticulum. *B,* Coronal reconstruction shows the posterior aortic arch (A) and descending aorta (DA). The origin of the left subclavian artery (S) from a diverticulum is visible.

there is a low frequency (5% to 10%) of associated congenital heart lesions, and they are usually simple, such as atrial septal defect. Mirror image right arch is relatively uncommon and is almost always (98%) associated with congenital heart disease (usually complex anomalies such as tetralogy of Fallot). The CT appearance of a mirror image arch is well described by its name—it is the mirror image of a normal left arch, with a left innominate artery being present (Fig. 3-4). With both types of right arch the

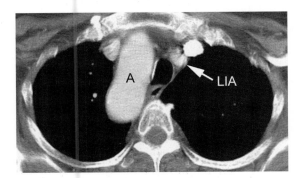

FIGURE 3-4 **Right aortic arch with mirror image branching.** A right aortic arch (A) and a left innominate artery (LIA) are present. There is no evidence of an aberrant left subclavian artery. This patient had no evidence of congenital heart disease.

descending aorta is usually left sided, crossing from right to left in the lower mediastinum.

Double Aortic Arch

Double aortic arch is relatively uncommon, but because the plain radiograph shows a mediastinal abnormality, it is often evaluated using CT. This anomaly is uncommonly associated with congenital heart disease, but because a complete vascular ring is present, symptoms of dysphagia are common. In this anomaly, the ascending aorta splits into right and left halves. The right arch, which is usually higher and larger than the left, passes to the right of the trachea and esophagus, crosses behind these structures, and rejoins the left arch, which occupies a relatively normal position (Fig. 3-5). Each arch is smaller than normal and smaller than the descending aorta. Also, each arch gives rise to a subclavian and carotid artery, and no innominate artery is present. This results in a symmetrical appearance to the great vessels in the supra-aortic mediastinum that is highly suggestive of the diagnosis.

Coarctation and Pseudocoarctation

Coarctation, and its variant pseudocoarctation, can be diagnosed using CT; but even if this is

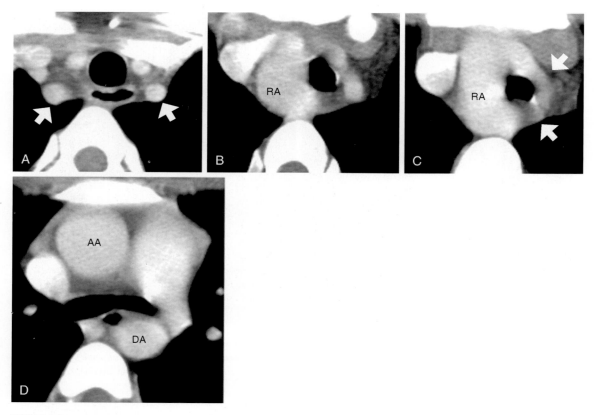

FIGURE 3-5 **Double aortic arch.** *A,* In the upper mediastinum, the subclavian *(arrows)* and carotid arteries appear bilaterally symmetrical. *B,* At a level below *A,* the right arch (RA) is visible to the right of the trachea. On the left side of the mediastinum, the left carotid and subclavian arteries, which arise from the left arch, are visible. The right arch is characteristically higher and larger than the left. *C,* At a level below *B,* the left arch *(arrows)* is now visible. It appears smaller than the right arch (RA). *D,* At a level below *C,* the ascending aorta (AA) and descending aorta (DA) appear normal.

possible, catheterization is usually necessary to measure intra-arterial pressures and, thus, the significance of the vascular obstruction. Some believe that use of the term *pseudocoarctation* is inappropriate; they consider this lesion to be a coarctation and not "pseudo," but the CT and clinical findings in these two entities are different. They are considered separately here if for no other reason than the term *pseudocoarctation* is in common usage.

The site of narrowing in coarctation is generally at the aortic isthmus, distal to the origin of the left subclavian artery and near the ligamentum arteriosum (juxtaductal coarctation). On CT, the narrowed segment is often visible, being decidedly smaller than the aorta above and below this level (Fig. 3-6). This size difference not only reflects the narrowed segment at the coarctation, but also some dilation of the prestenotic and poststenotic aorta. A long narrowing of the aortic arch (hypoplasia) is less common. Images reconstructed in the plane of the aortic arch can show the coarctation to better advantage. One word of caution: The degree of narrowing at the site of coarctation may be overestimated if the reformatted plane is slightly off the sagittal plane of the aorta. Dilatation of internal mammary arteries or intercostal arteries (usually the third through eighth) acting as collateral pathways can be seen.

In pseudocoarctation, the aortic arch is kinked anteriorly and its lumen is somewhat narrowed, but a significant pressure gradient across the kink and collateral vessels are not present. The CT appearance of this anomaly is characteristic but sometimes confusing (Fig. 3-7). The aortic arch is higher than normal and initially descends in an abnormally anterior position, well in front of the spine. At a level near the carina, however, the aorta again angles posteriorly, forming a second arch, and assumes its normal position anterolateral to the spine. This

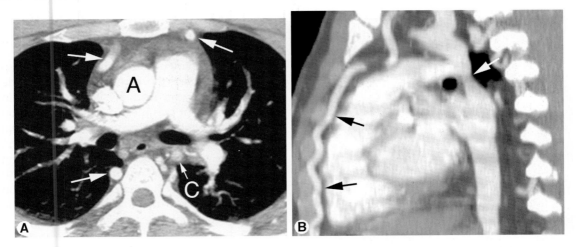

FIGURE 3-6 **Aortic coarctation.** CT scan with contrast enhancement in a patient with coarctation. *A,* The proximal descending aorta, at the level of the coarctation (C), is significantly smaller than the ascending aorta (A). Internal mammary and intercostal arteries *(arrows)* are dilated, serving as collateral pathways. *B,* Sagittal reconstruction along the plane of the aorta shows marked narrowing at the site of the coarctation *(white arrow).* A dilated internal mammary artery is visible anteriorly *(black arrows).*

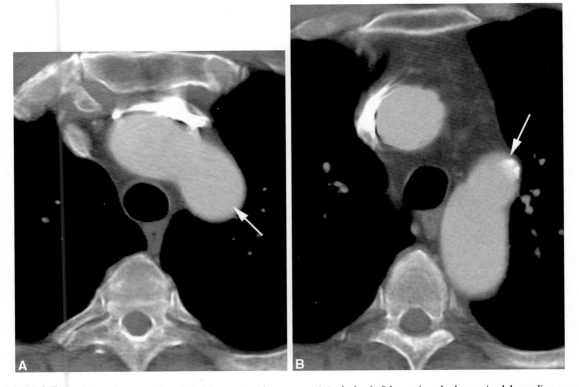

FIGURE 3-7 **Aortic pseudocoarctation.** CT with contrast enhancement. *A,* At the level of the aortic arch, the proximal descending aorta *(arrow)* is located well anterior to the spine. *B,* At the level of the kink *(arrow),* the aorta angles posteriorly and assumes its normal position adjacent to the spine.

Continued

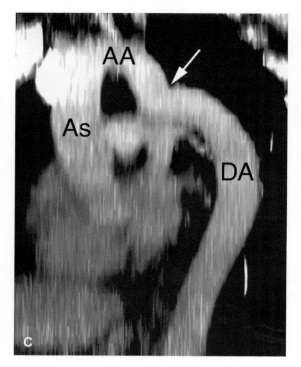

FIGURE 3-7 Cont'd *C,* A sagittal CT reconstruction through the heart and aorta shows the ascending aorta (As), aortic arch (AA), the anterior aortic kink *(arrow),* and the descending aorta (DA). This appearance is typical of pseudocoarctation.

anomaly is usually not associated with symptoms and is usually detected incidentally on chest radiographs. Its plain film appearance may be characteristic.

Both coarctation and pseudocoarctation are associated with congenital bicuspid aortic valve (30% to 85% of patients with coarctation); this may result in aortic stenosis. In some patients, CT shows aortic valve calcification, allowing this diagnosis to be suggested.

Aortic Aneurysm

If the ascending aorta measures more than 4 cm in diameter, it is usually referred to as dilated or ectatic. Although a diagnosis of "aortic dilatation" as opposed to "aortic aneurysm" is somewhat arbitrary, this chapter uses "aortic dilatation," or "ectasia," to refer to a generalized dilatation of relatively mild degree (4 cm), with the implication that it is not necessarily a serious problem. "Aneurysm," in contrast, refers to a more focal abnormality or more severe dilatation of the entire aorta (5 cm). If the aorta is more than 6 cm, treatment is usually necessary. In

other words, for the aorta, a diameter of 4 cm = aortic dilatation, 5 cm = aortic aneurysm, and 6 cm = surgery.

In some patients with an (atherosclerotic) aortic aneurysm, the diagnosis can be made and the aneurysm distinguished from a solid mass because of peripheral intimal calcification visible on unenhanced scans. Thrombus within an aneurysm or hematoma adjacent to a leaking aneurysm may appear higher in attenuation than aortic blood on unenhanced scans. With contrast infusion, the lumen of the aorta and the aneurysm and the thickness of the aortic wall can be defined clearly (Fig. 3-8).

With atherosclerotic aneurysms, the aortic wall is often thickened, and calcification is commonly visible. There may be visible areas of plaque or thrombus in the lumen of the aneurysm (Fig. 3-9); these may also calcify. Plaque often appears low in attenuation relative to soft tissue or aortic wall because of its fat content or because of some opacification of the aortic wall itself. Plaque can also be seen in patients with atherosclerosis who do not have aortic dilatation. Focal ulceration of plaque or thrombus (see Fig. 3-9) may occur and should be distinguished from penetrating atherosclerotic ulcer (see later).

Aneurysms are often described as fusiform or saccular, depending on their appearance. Aneurysms localized to the ascending aorta may occur with atherosclerosis, Marfan's syndrome, cystic medial necrosis, syphilis, or aortic valvular disease. An aneurysm near the ligamentum arteriosum may be atherosclerotic in origin, a ductus aneurysm (aneurysm at the site of the ductus arteriosus or a ductus diverticulum), mycotic, related to coarctation, or post-traumatic (i.e., a pseudoaneurysm). Mycotic aneurysms are usually focal, and they may be associated with periaortic inflammation or abscess; gas bubbles may be seen within soft tissues. Descending aortic aneurysms are usually atherosclerotic.

Aortic Trauma

Spiral CT has assumed an important role in the diagnosis of aortic injuries. Traumatic aortic laceration, rupture, or pseudoaneurysm occurs most commonly at the following areas: (1) aortic root, (2) level of the ligamentum arteriosum, or (3) diaphragm and aortic hiatus. Patients with aortic root injury often die at the scene of injury; in patients who reach the hospital, injuries at

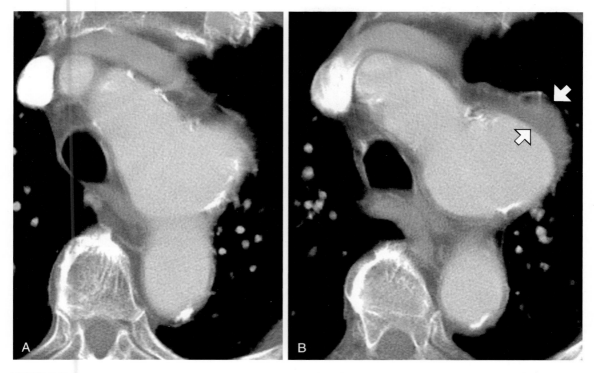

FIGURE 3-8 **Aortic aneurysm.** *A* and *B,* A focal, saccular aneurysm of the aortic arch shows some clot lining its lumen *(arrows).*

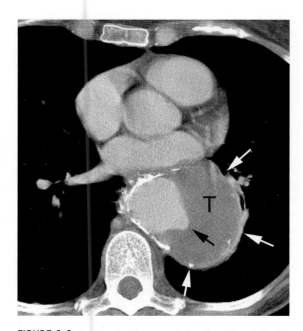

FIGURE 3-9 **Aortic aneurysm containing thrombus.** A focal, saccular aneurysm of the descending aorta *(white arrows)* shows calcification of its wall. The aneurysm contains a large thrombus (T) with focal ulceration *(black arrow).*

the level of the ligamentum are most common (Fig. 3-10).

Mediastinal hematoma (fluid with a density of about 50 H) contiguous with the aorta is invariably visible on CT in patients with aortic laceration or rupture (see Fig. 3-10); absence of hematoma effectively excludes this diagnosis. The presence of hematoma at the location of a sternal or vertebral fracture does not predict aortic injury.

Contrast-enhanced spiral CT with thin colli-mation (e.g., 2.5 mm) is highly sensitive in diag-nosing acute aortic laceration, with a sensitivity of nearly 100%. The site of rupture or tear may have the appearance of an irregular aortic wall, dissection, or focal false aneurysm (see Fig. 3-10); extravasation of contrast is rarely seen. It has been suggested that aortography is not needed if the following occur: (1) no medi-astinal hematoma is visible, or (2) no aortic ab-normality is seen in patients with a visible hematoma. Aortography may be necessary in some patients with inadequate CT studies or questionable CT findings.

Chronic post-traumatic pseudoaneurysm is usually located in the region of the ligamentum and aortopulmonary window, below the takeoff of the left subclavian artery (Fig. 3-11). Because

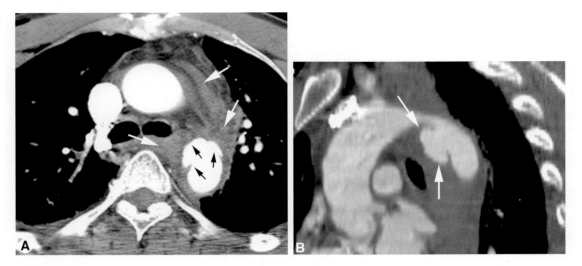

FIGURE 3-10 **Acute traumatic aortic rupture with pseudoaneurysm.** *A,* After a motor vehicle accident, contrast-enhanced CT shows mediastinal hematoma *(white arrows)* contiguous with the aorta. There is irregularity of the proximal descending aorta with a pseudoaneurysm anteriorly *(black arrows).* *B,* Sagittal reconstruction along the aorta shows a pseudoaneurysm *(arrows)* involving the proximal descending aorta. This location is most common.

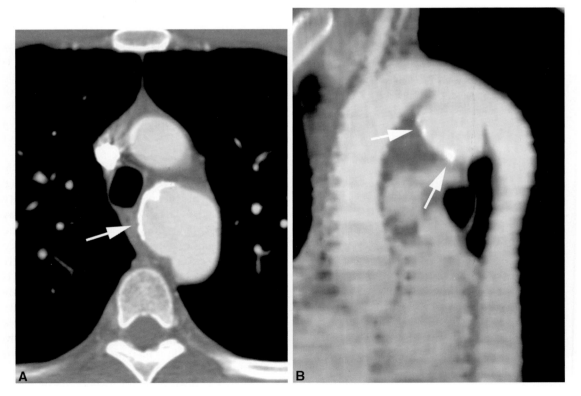

FIGURE 3-11 **Chronic post-traumatic pseudoaneurysm.** Contrast-enhanced CT scan in a patient who had previously been in a motor vehicle accident. *A,* A focal pseudoaneurysm extends anteriorly *(arrow)* with calcification of its wall. *B,* Sagittal reconstruction shows the pseudoaneurysm *(arrows)* in a typical location.

this represents a contained aortic rupture, not marginated by aortic wall, peripheral calcification is unusual.

Aortic Dissection

Aortic dissection often is associated with hypertension, weakness of the aortic wall (e.g., Marfan's syndrome or cystic medial necrosis), or trauma. Patients usually have acute chest pain. The goal in diagnosing dissection is the demonstration of an intimal flap, displaced inward from the edge of the aorta, separating the true and false channels. CT is ideally suited to this because of its cross-sectional format.

Two schemes for the classification of dissections have been proposed by Daily and DeBakey. Daily's classification, commonly known as the Stanford classification, is most frequently used because of its simplicity and relevance to treatment.

Using the Stanford classification, aortic dissections are divided into types A and B. Type A dissections involve the ascending aorta (Fig. 3-12); approximately two thirds of acute dissections are type A. Because of the possibility of retrograde dissection and rupture into the pericardium (resulting in tamponade) or occlusion of the coronary or carotid arteries, these dissections are usually treated surgically with grafting of the region of the tear. Type B dissections do not involve the aortic arch but typically arise distal to the left subclavian artery (Fig. 3-13). These are generally treated medically (by normalization of blood pressure) instead of surgically.

DeBakey's classification has three types. Type I (involvement of the entire aorta, both ascending and descending) is most common. Type II dissections, which are often associated with Marfan's syndrome, involve the ascending aorta only and, together with type I, correspond to Daily's type A. Type III dissections involve the descending aorta only and are related to hypertension or trauma; this type is equivalent to Daily's type B.

CT is highly sensitive and specific (>95%) in diagnosing dissection and in determining its

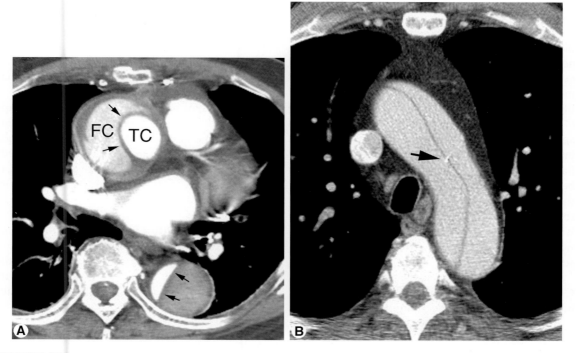

FIGURE 3-12 **Type A aortic dissection in two patients.** *A,* A patient with acute chest pain shows a type A dissection involving the ascending and descending aorta. The intimal flap *(black arrows)* is lower in attenuation than the contrast-opacified blood. In the ascending aorta, the true channel (TC) is more densely opacified and is smallest. The false channel (FC) is less densely opacified, more irregular in appearance, and contains thrombus. The ascending aorta is dilated. In the descending aorta, the true channel is more densely opacified and is most compressed, whereas the false channel is poorly opacified and is located lateral and posterior to the true channel. *B,* The intimal flap is visible in the aortic arch. Calcification of the intima *(arrow)* is visible.

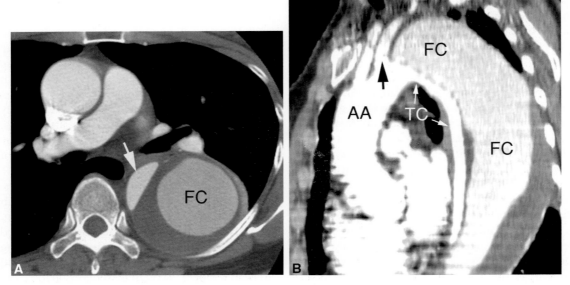

FIGURE 3-13 **Type B aortic dissection.** *A,* Enhanced spiral CT shows a dissection in the descending aorta. The false channel (FC) is largest, located posterolaterally, less opacified, and lined by thrombus. The true channel *(arrow)* is most compressed. The ascending aorta is normal in appearance. *B,* Sagittal reconstruction shows the large false channel (FC) originating distal to the left subclavian artery *(black arrow).* The true channel (TC) is small and most densely opacified; it is seen to communicate directly with the normal ascending aorta (AA). The intimal flap is visible separating the true and false channels.

location, type, and the aortic branches involved; consequently, it is an excellent screening and diagnostic procedure in patients with a suggestive clinical presentation. Transesophageal echocardiography may be performed in some patients with suspected acute dissection; it is highly sensitive, but has a lower specificity (70%). The accuracy of magnetic resonance imaging is similar to CT, and magnetic resonance imaging may be performed in patients unable to have radiographic contrast agents; also, it may be performed before surgery in patients shown to have a type A dissection. CT or magnetic resonance imaging can be used to follow up with patients with dissection after treatment to watch for redissection or extension of the dissection.

In patients with suspected dissection, CT should be performed with rapid contrast infusion. Using spiral technique, it is easy to scan through the great vessels, aortic arch, and descending aorta (3- to 5-mm collimation for single-detector CT or 2.5-mm detector width for multidetector CT [MDCT]) during rapid contrast infusion (at 2.5–3.5 mL/second) and to continue the scans to the level of the aortic bifurcation in the abdomen. A 30-second scanning delay should be used after the

start of injection, or scanning should be timed by the computer. Contrast-enhanced scans are usually preceded by unenhanced scans through the thorax (5-mm collimation or detector width) to look for intramural hematoma (see later).

In a patient with dissection, the intimal flap is usually delineated by contrast medium filling both the true and false channels. The true and false channels often may be distinguished based on the following CT findings (see Figs. 3-12*A* and 3-13), although this may be difficult or impossible in some cases:

1. In patients with a type B dissection, trace what you know to be the true channel (i.e., the ascending aorta) on adjacent images to see with which of the two distal channels it communicates (thus indicating the true lumen).
2. The false channel tends to be located lateral to the true channel at the level of the aortic arch and spirals posteriorly in the descending aorta. Because of this characteristic location, the left renal artery is the abdominal branch most likely to arise from the false channel.
3. The true lumen is usually smallest.

4. The false channel is usually most irregular in contour, and it may contain strands of tissue termed *cobwebs* within the contrast stream.
5. The false channel is more likely to contain thrombus.
6. Blood flow is slowest and opacification is often delayed in the false channel.
7. Aortic wall calcification may be seen lateral to the true channel.

Streak artifacts, arising because of cardiac motion or vascular pulsations, may mimic an intimal flap. They are commonly seen at the level of the aortic root and in the descending aorta, adjacent to the left heart border. Typically, they are less sharply defined than a true intimal flap, extend beyond the edges of the aorta, or are inconsistently seen from one level to the next.

Two abnormalities may closely mimic the clinical presentation of dissection. Consequently, these may be seen on CT scans obtained to exclude dissection. These are intramural hematoma and penetrating atherosclerotic ulcer.

Intramural Hematoma

Intramural hematoma results from hemorrhage into the aortic wall. Acute intramural hematoma may closely mimic the presentation of dissection (acute chest pain in a patient with hypertension). It is thought to occur because of bleeding from vasa vasorum, although, in some cases, it may represent a sealed-off dissection.

On contrast-enhanced scans, intramural hematoma appears as a smooth, crescentic, or less commonly, concentric thickening of the aortic wall (Fig. 3-14). On unenhanced scans, the intramural hematoma appears denser than unenhanced blood in the aortic lumen; because of this characteristic appearance, CT in a patient with suspected dissection should be preceded by unenhanced scans through the thorax. If unenhanced scans are not obtained prospectively,

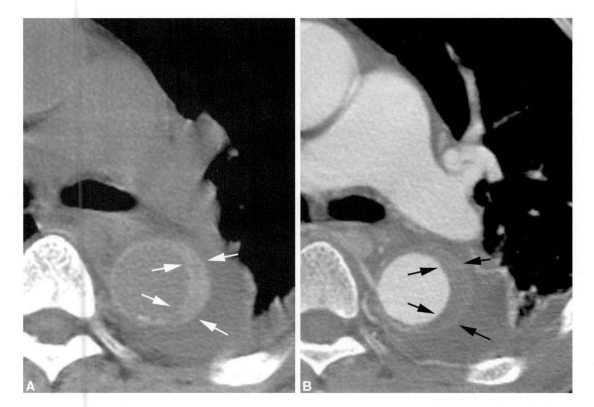

FIGURE 3-14 **Intramural hematoma (type B).** In a man with acute chest pain, unenhanced CT *(A)* shows crescentic thickening of the aortic wall *(arrows).* This is higher in attenuation than blood in the aortic lumen. *B,* Contrast-enhanced spiral CT shows crescentic thickening of the aortic wall *(arrows).* On the enhanced scan, the high attenuation of the hematoma is difficult to appreciate.

delayed unenhanced scans may be obtained. Inward displacement of intimal calcification can also be seen on unenhanced scans.

Keep in mind that the normal aortic wall is a few millimeters in thickness. On unenhanced scans, it appears the same density as blood in the aortic lumen in healthy subjects. In patients with anemia (hematocrit, ≤35%), the normal aortic wall may appear denser than blood. Do not confuse this with intramural hematoma. As a rough rule, the CT density of blood in the aortic lumen (in H) is about the same as the hematocrit.

The smooth crescentic or concentric wall thickening seen with intramural hematoma is usually different in appearance from dissection with a thrombosed channel. Thrombosed dissection uncommonly appears crescentic or concentric in shape. Thrombus lining an aneurysm can also mimic intramural hematoma, but it is usually more irregular in contour. The presence of acute chest pain as a presenting symptom also suggests an acute intramural hematoma rather than thrombus within a chronic dissection or aneurysm.

Intramural hematoma may progress to frank dissection (by rupture into the aortic lumen) or aneurysmal dilatation, or it may resolve. Treatment is similar to that of dissection occurring in the same location (i.e., type A or B). Type A intramural hematoma is treated surgically.

Penetrating Atherosclerotic Ulcer

In patients with atherosclerosis, ulceration of plaque may penetrate the aortic wall. The descending aorta is most often involved. This may lead to chest pain similar to dissection.

True penetrating ulcer penetrates the intima and extends into (or through) the aortic wall (Fig. 3-15); its appearance is similar to that of a penetrating gastric ulcer. Calcification of the aortic wall or enhancement of the wall after contrast infusion may help in diagnosing wall penetration. Ulceration of an atheroma or thrombus (see Fig. 3-9) may mimic the appearance of penetrating ulcer, but it is more superficial and does not involve the aortic wall itself. This abnormality may also be associated with intramural hematoma, dissection, or pseudoaneurysm. Surgical treatment may be necessary in some cases.

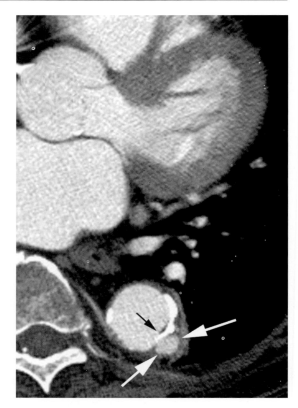

FIGURE 3-15 **Penetrating atherosclerotic ulcer.** Enhanced spiral CT in a man with chest pain shows contrast opacification of a focal ulceration extending into the aortic wall *(white arrows)*. Calcification *(black arrow)* shows the location of the intima.

☐ SUPERIOR VENA CAVA AND GREAT VEINS

Congenital Abnormalities

Azygos Lobe
An azygos lobe is a common anomaly and is present in about 1 in 200 patients. Azygos lobe results in a typical appearance on plain radiographs and CT that is easily recognized and produces a characteristic alteration in normal mediastinal anatomy. In patients with this anomaly, the azygos arch is located more cephalad than normal, at, near, or above the junction of the brachiocephalic veins. Above this level, the azygos fissure is visible within the lung, marginating the azygos lobe (Fig. 3-16).

Persistent Left Superior Vena Cava
The only other frequent venous anomaly is persistent left superior vena cava (SVC), which represents failure of the embryonic left anterior

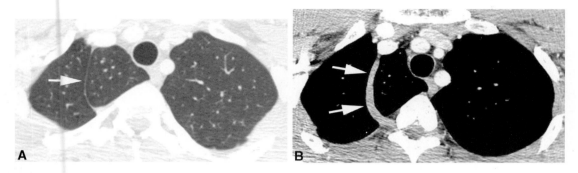

FIGURE 3-16 **Azygos lobe.** *A,* Within the upper lung, the azygos fissure *(arrow)* distinguishes the azygos lobe medially from the remainder of the upper lobe. *B,* At a lower level, the azygos arch *(arrows)* passes from anterior to posterior. In this patient, it arises from the right brachiocephalic vein.

cardinal vein to regress. This anomaly is difficult to recognize on plain films; however, in some patients, there is a slight prominence of the left superior mediastinum. It is present in 0.3% of healthy subjects, approximately the same frequency as an azygos lobe; it is usually without symptoms or associated abnormalities. It has a greater frequency (4.4%) in patients with congenital heart disease.

On CT in patients with this anomaly, the left SVC is positioned lateral to the left common carotid artery in the supra-aortic mediastinum (Fig. 3-17). It descends along the left mediastinum, passing downward, anterior to the left hilum, to enter the coronary sinus posterior to the left atrium. In most patients, a right vena cava is also present, and the two vessels are about the same size and in the same relative position, on opposite sides of the mediastinum. In 65% of patients, the left brachiocephalic vein is absent. However, if it is also present, joining the right and left superior venae cavae, the right SVC will be larger than the left.

A left SVC will densely opacify after contrast medium injection into the left arm. If contrast medium is injected on the right and the vein does not opacify, its tubular shape and characteristic position are usually enough for a definite diagnosis.

Azygos or Hemiazygos Continuation of the Inferior Vena Cava

The embryogenesis of the inferior vena cava is one of the most complicated sequences I know of, and several vessels must develop and regress in turn for it to form normally. During fetal development, the vessels that form the azygos and hemiazygos veins normally communicate with the suprarenal inferior vena cava, but this communication usually breaks down. If it does not, then azygos or hemiazygos continuation of the inferior vena cava is said to be present.

These lesions may be associated with other congenital anomalies, including polysplenia (in patients with hemiazygos communication) or asplenia (with azygos communication), or they may be isolated abnormalities. Typical findings include marked dilatation of the azygos arch and posterior azygos vein (Fig. 3-18). If hemiazygos continuation is present, the dilated azygos vein will be seen to cross the mediastinum, from right to left, behind the descending aorta, to communicate with a dilated hemiazygos vein. A normal-appearing inferior vena cava often is visible at the level of the heart and diaphragm, draining the hepatic veins. Either anomaly may be associated with duplication of the abdominal inferior vena cava. Rarely, a dilated hemiazygos vein drains into the left brachiocephalic vein instead of joining the azygos.

Superior Vena Cava Syndrome

Obstruction of the SVC, or either of the brachiocephalic veins, is a common clinical occurrence, and symptoms of venous obstruction may lead to CT. Also, in some patients undergoing CT for the diagnosis of mediastinal mass or lung cancer, CT will show findings of vena cava obstruction.

SVC obstruction can be seen in a variety of diseases, most commonly bronchogenic carcinoma, although in some parts of the United States, granulomatous mediastinitis as a result of histoplasmosis is a common cause. Other causes of SVC obstruction include sarcoidosis,

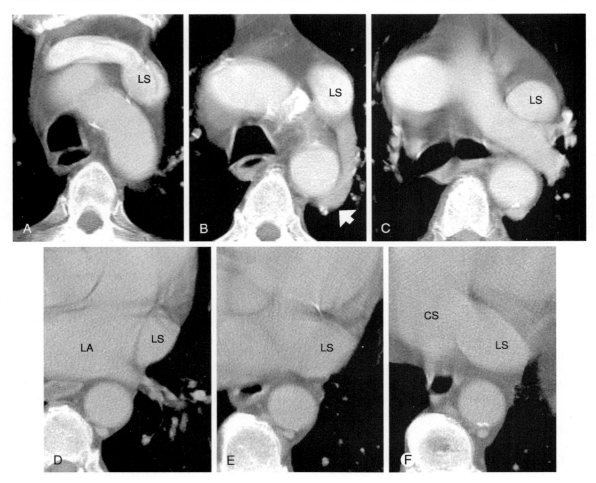

FIGURE 3-17 **Persistent left superior vena cava (SVC) with a hemiazygos arch.** The course of the left SVC is visible at six different levels. *A,* The right vena cava is absent, and injection into the right arm results in dense opacification of the left brachiocephalic vein, because its only drainage is by means of the left SVC (LS). *B,* At a lower level, the left SVC (LS) causes a hemiazygos arch *(arrow),* derived from the left superior intercostal vein. The azygos arch is absent, together with the right SVC. *C,* Inferior to *B,* the left SVC (LS) passes anterior to the left pulmonary artery. *D–F,* Adjacent to the heart, the left SVC (LS) passes anterior to the inferior pulmonary vein, lateral to the left atrium (LA), and enters the coronary sinus (CS).

fibrosing mediastinitis, tuberculosis, or mediastinal radiation for neoplasm. Because of the frequent use of subclavian catheters, venous thrombosis resulting in obstruction is not uncommon.

On CT in patients with SVC obstruction (Figs. 3-19 and 3-20), a number of characteristic findings are present. Beginning peripherally as the contrast medium bolus is injected, it is common to see opacification of a number of small venous collateral vessels in the shoulder, upper chest wall, and upper mediastinum. However, keep in mind that some filling of small veins in the chest wall and axilla can be seen in the absence of a venous abnormality (perhaps because of poor positioning of the patient's arm for injection). Unless other findings of venous obstruction (e.g., large collateral veins) are present, this finding should not be of great concern.

In patients with obstruction of the SVC, flow of contrast medium from the arm is delayed and the scan sequence must be delayed accordingly, or mediastinal vascular opacification will be poor. Some characteristic collateral vessels are often seen in patients with obstruction of the SVC. These include a number of veins that drain into the azygos system, thus bypassing the area of obstruction. These veins commonly include the internal mammary veins, left superior intercostal vein (which results in the "aortic nipple" sometimes visible on chest radiographs),

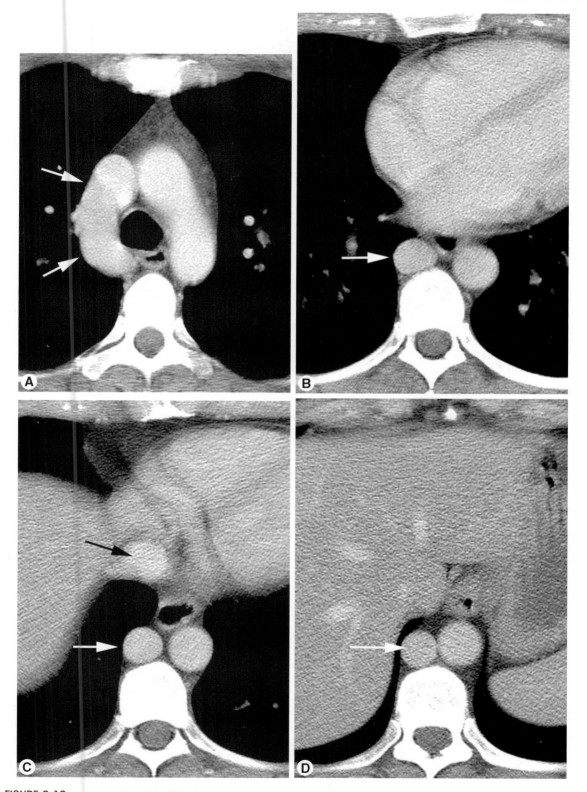

FIGURE 3-18 **Azygos continuation of the inferior vena cava.** The azygos arch *(white arrows, A)* and the posterior azygos vein *(white arrow, B–D)* are markedly dilated. A normal-appearing inferior vena cava is visible at the level of the heart and diaphragm *(black arrow, C)*, draining the hepatic veins, but it is not seen below that level.

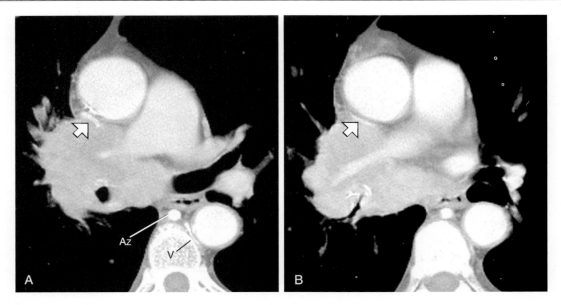

FIGURE 3-19 **Superior vena cava (SVC) obstruction in bronchogenic carcinoma.** *A* and *B,* In a patient with a large right hilar mass and mediastinal invasion, the SVC *(arrows)* is nearly obstructed. The azygos vein (AZ) and a left intercostal vein (V) are opacified, because they are serving as collateral pathways to bypass the obstruction.

intercostal veins, and the hemiazygos vein. In addition to dilatation of these veins because of increased flow, they opacify after contrast medium infusion in the presence of SVC obstruction.

In patients with thrombosis of the SVC or brachiocephalic veins, thrombus is sometimes visible in the vessel lumen, outlined by contrast medium. One word of caution, however: If con-

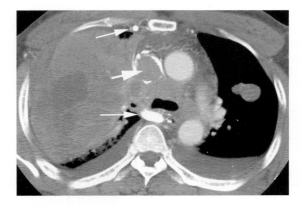

FIGURE 3-20 **Superior vena cava syndrome in metastatic carcinoma.** CT with contrast enhancement in a patient with metastatic carcinoma and symptoms of superior vena cava syndrome. The superior vena cava contains a large tumor thrombus *(large arrow).* Internal mammary vein and azygos vein *(small arrows)* are opacified because they are serving as collateral pathways. The right upper lobe is consolidated because of postobstructive pneumonia. Pleural effusions are present.

trast medium is injected into only one arm, as is typical, streaming of unopacified blood from one brachiocephalic vein into the SVC can mimic the appearance of vena cava clot.

☐ PULMONARY ARTERIES

Pulmonary artery anomalies are rare. Dilatation of the pulmonary artery as a result of pulmonic stenosis or pulmonary hypertension is much more common than congenital lesions. A main pulmonary artery diameter measuring 3.0 cm or more (lateral to the ascending aorta), or exceeding the diameter of the ascending aorta, suggests pulmonary hypertension (see Fig. 3-16). With pulmonic stenosis, the main and left pulmonary arteries are dilated, whereas the right pulmonary artery is relatively normal in size. With pulmonary hypertension, both pulmonary arteries are large.

Pulmonary artery aneurysms are rare; they may be mycotic aneurysms or caused by catheter-related complications, Takayasu's arteritis, Williams syndrome, prenatal varicella, or Behçet's syndrome.

Pulmonary Embolism

Contrast medium–enhanced CT is commonly used to diagnose pulmonary embolism (PE;

Figs. 3-21 and 3-22). Use of radionuclide imaging and pulmonary arteriography have decreased significantly in clinical practice.

An appropriate CT technique using single-detector CT includes: (1) 3-mm collimation; (2) a pitch of 1.7 to 2; (3) a single breath hold of 20 seconds; (4) coverage of the main and segmental pulmonary artery branches (volume of about 10–12 cm); (5) contrast medium injection at a rate of 3 to 4 mL/second, with the injection started 20 seconds before scanning or timed by the scanner; and (6) reconstruction at 2-mm intervals.

MDCT is highly advantageous because of the thin slices and rapid scanning possible. With MDCT, an appropriate technique is: (1) 1.25-mm detector rows; (2) a pitch of 1.6; (3) a single breath hold of 5 seconds; (4) coverage of the entire thorax (volume of 20–25 cm); (5) contrast medium injection at a rate of 4 mL/second, with the injection started 20 seconds before scanning or timed by the scanner; and (6) reconstruction at 1.25-mm intervals.

A filling defect visible within a pulmonary artery is usually diagnostic of PE (see Figs. 3-21 to 3-23); large intraluminal pulmonary artery masses also can be seen with pulmonary artery sarcoma or tumor embolism, but are much less common.

An acute PE is usually centered in the lumen of the artery, being outlined by the injected contrast agent (see Figs. 3-21 and 3-22). If the vessel is seen in cross section, this appearance is termed the *doughnut sign.* If the vessel is visible along its length, it is termed the *railroad track sign.* Some clots may completely obstruct an artery. The clot usually measures 60 H or less in attenuation; the opacified blood outlining it measures considerably more (i.e., 200 H). Pulmonary emboli are usually long or "worm-shaped," and they are usually visible on a number of scans when oriented perpendicular to the scan plane or along the length of an artery lying in the scan plane. An apparent filling defect that is seen on only one or two scans is likely an artifact.

A chronic PE is usually adherent to the vessel wall and is located peripherally, with contrast in the center of the vessel lumen (see Fig. 3-23). This is the opposite of what is seen with acute PE. Pulmonary artery webs can indicate prior emboli. Enlargement of the main pulmonary artery may be seen because of pulmonary hypertension.

The sensitivity and specificity of spiral CT in diagnosing acute PE in the main pulmonary artery branches is nearly 100%; its overall sensitivity and specificity exceeds 90% for segmental emboli. Although MDCT may show subsegmental emboli quite clearly, the sensitivity of CT for detecting these small clots is less. It should be kept in mind, however, that isolated subsegmental emboli are relatively uncommon (other large clots are usually also seen); arteriography is not good for diagnosing these small clots either, and small subsegmental clots, in and of themselves, are not usually significant from a hemodynamic point of view. Several studies have shown that if a CT is read as "no PE,"

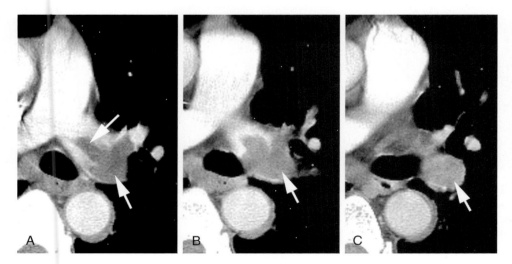

FIGURE 3-21 **Acute pulmonary embolism in the left main pulmonary artery.** *A–C,* Clot fills the left main and interlobar pulmonary artery *(arrows)* and is outlined by contrast medium in *A.*

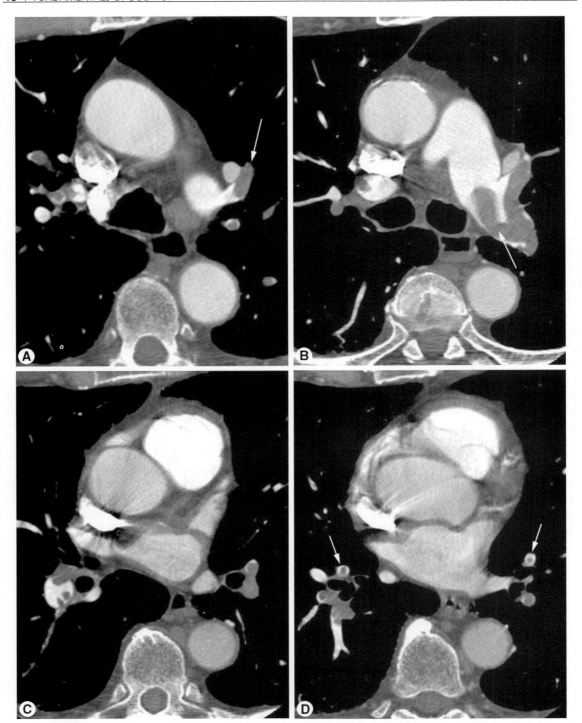

FIGURE 3-22 **Multidetector CT (1.25 mm) in acute pulmonary embolism.** *A–D,* Multiple clots *(arrows)* are visible within large central, lobar, segmental, and subsegmental pulmonary artery branches. They are outlined by contrast medium, showing examples of the "railroad track sign" *(arrow, B)* and the "doughnut sign" *(arrows, D).* Some vessels are completely obstructed and the clots are not outlined by contrast *(arrow, A).*

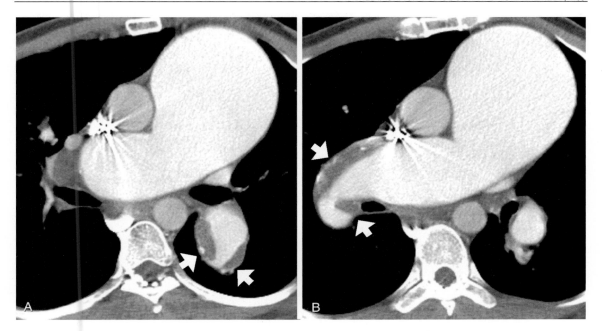

FIGURE 3-23 **Chronic pulmonary embolism and pulmonary hypertension in a patient with Marfan's syndrome.** *A* and *B,* The main pulmonary artery is dilated because of pulmonary hypertension. Thrombus *(arrows)* is adherent to the vessel wall. Some calcification of the vessel wall is also seen.

patient outcome is as good as with a negative radionuclide scan, regardless of whether small clots are being missed.

Only about 5% of patients having CT for possible PE actually have PE. The remainder of these patients has other abnormalities associated with acute chest pain, dyspnea, and hypoxemia. These include atelectasis, pneumonia, pulmonary edema, pleural effusions, and many others. Radionuclide imaging and arteriography are not helpful in diagnosing these abnormalities. In contrast CT is helpful. Because MDCT encompasses the entire thorax, it is advantageous in assessing other diseases in patients being imaged for possible PE.

SUGGESTED READING

BATRA P, BIGONI B, MANNING J, et al: Pitfalls in the diagnosis of thoracic aortic dissection at CT angiography. Radiographics 20:309-320, 2000.

BECHTOLD RE, WOLFMAN NT, KARSTAEDT N, CHOPLIN RH: Superior vena caval obstruction: Detection using CT. Radiology 157:485-487, 1985.

CASTANER E, ANDREU M, GALLARDO X, et al: CT in nontraumatic acute thoracic aortic disease: Typical and atypical features and complications. Radiographics 23:S93-S110, 2003.

DILLON EH, VAN LEEUWEN MS, FERNANDEZ MA, MALI WPTM: Spiral CT angiography. AJR Am J Roentgenol 160:1273-1278, 1993.

GAVANT ML, FLICK P, MENKE P, GOLD RE: CT aortography of thoracic aortic rupture. AJR Am J Roentgenol 166:955-961, 1996.

GAVANT ML, MENKE PG, FABIAN T, et al: Blunt traumatic aortic rupture: Detection with helical CT of the chest. Radiology 197:125-133, 1995.

GEFTER WB, HATABU H, HOLLAND GA, et al: Pulmonary thromboembolism: Recent developments in diagnosis with CT and MR imaging. Radiology 197:561-574, 1995.

GOODMAN LR, LIPCHIK RJ: Diagnosis of pulmonary embolism: Time for a new approach [editorial]. Radiology 199:25-27, 1996.

GOTWAY MB, PATEL RA, WEBB WR: Helical CT for the evaluation of suspected acute pulmonary embolism: Diagnostic pitfalls. J Comput Assist Tomogr 24:267-273, 2000.

HAYASHI H, MATSUOKA Y, SAKAMOTO I, et al: Penetrating atherosclerotic ulcer of the aorta: Imaging features and disease concept. Radiographics 20:995-1005, 2000.

MAYO JR, REMY-JARDIN M, MÜLLER NL, et al: Pulmonary embolism: Prospective comparison of spiral

CT with ventilation-perfusion scintigraphy. Radiology 205:447–452, 1997.

Tello R, Costello P, Ecker C, et al: Spiral CT evaluation of coronary artery bypass graft patency. J Comput Assist Tomogr 17:253–259, 1993.

Trerotola SO: Can helical CT replace aortography in thoracic trauma [editorial]? Radiology 197:13–15, 1995.

Webb WR, Gamsu G, Speckman JM, et al: CT demonstration of mediastinal aortic arch anomalies. J Comput Assist Tomogr 6:445–451, 1982.

Webb WR, Gamsu G, Speckman JM, et al: CT demonstration of mediastinal venous anomalies. AJR Am J Roentgenol 159:157–161, 1982.

Zeman RK, Berman PM, Silverman PM, et al: Diagnosis of aortic dissection: Value of helical CT with multiplanar re-formations and three-dimensional rendering. AJR Am J Roentgenol 164:1375–1380, 1995.

4

Mediastinum: Lymph Node Abnormalities and Masses

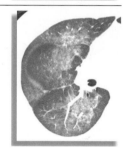

W. Richard Webb, M.D.

☐ LYMPH NODE GROUPS

Mediastinal lymph nodes are generally classified by location, and most descriptive systems are based on a modification of Rouvière's classification of lymph node groups.

Anterior Mediastinal Nodes

Internal mammary nodes are located in a retrosternal location near the internal mammary artery and veins (Fig. 4-1). They drain the anterior chest wall, anterior diaphragm, and medial breasts.

Paracardiac nodes (diaphragmatic, pericardial) surround the heart on the surface of the diaphragm and communicate with the lower internal mammary chain (Fig. 4-2). Like internal mammary nodes, they are most commonly enlarged in patients with lymphoma and metastatic carcinoma, particularly breast cancer.

Prevascular nodes lie anterior to the great vessels (see Figs. 4-1, 4-3, and 4-4A). They may be involved in a variety of diseases, notably lymphoma, but their involvement in lung cancer is unusual.

Middle Mediastinal Nodes

Lung diseases (e.g., lung cancer, sarcoidosis, tuberculosis, fungal infections) that secondarily involve lymph nodes typically involve middle mediastinal lymph nodes.

Pretracheal or *paratracheal nodes* occupy the pretracheal (or anterior paratracheal) space (see Figs. 4-1, 4-3, and 4-4A). The most inferior node in this region is the so-called azygos node. These nodes form the final pathway for lymphatic drainage from most of both lungs (except the left upper lobe). Because of this, they are commonly abnormal regardless of the location of the lung disease.

Aortopulmonary nodes are considered by Rouvière to be in the anterior mediastinal group, but because they serve the same function as right paratracheal nodes, they are considered here (see Figs. 4-3C, 4-4B, and 4-4C). The left upper lobe is drained by this node group.

Subcarinal nodes are located in the subcarinal space, between the main bronchi (see Fig. 4-4B to D), and drain the inferior hila and both lower lobes. They communicate in turn with the right paratracheal chain.

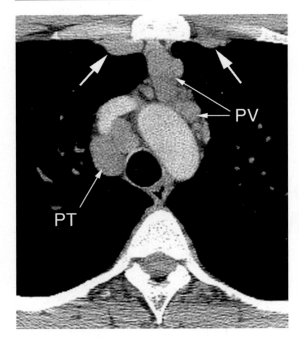

FIGURE 4-1 **Internal mammary node enlargement in sarcoidosis.** Bilateral internal mammary nodes *(large arrows)* are enlarged, as are pretracheal (PT) and prevascular (PV) nodes.

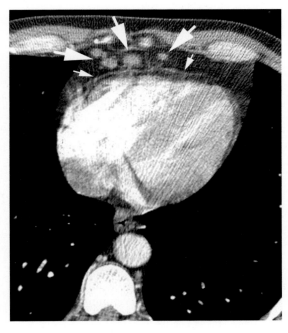

FIGURE 4-2 **Paracardiac node enlargement.** In a patient with lymphoma, enlargement of paracardiac nodes *(large arrows)* is visible. These lie anterior to the pericardium *(small arrows)*.

Peribronchial nodes surround the main bronchi on each side (see Fig. *4-4B* and *C*). They communicate with bronchopulmonary (hilar; see Fig. 4-4*C* and *D*), subcarinal, and paratracheal nodes.

Posterior Mediastinal Nodes

Paraesophageal nodes lie posterior to the trachea or are associated with the esophagus, or both (Fig. 4-5). Subcarinal nodes are not included in this group.

Inferior pulmonary ligament nodes are located below the pulmonary hila, medial to the inferior pulmonary ligament. On CT, they are usually seen adjacent to the esophagus on the right and descending aorta on the left. Below the hila, they are difficult to distinguish from paraesophageal nodes. Together with the paraesophageal nodes, they drain the medial lower lobes, esophagus, pericardium, and posterior diaphragm.

Paravertebral nodes lie lateral to the vertebral bodies, posterior to the aorta on the left (see Fig. 4-5). They drain the posterior chest wall and pleura. They are most commonly involved, together with retrocrural or retroperitoneal abdominal nodes, in patients with lymphoma or metastatic carcinoma.

Lymph Node Stations

In the 1970s, the American Joint Committee on Cancer (AJCC) and the Union Internationale Contre le Cancer (UICC) introduced a numeric system for localization of intrathoracic lymph nodes for the purpose of lung cancer staging. Lymph nodes were described relative to regions in the mediastinum termed *lymph node stations.* The AJCC/UICC node mapping system was modified in 1983 by the American Thoracic Society to more precisely define anatomic and CT criteria for each station, and the American Thoracic Society classification system has been in common usage since its development. In 1997, the AJCC/UICC published a further revision intended to be a compromise between the AJCC and American Thoracic Society classifications (Fig. 4-6). A detailed knowledge of "lymph node stations" is not necessary in clinical practice, but a passing familiarity with this classification is encouraged (Table 4-1).

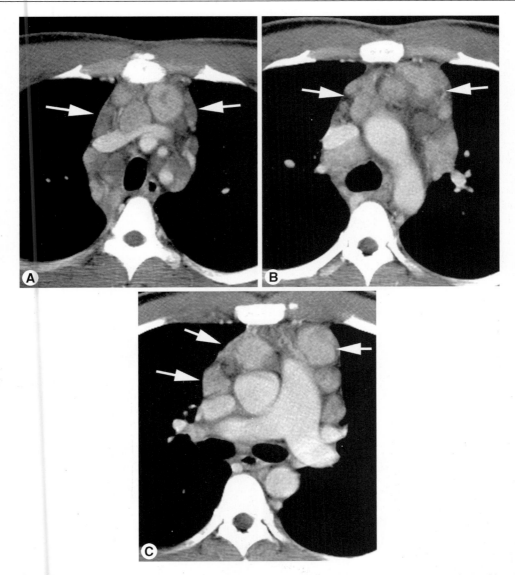

FIGURE 4-3 **Prevascular lymph node enlargement in Hodgkin's lymphoma.** Enlarged prevascular or anterior mediastinal lymph nodes *(arrows)* are seen anterior to the brachiocephalic veins and great vessels *(A),* anterior to the aortic arch and superior vena cava *(B),* and anterior to the superior vena cava, aortic root, and main pulmonary artery *(C).* Enlarged pretracheal lymph nodes are also visible at all three levels. In *C,* prevascular nodes are contiguous with nodes lateral to the main pulmonary artery, usually considered to be in the aortopulmonary window. Some nodes appear low in attenuation and are probably necrotic.

☐ CT APPEARANCE OF LYMPH NODES

Lymph nodes are generally visible as discrete, round, or elliptical soft-tissue attenuation structures surrounded by mediastinal fat and distinguishable from vessels by their location. They often occur in clusters (Fig. 4-7). In some locations, nodes that contact vessels may be difficult to identify without contrast infusion.

Internal mammary nodes, paracardiac nodes, and paravertebral nodes are not usually seen on CT in healthy subjects, but in other areas of the mediastinum, normal nodes are often visible. The expected size of normal nodes varies with their location, and a few general rules apply. Subcarinal nodes (AJCC/UICC station 7) can be quite large in healthy subjects. Pretracheal nodes are also commonly visible, but these nodes are typically smaller than

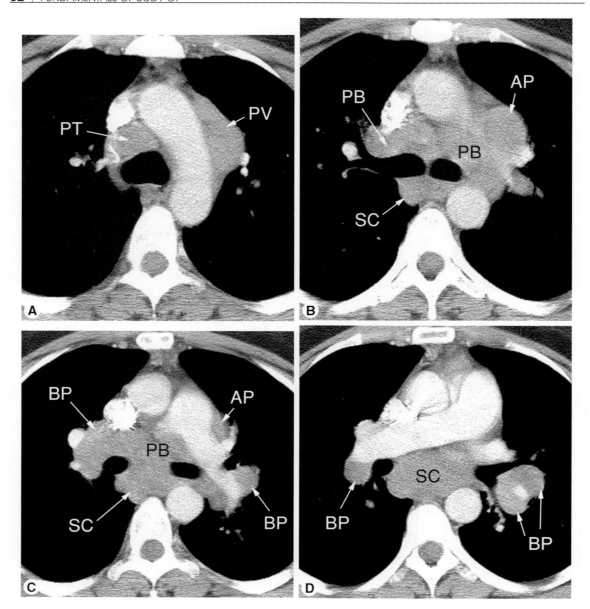

FIGURE 4-4 Lymph node enlargement in a patient with sarcoidosis. *A,* At the aortic arch level, enlarged pretracheal (PT) and prevascular (PV) nodes are visible. *B,* At the level of the tracheal carina, lymph nodes lateral to the left pulmonary artery are termed *aortopulmonary* (AP). Lymph nodes adjacent to the main bronchi are termed *peribronchial* (PB). Subcarinal (SC) lymph nodes are located posterior to the carina. *C,* At a lower level, aortopulmonary (AP), peribronchial (PB), and subcarinal (SC) nodes are again visible. Hilar lymph nodes are termed *bronchopulmonary* (BP). *D,* Below *C,* large subcarinal (SC) nodes and bronchopulmonary (BP) nodes are again visible.

normal subcarinal nodes. Nodes in the supra-aortic mediastinum (AJCC/UICC stations 1-3) are usually smaller than lower pretracheal nodes, and left paratracheal nodes are usually smaller than right paratracheal nodes.

Measurement of Lymph Node Size

The *short axis* or *least diameter* (i.e., the smallest node diameter seen in cross section) is generally used when measuring the size of a lymph

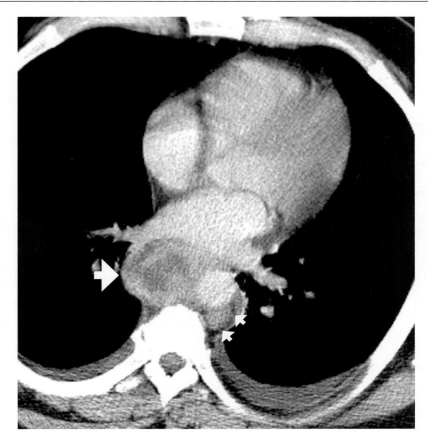

FIGURE 4-5 **Paravertebral lymph node enlargement in metastatic testicular carcinoma.** Large lymph nodes on the right *(large arrow)* can be considered paraesophageal or inferior pulmonary ligament. They appear inhomogeneous and are necrotic. An enlarged left paravertebral lymph node *(small arrows)* is also visible posterior to the aorta.

node. Measuring the short axis is better than measuring the *long axis* or *greatest diameter* because it more closely reflects actual node diameter when nodes are obliquely oriented relative to the scan plane and shows less variation among healthy subjects. Different values for the upper limits of normal short-axis node diameter have been found for different mediastinal node groups (Table 4-2). However, except for the subcarinal regions, a short-axis node diameter of 1 cm or less is generally considered normal for clinical purposes. In the subcarinal region, 1.5 cm is usually considered to be the upper limits of normal.

Lymph Node Enlargement

Except in the subcarinal space, lymph nodes are considered to be enlarged if they have a short-axis diameter greater than 1 cm. In most cases, they are outlined by fat and are visible as discrete structures (see Fig. 4-3). However, in the pres-

ence of inflammation or neoplastic infiltration, abnormal nodes can be matted together, giving the appearance of a single large mass or resulting in infiltration and replacement of mediastinal fat by soft-tissue opacity.

The significance given to the presence of an enlarged lymph node must be tempered by knowledge of the patient's clinical situation. For example, if the patient is known to have lung cancer, then an enlarged lymph node has a 70% likelihood of being involved by tumor. However, the same node in a patient without lung cancer is much less likely to be of clinical significance. In the absence of a known disease, an enlarged node must be regarded as likely to be hyperplastic or postinflammatory. Also, the larger a node is, the more likely it is to represent a significant abnormality. Mediastinal lymph nodes larger than 2 cm are often involved by tumor, although this may also be seen in patients with sarcoidosis or other granulomatous diseases.

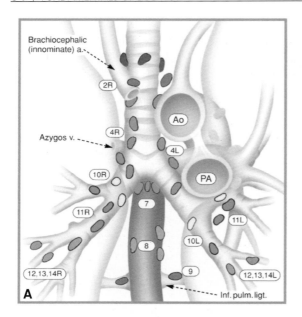
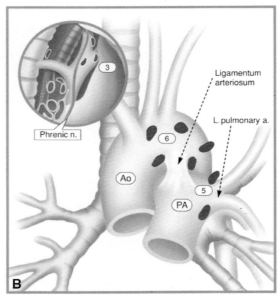

FIGURE 4-6 American Joint Committee on Cancer and the Union Internationale Contre le Cancer lymph node stations. *A* and *B*, Ao, aorta; PA, pulmonary artery. (Reproduced from Mountain CF, Dresler CM: Regional lymph node classification for lung cancer staging. Chest 111:1718–1723, 1997, with permission.)

Lymph Node Calcification

Calcification can be dense, involving the node in a homogeneous fashion, stippled, or "egg shell" in appearance. The abnormal nodes are often enlarged but can also be of normal size. Multiple calcified lymph nodes are often visible, usually in contiguity.

Lymph node calcification usually indicates prior granulomatous disease, including tuberculosis, histoplasmosis and other fungal infections, and sarcoidosis (Fig. 4-8). The differential diagnosis also includes silicosis, coal workers' pneumoconiosis, treated Hodgkin's disease, metastatic neoplasm, typically mutinous adenocarcinoma, thyroid carcinoma, or metastatic osteogenic sarcoma. Egg-shell calcification is most often seen in patients with silicosis or coal workers' pneumoconiosis, sarcoidosis, and tuberculosis.

Low-Attenuation or Necrotic Lymph Nodes

Enlarged lymph nodes may appear to be low in attenuation (see Fig. 4-5), often with an enhancing rim if contrast has been injected. Typically, low-attenuation nodes reflect the presence of necrosis. They are commonly seen in patients with active tuberculous, fungal infections, and neoplasms, such as metastatic carcinoma and lymphoma.

Lymph Node Enhancement

Healthy lymph nodes may show some increase in attenuation after intravenous contrast infusion. Pathologic lymph nodes with an increased vascular supply may increase significantly in attenuation. The differential diagnosis of densely enhancing mediastinal nodes is limited and includes Castleman's disease (see Fig. 4-15), angioimmunoblastic lymphadenopathy, vascular metastases (e.g., renal cell carcinoma, papillary thyroid carcinoma, lung carcinoma, sarcoma, and melanoma), tuberculosis, and sometimes sarcoidosis.

☐ DIFFERENTIAL DIAGNOSIS OF MEDIASTINAL LYMPH NODE ENLARGEMENT

Lung Cancer

Approximately 35% of patients diagnosed with lung cancer have mediastinal node metastases (Fig. 4-9). Lung cancer most often involves the

TABLE 4-1

American Joint Committee on Cancer/Union Internationale Contre le Cancer 1997 Lymph Node Stations

Node Group	AJCC/UICC Station	AJCC/UICC Designation	AJCC/UICC Anatomic Criteria
Paratracheal	1	Highest mediastinal	Cranial to the superior aspect of L brachiocephalic vein
Paratracheal	2	Upper paratracheal	Below station 1 and cranial to superior aspect of the aortic arch
Prevascular	3	Prevascular	Anterior to the great vessel branches and cranial to aortic arch
Paraesophageal		Retrotracheal	Posterior to the trachea and cranial to the inferior aspect of azygos arch
Paratracheal	4R	R lower paratracheal	R of tracheal midline, below 2, and cranial to the RUL bronchus
	4L	L lower paratracheal	L of the tracheal midline, below 2, and cranial to the LUL bronchus
Aortopulmonary	5	Subaortic or Aortopulmonary	Lateral to the ligamentum arteriosum, aorta, or LPA, proximal to the first branch of the LPA within the mediastinal pleural envelope
Prevascular	6	Para-aortic (ascending aortic or phrenic)	Anterior and lateral to the ascending aorta and the aortic arch and innominate artery, caudal to the superior aspect of aortic arch
Subcarinal	7	Subcarinal	Caudal to the carina but not associated with the lower lobe bronchi or pulmonary arteries within the lung
Paraesophageal	8	Paraesophageal	Adjacent to the wall of the esophagus and to the right or left of esophagus
Inferior pulmonary ligament	9	Pulmonary ligament	Within the pulmonary ligament, including those in the posterior wall and lower part of the inferior pulmonary vein
Peribronchial (hilar)	10R	R hilar	Adjacent to the R main bronchus or proximal bronchus intermedius
	10L	L hilar	Caudal to the superior LUL bronchus, adjacent to L main bronchus
Bronchopulmonary (hilar)	11	Interlobar	Between lobar bronchi and adjacent to proximal lobar bronchi
Lobar	12	Lobar	Adjacent to distal lobar bronchi
Segmental	13	Segmental	Adjacent to segmental bronchi
Subsegmental	14	Subsegmental	Adjacent to subsegmental bronchi

AJCC, American Joint Committee on Cancer; L, left; LPA, left pulmonary artery; LUL, left upper lobe; R, right; RUL, right upper lobe; UICC, Union Internationale Contre le Cancer.

middle mediastinal node groups. Left upper lobe cancers typically metastasize to aortopulmonary window nodes, whereas tumors involving the lower lobes on either side tend to metastasize to the subcarinal and right paratracheal groups. Right upper lobe tumors typically involve paratracheal nodes.

Lung Cancer Staging

In patients with non–small-cell bronchogenic carcinoma, although the cell type and histologic characteristics of the tumor affect prognosis, the anatomic extent of the tumor (tumor stage) is usually most important in determining the thera-peutic approach. The most widely used anatom-ic staging classification is the TNM classification of the AJCC.

This classification is based on a consider-ation of the following characteristics: (1) the location and extent of the primary tumor (T); (2) the presence or absence of lymph node metastases (N); and (3) the presence or absence of distant metastases (M) (Table 4-3). Based on this classification, excellent correlations are found between tumor stage and survival after treatment.

For radiologic purposes, precise classifica-tion of tumor stage is not usually necessary.

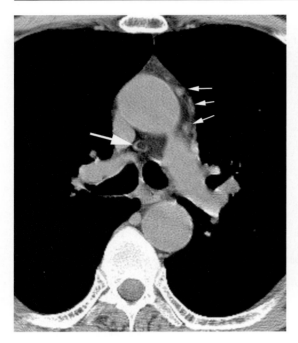

FIGURE 4-7 **Normal mediastinal nodes.** Small lymph nodes are visible in the aortopulmonary window *(small arrows)*, with a short-axis diameter of less than 1 cm. A normal-sized pretracheal lymph node *(large arrows)* has a fatty hilum and contains a large amount of fat. This is a benign appearance.

However, differentiation of resectable disease (stages I–IIIa) and unresectable disease (stages IIIb–IV) is important (see Table 4-3). The criteria for resectability listed in Table 4-3 are generally accepted but are not absolute; different surgeons may have different criteria as to what is resectable. In particular, the resectability of some stage IIIa tumors is controversial.

TABLE 4-2

Upper Limits of Normal for Short-Axis Node Diameter

Node Group	AJCC/UICC Node Station	Short-Axis Node Diameter* (mm)
Supraaortic paratracheal	2	7
Subaortic paratracheal	4	9
Aortopulmonary window	5	9
Prevascular	6	8
Subcarinal	7	12
Paraesophageal	8	8

*Mean normal node diameter plus two standard deviations.
AJCC, American Joint Committee on Cancer; L, left; R, right; UICC, Union Internationale Contre le Cancer.

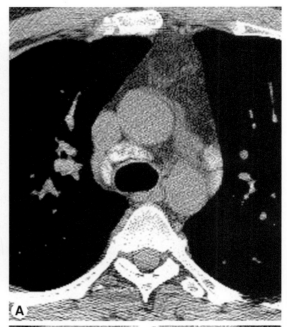

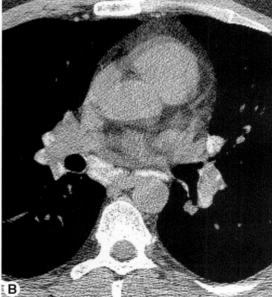

FIGURE 4-8 **Lymph node calcification in sarcoidosis.** *A* and *B,* Enlarged lymph nodes show homogeneous and stippled calcification. Pretracheal, aortopulmonary, subcarinal, and hilar lymph nodes are involved.

The next section discusses the impact of mediastinal lymph node metastases and mediastinal invasion on lung cancer staging. Chapters 5 and 7 discuss other aspects of lung cancer staging.

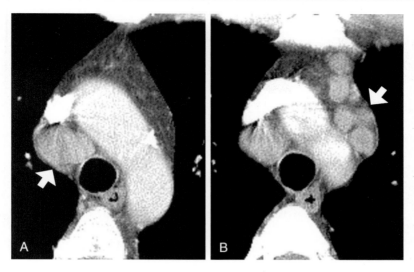

FIGURE 4-9 **Lymph node enlargement in a patient with a right-sided bronchogenic carcinoma.** *A,* Lymph node enlargement in the pretracheal space *(arrow)* is ipsilateral, N2, and potentially resectable. These nodes are large, and thus are likely involved by tumor. *B,* Lymph node enlargement in the prevascular space *(arrow)* is contralateral, N3, and is considered unresectable.

Mediastinal Node Metastases in Lung Cancer

In the TNM lung cancer staging system, ipsilateral mediastinal node metastases and subcarinal node metastases are termed *N2* and are considered potentially resectable (although this is not always the case); contralateral nodes are termed *N3* and are considered unresectable (see Fig. 4-9).

In patients with lung cancer, the likelihood that a mediastinal node is involved by tumor is directly proportional to its size. However, although large nodes are most likely to be involved by tumor (see Fig. 4-9), they can be benign; similarly, although small nodes are usually normal, they can harbor metastases. Although a short-axis measurement of greater than 1 cm is used in clinical practice to identify abnormally enlarged nodes, it is important to realize that no node diameter clearly separates benign nodes from those involved by tumor.

Using a short-axis node diameter of 1 cm as the upper limit of node size, CT will detect mediastinal lymph node enlargement in about 60% of patients with node metastases (its sensitivity), whereas about 70% of patients with normal nodes will be classified normal on CT (its specificity). Although CT is not highly accurate in diagnosing node metastases, it is commonly used to guide subsequent procedures or treatment.

In patients without node enlargement on CT, thoracotomy may be performed without prior mediastinoscopy, although this varies with the surgeon. Although some such patients will be found to have microscopic or small intranodal metastases, their presence does not necessarily indicate that surgery was inappropriate. Some patients with ipsilateral intranodal mediastinal metastases (N2) can have successful treatment results after surgical excision of nodes and radiation or chemotherapy.

In contrast, if mediastinal lymph node enlargement is seen on CT, about 70% of patients will have node metastases; benign hyperplasia of mediastinal lymph nodes accounts for the other 30%. Patients with large mediastinal nodes usually have node sampling at mediastinoscopy or by CT-guided needle biopsy before surgery. If node metastases are found at mediastinoscopy, surgery is not generally performed, even though the nodes would be classified as N2; it has been shown that patients with node metastases diagnosed at mediastinoscopy have a poor prognosis after surgery. It should be kept in mind that in patients with enlarged nodes on CT and mediastinal lymph node metastases, the metastases are not always in the nodes that appear large; that is, in some cases, CT can be right for the wrong reason.

Positron emission tomography scanning is more accurate than CT in the assessment of mediastinal lymph nodes in lung cancer and has assumed a significant role. Positron emission tomography has a sensitivity of about 80%

TABLE 4-3

TNM Staging of Lung Cancer

T (Primary Tumor)

T0   No evidence of a primary tumor

T1   A tumor that is:

         a. 3 cm or less in greatest diameter

         b. surrounded by lung or visceral pleura

         c. without invasion proximal to a lobar bronchus (i.e., involving main bronchus)

T2   A tumor with any of the following features:

         a. greater than 3 cm in largest diameter

         b. involving a main bronchus $\geq$2 cm distal to the carina

         c. invading the visceral pleura

         d. producing atelectasis or obstructive pneumonia, extending to the hilum, but involving less than the entire lung

T3   A tumor of any size that either:

         a. invades any chest wall, diaphragm, mediastinal pleura, or parietal pericardium, or

         b. is located <2 cm distal to the carina without involvement of the carina or is associated with atelectasis or obstructive pneumonia of an entire lung

T4   *A tumor of any size with any of the following features:*

         a. invading the mediastinum, heart, great vessels, trachea, esophagus, vertebral body, or carina

         b. producing malignant pleural or pericardial effusion (pleural effusion not obviously associated with metastases has no effect on stage)

         c. associated with satellite tumor nodules in the same lobe as the primary tumor (nodules in a different lobe are considered metastases or M1)

N (Nodal Involvement)

N0   No regional node metastases

N1   Metastases to ipsilateral peribronchial, hilar, and/or intrapulmonary nodes

N2   Metastases to ipsilateral mediastinal nodes, subcarinal nodes, or both

N3   *Metastases to contralateral hilar or mediastinal lymph nodes, or scalene or supraclavicular lymph nodes*

M (Distant Metastases)

M0   Metastases absent

M1   *Metastases present*

Resectable Stages

IA   T1N0M0

IB   T2N0M0

IIA   T1N1M0

IIB   T2N1M0

        T3N0M0

IIIA   T1N2M0

        T2N2M0

        T3N1M0

        T3N2M0

Unresectable Stages

IIIB   *T1N3M0*

        T2N3M0

        T3N3M0

IV   *M1*

Findings that usually indicate unresectability in most situations are in italics.

for diagnosis of mediastinal node metastases (vs. 60% for CT) and a specificity of about 90% (vs. 70% for CT). Positron emission tomography is usually combined with CT, because of the poor anatomic detail provided by positron emission tomography.

Mediastinoscopy is slightly more sensitive than CT, has a much higher specificity (100%; that is, no normal nodes are called abnormal based on mediastinoscopy), and has a higher accuracy for diagnosing mediastinal node metastases. However, the mediastinoscopist cannot evaluate all mediastinal compartments or lymph node groups, and a significant percentage (up to 25%) of patients with bronchogenic carcinoma who have a negative mediastinoscopy result are found to have mediastinal nodal metastases at surgery. Through a standard transcervical approach, the mediastinoscopist can only evaluate pretracheal lymph nodes, nodes in the anterior subcarinal space, and lymph nodes extending anterior to the right main bronchus. Lymph nodes in the anterior mediastinum (prevascular space), aortopulmonary window, and posterior portions of the mediastinum (e.g., posterior subcarinal space, azygoesophageal recess) are inaccessible using this technique, although some can be evaluated using a left

parasternal mediastinoscopy (Chamberlain procedure). CT, in contrast, allows evaluation of all these areas, shows where any enlarged nodes are, and can serve to guide needle aspiration biopsy or parasternal mediastinotomy if enlarged lymph nodes are visible in areas that cannot be evaluated using a standard approach.

In patients with small peripheral lung nodules, mediastinal metastases are uncommon, and thoracotomy may be warranted without prior CT or mediastinoscopy; but this is controversial. Most surgeons obtain CT in this situation.

Mediastinal Invasion by Lung Cancer

In addition to mediastinal node metastasis, bronchogenic carcinoma can involve the mediastinum by direct extension, so-called mediastinal invasion. In current surgical practice, invasion of the mediastinal pleura, termed *T3* in the lung cancer staging system, does not prevent surgery. However, significant invasion of mediastinal fat or other mediastinal structures, such as the trachea or esophagus, does prevent resection; such lesions are termed *T4* (Fig. 4-10).

How accurate is CT in predicting mediastinal invasion? Obviously, you can be sure that

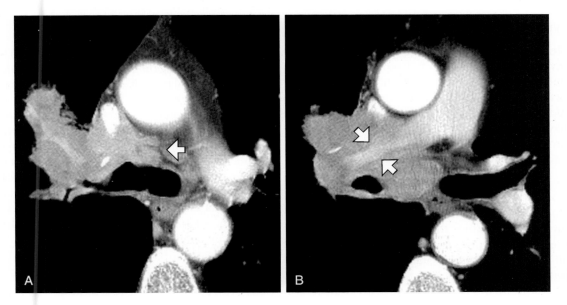

FIGURE 4-10 **Mediastinal invasion by bronchogenic carcinoma.** A right hilar tumor has resulted in extensive mediastinal invasion, anterior to the carina *(arrow, A)* and surrounding and narrowing the right pulmonary artery *(arrows, B)*. There is extensive replacement of fat by tumor, the tumor surrounds and compresses the pulmonary artery and compresses the vena cava, and fat planes are invisible adjacent to the great vessels.

a lung mass not contacting the mediastinum is not invasive, and this is an important use of CT.

CT findings of mediastinal invasion (see Fig. 4-10) include:

1. Replacement of mediastinal fat by soft-tissue attenuation tumor
2. Compression or displacement of mediastinal vessels by tumor
3. Tumor contacting more than 90 degrees of the circumference of a structure, such as the aorta, pulmonary artery, and so on (the greater the extent of circumferential contact, i.e., 180 degrees, the greater the likelihood of invasion)
4. Obliteration of the mediastinal fat plane normally seen adjacent to most mediastinal structures
5. Tumor contacting more than 3 cm of the mediastinum
6. Obtuse angles where tumor contacts the mediastinum
7. Mediastinal pleural or pericardial thickening

A definite diagnosis of invasion can be made if tumor is visible infiltrating mediastinal fat. Other findings of mediastinal invasion are less accurate. If none of these findings is present, the tumor is likely resectable.

Lymphoma and Leukemia

Mediastinal lymph nodes are commonly involved in patients with lymphoma. A small percentage of patients are first recognized because of mediastinal masses noted on chest radiographs, but these patients will often have systemic signs and symptoms, including fever, night sweats, weight loss, weakness, and fatigue.

Hodgkin's Disease

Hodgkin's disease has a predilection for thoracic involvement, both at the time of diagnosis and if the disease recurs. Hodgkin's disease occurs in all ages but peaks in incidence in the third and fifth decades of life.

More than 85% of patients with Hodgkin's disease eventually experience development of intrathoracic disease, typically involving the superior mediastinal (prevascular, pretracheal, and aortopulmonary) lymph nodes (Figs. 4-3 and 4-11). An important rule is that intrathoracic

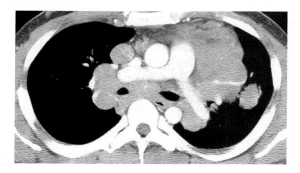

FIGURE 4-11 **Hodgkin's lymphoma.** Extensive enlargement of mediastinal and hilar lymph nodes is visible. A left lung nodule reflects pulmonary involvement.

lymphadenopathy not associated with superior mediastinal node enlargement is unlikely to be Hodgkin's lymphoma.

In one study, it was uncommon for CT to show evidence of mediastinal adenopathy if the chest radiograph was normal; but if the chest radiograph was abnormal, CT detected additional sites of adenopathy in many cases (Table 4-4). CT was most helpful in diagnosing subcarinal, internal mammary, and aorto-pulmonary window node enlargement. Cardiophrenic angle (paracardiac) lymph nodes are present in about 10% of patients and are seen well on CT (see Fig. 4-2). Adenopathy in this location is less common in other diseases. In a significant percentage of patients, the additional node involvement shown by CT changes therapy.

Enlargement of a single node group can be seen with Hodgkin's disease, most commonly in the prevascular mediastinum. This often indicates the presence of nodular sclerosing histology, which accounts for 50% to 80% of adult Hodgkin's disease. In patients with lymphoma, mediastinal lymph nodes may become matted, being visible as a single large mass (Fig. 4-12), rather than individual discrete nodes. Mediastinal nodes or masses in patients with Hodgkin's lymphoma can appear cystic or fluid filled on CT (see Fig. 4-12). Calcification is unusual and of limited extent, except after treatment.

Non–Hodgkin's Lymphoma

Non–Hodgkin's lymphoma is a diverse group of diseases that vary in radiologic manifestation, clinical presentation, course, and prognosis. In comparison with Hodgkin's disease, these tumors are less common and occur in an older group of patients (40-70 years old). At the time

TABLE 4-4

Mediastinal Lymph Node Enlargement in Hodgkin's Disease

Site	Abnormal (%)	Visible on CT (%)	Visible on Radiographs (%)
Pretracheal	64	64	57
Aortopulmonary window	62	62	48
Subcarinal	46	44	9
Internal mammary	38	38	4
Posterior medial	18	12	11
Paracardiac	13	10	7

of presentation, the disease is often generalized (85% are stages III or IV), and chemotherapy is most appropriate. For this reason, precise anatomic staging is less crucial than with Hodgkin's disease.

In one series, 43% had intrathoracic disease and 40% had involvement of only one node group, which is much more common than in patients with Hodgkin's disease (Fig. 4-13). Also, posterior mediastinal nodes were more frequently involved. Lung involvement was present in only 4%; in some patients, lung infiltration may be rapid.

CT, as in patients with Hodgkin's disease, can show evidence of intrathoracic disease when it is unrecognizable on plain radiographs and can affect management in patients with localized (stage I or II) disease.

Leukemia

Leukemia, particularly the lymphocytic varieties, can cause hilar or mediastinal lymph node enlargement, pleural effusion, and occasionally infiltrative lung disease. Lymphadenopathy is generally confined to the middle mediastinum, and the larger masses seen with some lymphomas generally do not occur.

Metastases

Extrathoracic primary tumors can result in mediastinal node enlargement, either with or without hilar or lung metastases (see Figs. 4-5 and 4-14). Node metastases can be present because of inferior extension from neck masses (thyroid carcinoma, head and neck tumors), extension along lymphatic channels from below the diaphragm (testicular carcinoma, renal cell carcinoma, gastrointestinal malignancies), or dissemination by other routes (breast carcinoma, melanoma). Middle mediastinal

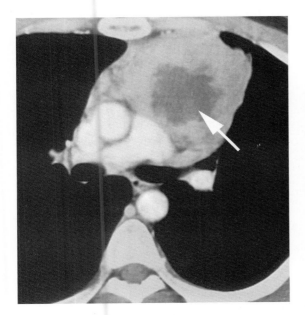

FIGURE 4-12 **Anterior mediastinal Hodgkin's lymphoma with necrosis.** The anterior mediastinal mass contains an irregular area of cystic necrosis *(arrow)*.

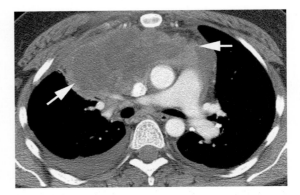

FIGURE 4-13 **Non–Hodgkin's lymphoma involving the anterior mediastinum.** A bulky mediastinal mass *(arrows)* contains areas of low attenuation, likely caused by necrosis. Mediastinal vascular structures are displaced posteriorly. Bilateral pleural effusions are present. Involvement of a single lymph node group is common with non–Hodgkin's lymphoma.

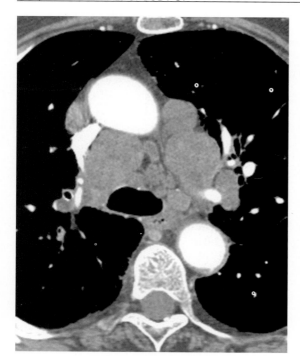

FIGURE 4-14 Extensive mediastinal lymph node metastases in colon carcinoma. Enlarged lymph nodes are visible in the pretracheal space, prevascular space, and aortopulmonary window. Hilar lymph nodes are also enlarged.

(paratracheal) or paravertebral mediastinal nodes are most commonly involved when the tumor is subdiaphragmatic. With breast carcinoma, internal mammary node metastases occur.

Sarcoidosis

Mediastinal lymph node enlargement is common in patients with sarcoidosis, occurring in 60% to 90% of cases. Typically, node enlargement is extensive, involving the hila, as well as the mediastinum, and masses appear bilateral and symmetrical in most patients (see Figs. 4-1, 4-4, and 4-8); this sometimes allows the differentiation of sarcoid from lymphoma, which is more typically asymmetrical. Also, lymph nodes can be quite large in patients with sarcoidosis, but large isolated masses, as seen in some patients with lymphoma, are uncommon. Paratracheal lymph nodes are typically involved. Even though it is commonly stated that sarcoidosis does not involve anterior mediastinal lymph nodes, this is often visible on CT; paravertebral node enlargement is seen occasionally (Table 4-5).

Infections

A variety of infectious agents can cause mediastinal lymph node enlargement during the acute stage of the infection. These include a number of fungal infections (commonly histoplasmosis and coccidioidomycosis), tuberculosis, bacterial infections, and viral infections. Typically, there will be symptoms and signs of acute infection, and chest radiographs will show evidence of pneumonia.

The lymph node enlargement will often be asymmetrical, involving hilar and middle mediastinal nodes. In patients with tuberculosis, enlarged nodes typically show rim enhancement and central necrosis after contrast medium injection; this appearance is nearly diagnostic in patients with an appropriate history. Lymph node calcification occurs in patients with chronic fungal or tuberculous infection.

Castleman's Disease (Angiofollicular Lymph Node Hyperplasia)

An unusual disease of unknown cause, Castleman's disease occurs in two forms. The more common localized form is characterized by enlargement of hilar or mediastinal lymph nodes, with mediastinal nodes, usually middle or posterior. A single smooth or lobulated mass, which can be large, is typically visible on CT, and dense opacification after contrast medium infusion is commonly visible. Localized Castleman's disease is usually asymptomatic and has a benign course.

The rare diffuse form of Castleman's disease results in generalized lymph node enlargement, involving mediastinal and hilar nodes, and often axillary, abdominal, and inguinal node groups (Fig. 4-15). It is often associated with systemic

TABLE 4-5

Sarcoidosis: Frequency of Enlarged Nodes Seen on CT in Patients with Nodes

Node Group	Frequency (%)
Hilar	90
Right paratracheal	100
Aortopulmonary window	90
Subcarinal	65
Anterior mediastinal	50
Posterior mediastinal	15

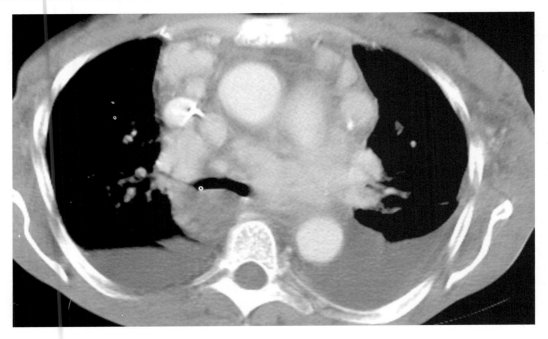

FIGURE 4-15 **Diffuse Castleman's disease.** Extensive, enhancing mediastinal lymphadenopathy in a patient with the diffuse form of Castleman's disease. The enhancement is typical. Enlarged axillary, abdominal, and inguinal lymph nodes were also visible. Bilateral pleural effusions are also present.

symptoms and has a progressive course despite treatment. As with the localized form, marked node enhancement can be seen.

☐ DIAGNOSIS OF MEDIASTINAL MASSES

The differential diagnosis of a mediastinal mass on CT is usually based on several characteristics of the mass and on the presence or absence of several findings. These include the mass's location, whether it is single or multifocal (i.e., involves several areas of the mediastinum), its shape (round or lobulated), whether it appears cystic, its attenuation (fat, fluid, tissue, or a combination of these; the presence of calcification and its character and amount), and additional findings such as pleural effusion.

Attenuation

The attenuation of a mass can be helpful in differential diagnosis. The variety of densities that can be seen in a mediastinal mass and their frequency are shown in Table 4-6.

Localization of Mediastinal Masses

Mediastinal masses result in alterations of normal mediastinal contours and displacement or compression of mediastinal structures. Recognizing these findings can be valuable in diagnosis and in suggesting the site of origin of the mass. Although most mediastinal masses can occur in different parts of the mediastinum, most have characteristic locations.

☐ PREVASCULAR SPACE MASSES

Masses in the prevascular space, when large, tend to displace the aorta and great arterial branches posteriorly (see Fig. 4-13), but distinct compression or narrowing of these relatively thick-walled structures is unusual. Within the supra-aortic mediastinum, displacement, compression, or obstruction of the brachiocephalic veins is not uncommon. In the subaortic mediastinum, posterior displacement or compression of the superior vena cava is typical only with right-sided masses. On the left, compression of the main pulmonary artery can be seen.

Although you are taught that the differential diagnosis of anterior mediastinal masses

TABLE 4-6

Attenuation Characteristics of Mediastinal Masses

Mass	Air	Fat	Water	Tissue	>Tissue	Calcium
Thymoma	N	N	O	A	N	O
Thymolipoma	N	A	N	C	N	N
Lymphoma (thymic)	N	N	O	A	N	R
Dermoid/teratoma	N	O	O	A	N	O
Germ-cell tumor	N	N	R	A	N	R
Thyroid tumor	N	N	O	A	C	C
Lipoma	N	A	N	N	N	N
Hygroma	N	C	C	C	N	N
Cysts (congenital)	R	N	C	O	N	R
Hernia	O	O	N	O	N	N
Lung cancer (nodes)	N	N	O	A	N	N
Tuberculosis (nodes)	N	N	C	A	N	C
Sarcoid (nodes)	N	N	R	A	N	O
Castleman's (nodes)	N	N	N	A	N	O
Neurogenic tumor	N	O	C	C	N	O
Neurenteric cyst	R	N	A	N	N	N
Meningocele	N	N	A	N	N	N
Hematopoiesis	N	O	N	A	N	N

"ACORN": A, always; C, common; O, occasionally; R, rare; N, never ("never" does not mean it never happens, but rather that it is so unlikely that practically you should "never" consider the diagnosis, and if you turn out to be wrong, you will "never" be blamed).

includes the "4 Ts" (thymoma, teratoma, thyroid tumor, and terrible lymphoma), the differential diagnosis should be extended to include: (1) thymoma and *other thymic tumors*; (2) teratoma and *other germ-cell tumors*; (3) thyroid masses; (4) lymphoma and *other lymph node masses*; and (5) parathyroid masses, cysts, fatty masses, and lymphangioma (hygroma).

☐ THYMIC TUMORS

Tumors of various histology arise from cells of thymic origin, including thymoma, thymic carcinoma, thymic carcinoid tumor, thymolipoma, thymic cyst, lymphoma, and leukemia. Thymic hyperplasia may mimic a mass.

Thymoma

Thymoma is a tumor of thymic epithelial origin, and it is a common cause of anterior mediastinal mass in adults. Occasionally, these lesions arise in the middle or posterior mediastinum. It is extremely difficult to determine if thymomas are benign or malignant by histologic criteria. Local invasion at surgery is a much more reliable sign,

and the terms *invasive thymoma* or *noninvasive thymoma* are preferable to malignant or benign thymoma, respectively. Approximately 30% of thymomas are pathologically and surgically invasive. Invasion of mediastinal structures or the pleural space is most typical. Distant metastases are not common with invasive thymoma.

From 10% to 30% of patients with myasthenia gravis will be found to have a thymoma, whereas a larger percentage of patients with thymoma (30% to 50%) have myasthenia. Other syndromes associated with thymoma include red blood cell hypoplasia and hypogammaglobulinemia.

On CT, thymomas are usually visible in the prevascular space (Fig. 4-16), but they can also be seen in a paracardiac location. They are detected as a localized mass distorting or replacing the normally arrowhead-shaped thymus. Typically, they are unilateral. Calcification and cystic degeneration can be present. On CT, bilaterality, large size, lobulated contour, poor definition of the tumor's margin, and associated pleural effusion or nodules suggest the presence of an invasive thymoma, but a definite diagnosis is difficult to make.

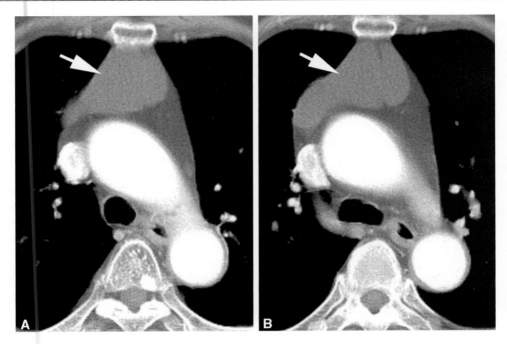

FIGURE 4-16 **Thymoma.** *A* and *B,* At two levels, a large but well-marginated mass involves the right thymic lobe *(arrows).* A noninvasive thymoma was found at surgery. The left thymic lobe is replaced by fat.

In patients suspected of having a thymoma because of myasthenia gravis, CT can demonstrate tumors that are invisible using plain radiographs. However, small thymic tumors may not be distinguishable from a normal or hyperplastic gland with CT.

Thymic Carcinoma

Similar to invasive thymoma, thymic carcinoma arises from thymic epithelial cells. However, unlike invasive thymoma, thymic carcinoma can be diagnosed as malignant on the basis of histology. This tumor is aggressive and is more likely to result in distant metastases than invasive thymoma. Thymic carcinoma cannot be distinguished from thymoma on CT.

Thymic Carcinoid Tumor

Thymic carcinoid tumors are usually malignant and aggressive. This lesion does not differ significantly from thymoma in its CT appearance, but it has a worse prognosis. Approximately 40% of patients have Cushing's syndrome as a result of tumor secretion of adrenocorticotropic hormone, and nearly 20% have been associated with multiple endocrine neoplasia syndromes I and II.

Thymolipoma

Thymolipoma is a rare, benign thymic tumor, consisting primarily of fat but also containing strands or islands of thymic tissue. The tumor is generally unaccompanied by symptoms and can be large when first detected, usually on chest radiographs. Because of its fatty content and pliability, it tends to drape around the heart and can simulate cardiac enlargement. On CT, its fatty composition, with wisps of soft tissue within it, can permit a preoperative diagnosis (Fig. 4-17).

Thymic Cyst

Thymic cysts are either congenital or acquired and can be diagnosed using CT if they are thin walled and their contents have an attenuation close to that of water. In some cases, they will show soft-tissue attenuation. Calcification of the cyst margin can occur. Notably, thymoma can have cystic components but also demonstrates solid areas or a thick or irregular wall.

An important general rule in diagnosing mediastinal masses is that cysts can appear solid, and solid (malignant) masses can have cystic or necrotic components. A true cyst has a thin wall;

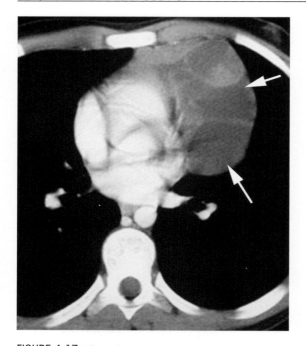

FIGURE 4-17 **Thymolipoma.** A large, low-attenuation, anterior mediastinal mass *(arrows)* is composed primarily of fat but also contains strands of soft tissue. The mass is somewhat droopy in appearance.

a mass with cystic degeneration usually has a thick, irregular wall.

Thymic Hyperplasia and Thymic Rebound

Thymic hyperplasia may result in thymic enlargement or a focal thymic mass. It is associated with myasthenia gravis. Distinction from thymoma on CT may be impossible.

The thymus may appear enlarged and relatively dense (containing little fat) in patients with thymic hyperplasia. In young patients, the thymus may show a significant rebound hyperplasia 3 months to a year after cessation of chemotherapy for malignancy. This can result in a distinctly enlarged thymus.

Lymphoma

Anterior mediastinal lymph node enlargement (see Figs. 4-3 and 4-9) or thymic involvement (Fig. 4-18) is present in more than half of patients with Hodgkin's disease. In patients with thymic involvement, lymphoma can present as a single spherical or lobulated mass, or as thymic enlargement. In such cases, lymphoma can be indistinguishable from thymoma or other causes of prevascular mass. However, if the abnormality is multifocal (indicating its origin from

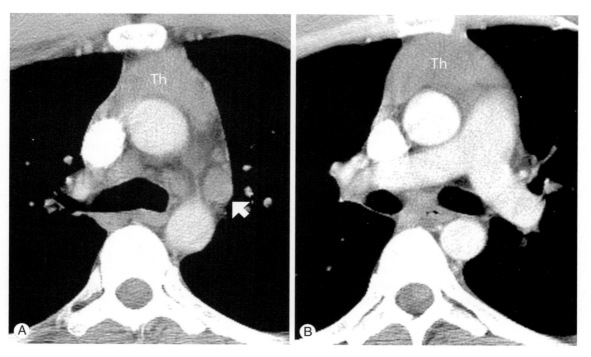

FIGURE 4-18 **Lymphoma with thymic and mediastinal lymph node enlargement.** *A* and *B,* The thymus (Th) is symmetrically enlarged. This appearance could represent thymoma or other primary thymic tumor. However, enlarged lymph nodes in the aortopulmonary window *(arrow, A)* and pretracheal space are a clue to the diagnosis.

nodes) or is associated with other sites of lymph node enlargement, the diagnosis is made more easily (see Fig. 4-18). Cystic areas of necrosis may be visible at CT in patients with lymphoma (see Fig. 4-12). Except in rare cases, calcification does not occur in the absence of radiation. Hodgkin's disease limited to the prevascular mediastinum is typically the nodular sclerosing cell type.

Germ-Cell Tumors

Several different tumors, originating from rests of primitive germ cells, can occur in the anterior mediastinum. These include teratoma, dermoid cysts, seminoma, choriocarcinoma, and endodermal sinus tumor. These tumors are less common than thymoma. Approximately 80% of germ-cell tumors are benign. Germ-cell tumors are usually considered in three categories: teratoma and dermoid cyst, seminoma, and nonseminomatous germ-cell tumors.

Teratoma and Dermoid Cyst

Teratomas can be cystic or solid and are most commonly benign. A teratoma contains tissues of ectodermal, mesodermal, and endodermal origins. A dermoid cyst is a specific type of tumor derived primarily from epidermal tissues, although other tissues are usually present. Teratomas are classified histologically as mature or immature. Mature teratomas are benign; immature teratoma usually behaves in a malignant fashion in adults, but may be benign in children.

Teratomas occur in a distribution similar to that of thymomas; they rarely originate in the posterior mediastinum. Benign lesions are often round, oval, and smooth in contour; as with thymoma, an irregular, lobulated, or ill-defined margin suggests malignancy. On average, these tumors are larger than thymomas, but they can be any size. Calcification can be seen (Fig. 4-19) but is nonspecific except in the unusual instance when a bone or tooth is present within the mass. They may appear cystic or contain visible fat, a finding of great value in differential diagnosis (see Fig. 4-19). A fat–fluid level can also be seen.

Seminoma

Seminoma occurs almost entirely in young men. It is the most common malignant mediastinal germ-cell tumor, accounting for 30% of such cases. On CT, seminoma presents as large,

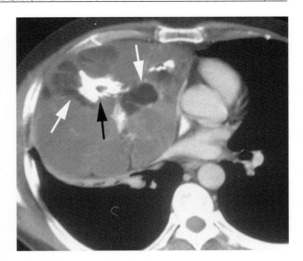

FIGURE 4-19 **Mature teratoma.** A lobulated anterior mediastinal mass contains low-attenuation fat *(white arrows),* an important finding in diagnosis, and calcium *(black arrow).*

smooth, or lobulated, homogeneous soft-tissue mass, although small areas of low attenuation can be seen. Obliteration of fat planes is common, and pleural or pericardial effusion may be present. Seminomas are radiosensitive, and the 5-year survival rate of affected patients is 50% to 75%.

Nonseminomatous Germ-Cell Tumors

Nonseminomatous germ-cell tumors, namely embryonal carcinoma, endodermal sinus (yolk sac) tumor, choriocarcinoma, and mixed types, are often grouped together because of their rarity, similar appearance, aggressive behavior, and poor prognosis. The tumors are usually unresectable at the time of diagnosis because of local invasion or distant metastasis. Unlike seminoma, radiotherapy is of limited value.

On CT, these tumors often show heterogeneous opacity, including ill-defined areas of low attenuation secondary to necrosis and hemorrhage or cystic areas. They often appear infiltrative, with obliteration of fat planes, and may be spiculated. Calcification may be seen.

Thyroid Masses

A small percentage of patients with a thyroid mass have some extension of the mass into the superior mediastinum, and, rarely, a completely intrathoracic mass can arise from ectopic mediastinal thyroid tissue. In most patients, such masses represent a goiter (Fig. 4-20), but other diseases (Graves' disease,

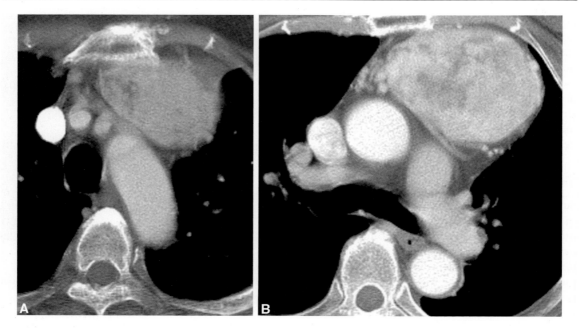

FIGURE 4-20 **Mediastinal goiter.** *A,* A large inhomogeneous mass is visible in the anterior mediastinum. *B,* It shows enhancement after contrast medium infusion. At higher levels, the mass was contiguous with the inferior thyroid.

thyroiditis) and neoplasms can result in an intrathoracic mass. Masses are often asymmetrical.

Most patients with intrathoracic goiter are asymptomatic, but symptoms of tracheal or esophageal compression can be present. CT usually shows anatomic continuity of the visible mass with the cervical thyroid gland. The location of the mass at CT is somewhat variable, and it can be anterior or posterior to the trachea. Masses anterior to the trachea splay the brachiocephalic vessels, whereas masses that are primarily posterior and lateral to the trachea displace the brachiocephalic vessels anteriorly. A location anterior to the great vessels is somewhat unusual (see Fig. 4-20). Calcifications and low-attenuation cystic areas are common in patients with goiter. Also, because of their high iodine content, the CT attenuation of goiters, Graves' disease, and thyroiditis can be greater than that of soft-tissue and thyroid tumors, but less dense than normal thyroid tissue.

As a rule, if a thyroid mass is suspected clinically, CT should be performed without contrast injection. This allows subsequent injection of radioactive iodine for diagnosis. The injection

of iodinated radiographic contrast agents delays radionuclide imaging.

Mesenchymal Masses

Lipomatosis and Lipoma

A diffuse accumulation of unencapsulated fat in the mediastinum, so-called mediastinal lipomatosis, can occur in patients with Cushing's syndrome, after long-term corticosteroid therapy, or as a result of exogenous obesity. It produces no symptoms. CT shows a generalized increase in anterior mediastinal fat surrounding the great vessels, with some lateral bulging of the mediastinal pleural reflections. On CT, fat has a characteristic low attenuation, measuring from -50 to -100 H.

As with other mesenchymal tumors, lipomas can occur in any part of the mediastinum but are most common anteriorly. Because of their pliability, they rarely cause symptoms. A lipoma, although of the same attenuation as lipomatosis, is localized. Most fatty masses are benign. Liposarcoma, teratoma, and thymolipoma, which are other masses that can contain fat, also contain soft-tissue elements, and thus can be distinguished from lipoma or lipomatosis.

Lymphangioma (Hygroma)

Lymphangiomas are classified histologically as simple, cavernous, and cystic. Simple lymphangiomas are composed of small, thin-walled lymphatic channels with considerable connective tissue stroma. Cavernous lymphangiomas consist of dilated lymphatic channels, whereas cystic lymphangiomas (hygromas) contain single or multiple cystic masses filled with serous or milky fluid and having little, if any, communication with normal lymphatics. Most commonly, these lesions are detected in children and may extend into the neck. However, they can be seen in adults as well. On CT, the mass can appear as a single cyst, can be multicystic, or can envelop, rather than displace, mediastinal structures. Discrete cysts may not be visible; calcification does not occur.

☐ PRETRACHEAL SPACE MASSES

Masses that occupy the pretracheal compartment characteristically replace or displace normal pretracheal fat. Because the pretracheal space is limited by the relatively immobile aortic arch anteriorly and to the left, large masses extend preferentially to the right, displacing and compressing the superior vena cava anteriorly and laterally. In the presence of a pretracheal mass, the superior vena cava appears crescentic and convex laterally. Lateral displacement of the superior vena cava results in most of the mediastinal widening visible on plain films. Large masses also displace the trachea posteriorly, but tracheal cartilage usually prevents significant tracheal narrowing. Masses in this compartment are almost always of lymph node origin.

The Trachea

The trachea extends inferiorly from the thoracic inlet for a distance of 8 to 10 cm before bifurcating into the right and left main bronchi. The trachea is usually round or oval in shape and is approximately 2 cm in diameter. In some patients, the trachea appears somewhat triangular, with the apex of the triangle directed anteriorly. This appearance is particularly common at the level of the carina and proximal main bronchi. In some patients, the tracheal cartilage is visible as a relatively dense horseshoe-shaped structure within the tracheal wall, with the open part of the horseshoe being posterior; calcification is common in older patients, particularly women. The tracheal wall measures no more than 2 or 3 mm in thickness.

Tracheal abnormalities are uncommon and may be asymptomatic unless the tracheal lumen is reduced to a few millimeters in diameter. Spiral CT, usually with narrow (1–3 mm) collimation or detector width is advantageous in imaging tracheal abnormalities.

Saber-sheath trachea is a relatively common tracheal abnormality, occurring in patients with chronic obstructive pulmonary disease. In this condition, there is side-to-side narrowing of the intrathoracic trachea, probably because of the repeated trauma of coughing, with the anterior-to-posterior tracheal diameter being preserved or increased (Fig. 4-21); the extrathoracic trachea is normal. A focal segment of the trachea at the thoracic inlet may be involved first. In severe cases, the opposite tracheal walls may touch each other.

Saber-sheath trachea should be distinguished from several diseases that produce concentric tracheal narrowing and involve the extrathoracic trachea as well. These include polychondritis (Fig. 4-22), Wegener's granulomatosis, amyloidosis, and tracheobronchopathia osteochondroplastica. These conditions are rare.

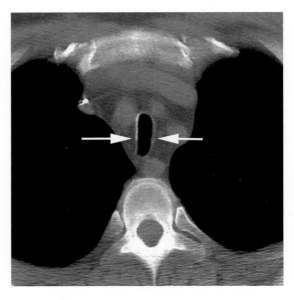

FIGURE 4-21 Saber-sheath trachea. The trachea is narrowed from side to side *(arrows),* whereas the sagittal diameter is normal or increased.

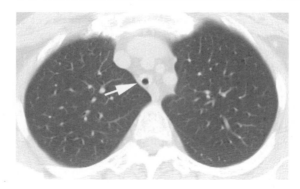

FIGURE 4-22 **Tracheal narrowing caused by polychondritis.**
The trachea is markedly narrowed *(arrow)* in a concentric
fashion. This appearance is distinctly different from that of saber-
sheath trachea. In this patient, the trachea was diffusely
narrowed, as were the main bronchi.

Tracheal stenosis occurring because of previous intubation is a relatively common abnormality. Narrowing of the tracheal lumen may be
associated with intratracheal soft-tissue masses
of reactive (granulation) tissue or collapse of the
tracheal wall because of destruction of the tracheal rings and associated fibrosis. Identifying
the shapes of the tracheal cartilages may be
helpful in distinguishing these two types of
tracheal stenosis.

Primary tracheal tumors are rare. The most
common primary malignancies, occurring in
approximately equal numbers, are squamous
cell carcinoma and cylindroma (adenoid cystic
carcinoma) (Fig. 4-23). In patients with either
of these, CT can be helpful in choosing treatment. If there is no mediastinal invasion
(as evidenced by a mediastinal mass), then the

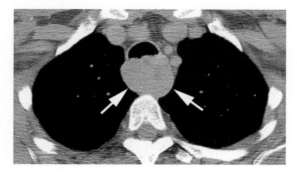

FIGURE 4-23 **Tracheal carcinoma (adenoid cystic carcinoma).**
The tumor is arising from the posterior tracheal wall and narrows
the tracheal lumen. An extrinsic mass *(arrows)* is present.

lesion may be curable with a partial tracheal
resection.

The trachea may be compressed, displaced,
or invaded by a variety of malignant mediastinal
tumors. Unless tumor can be seen within the
tracheal lumen, tracheal invasion is difficult to
diagnose. The trachea can be involved by lung
cancer as a result of direct extension from
a tumor arising in a main bronchus; bronchogenic carcinomas involving the trachea or carina
are usually considered unresectable (T4).
Thickening of the carina or tracheal wall contiguous with a bronchial lesion suggests this
diagnosis, but bronchoscopy is usually required
for a definite diagnosis.

☐ SUBCARINAL SPACE

Large masses in the subcarinal space can: (1)
produce a convexity of the azygoesophageal recess, (2) splay the carina, (3) displace the carina
anteriorly, (4) displace the esophagus to the left,
and/or (5) displace the right pulmonary artery
anteriorly and compress its lumen. The most
common masses involving this compartment
are lymph node masses, cysts, and esophageal
lesions.

Bronchogenic and Esophageal Duplication Cysts

Congenital bronchogenic cysts result from
anomalous budding of the foregut during development. Most commonly, they are visible in the
subcarinal space, but they can occur in any part
of the mediastinum. They appear as single,
smooth, round, or elliptical masses (Fig. 4-24)
and occasionally show calcification of their walls
or contents. Air–fluid levels occurring because
of communication with the trachea or bronchi
are rare. When large, bronchogenic cysts can
produce symptoms by compression of mediastinal structures. A rapid increase in size can occur
because of infection or hemorrhage.

Esophageal duplication cysts are indistinguishable from bronchogenic cysts, but they
always contact the esophagus. They usually appear as well-defined solitary masses and occasionally contain an air–fluid level when they
communicate with the esophagus.

CT can be of great value in diagnosing a
mediastinal cyst. If a mass is thin walled and is
of fluid attenuation (approximately 0 H), it can

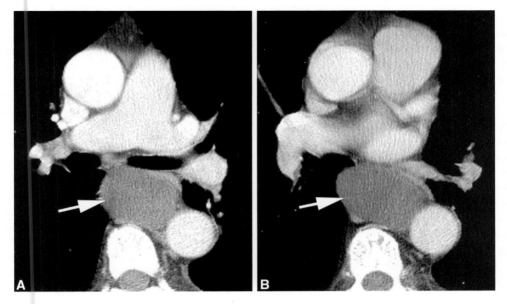

FIGURE 4-24 **Bronchogenic cyst.** *A* and *B,* A large, oval, low-attenuation cyst *(arrows)* is visible in the subcarinal region and azygoesophageal recess. This location is typical.

be assumed to represent a benign cyst. However, high CT numbers (20–40 H), suggesting a solid mass, can also be found in patients with foregut duplication cysts. These cysts contain a thick, gelatinous material or blood. In such patients, surgery is usually required for diagnosis, but magnetic resonance imaging may sometimes help.

Esophageal Lesions

Esophageal lesions are discussed in Chapter 17.

☐ AORTOPULMONARY WINDOW MASSES

Masses in the aortopulmonary region typically replace mediastinal fat; when large, they displace the mediastinal pleural reflection laterally. Displacement or compression of the aorta, pulmonary artery, and trachea are sometimes seen.

Aortopulmonary window masses are almost always the result of lymph node enlargement (see Figs. 4-3 and 4-4). Other masses occurring in this region include aortic abnormalities (aneurysm or pseudoaneurysm) and chemodectoma.

☐ RETROSTERNAL MEDIASTINUM

Enlargement of internal mammary nodes results in a convexity in the expected position of this node chain (see Fig. 4-1). Other than lymph node enlargement, masses in this region are unusual.

☐ PARAVERTEBRAL MASSES

Paravertebral masses may be seen to replace paravertebral fat. On the left, the normal concave mediastinal pleural reflection, posterior to the aorta, becomes convex in the presence of a significant mass. On the right, a paravertebral convexity is visible in a region where little tissue normally exists (see Fig. 4-5).

Neurogenic Tumors

Neurogenic tumors are divided into three groups, arising from (1) peripheral nerves or nerve sheath (neurofibroma, neurilemmoma), (2) sympathetic ganglia (ganglioneuroma, neuroblastoma), and (3) paraganglionic cells (pheochromocytoma, chemodectoma). Tumors in each of these three groups may be benign or malignant. Although neurogenic tumors can occur at any age, they are most common in young patients. Neuroblastoma and ganglioneuroma are most common in children, whereas neurofibroma and neurilemmoma more frequently affect young adults.

Radiographically, neurogenic tumors appear as well-defined, round or oval soft-tissue masses, typically in a paravertebral location (Fig. 4-25). Although the different tumors are by no means always distinguishable, ganglioneuroma tends to be elongated, lying adjacent to the spine, whereas neurofibroma and neurilemmoma are smaller and more spherical in shape. Although neural tumors are frequently of soft-tissue attenuation, they can be low in attenuation because of the presence of lipid-rich Schwann cells, fat, or cystic regions. Although benign tumors tend to be sharply marginated and fairly homogeneous, and malignant tumors tend to be infiltrating and irregular, these findings are not sufficiently reliable for diagnosis. Calcification can occur, particularly in neuroblastoma; the presence of calcium does not help in distinguishing benign from malignant lesions.

A neurofibroma arising in a nerve root can be dumbbell-shaped, that is, partially inside and partially outside the spinal canal. In such cases, the intervertebral foramen may be enlarged. CT can be helpful in determining the extent of the mass and associated vertebral abnormalities and can distinguish the mass from an aortic aneurysm or other vascular lesion if an intravenous contrast agent is given. CT after injection of myelographic contrast medium may be useful in demonstrating intraspinal extension.

Anterior or Lateral Thoracic Meningocele

A thoracic meningocele represents anomalous herniation of the spinal meninges through an intervertebral foramen or a defect in the vertebral body. It results in a soft-tissue mass visible on chest radiographs. In most patients, this abnormality is associated with neurofibromatosis; most are detected in adults. It is said that meningocele is the most common cause of a posterior mediastinal mass in patients with neurofibromatosis.

Meningoceles are described as lateral or anterior, depending on their relationship to the spine. They are slightly more common on the right. Findings that suggest the diagnosis include rib or vertebral anomalies at the same level or an association with scoliosis. The mass is often visible at the apex of the scoliotic curve. CT after intraspinal contrast medium injection shows filling of the meningocele and is diagnostic (Fig. 4-26); MRI may also be diagnostic.

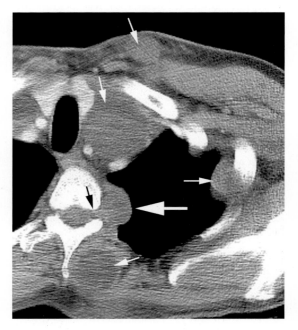

FIGURE 4-25 **Neurofibromas in neurofibromatosis.**
A smooth, paravertebral, posterior mediastinal mass is visible *(large white arrow)*. The neural foramen is slightly enlarged *(black arrow)*. Multiple other neurofibromas are also present, some relatively low in attenuation *(small white arrows)*.

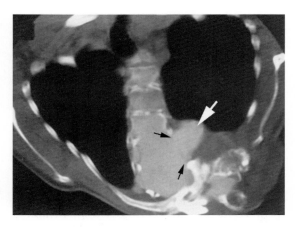

FIGURE 4-26 **Lateral thoracic meningocele.** In a patient with neurofibromatosis and scoliosis, a meningocele *(white arrow)* is associated with a large foraminal defect *(black arrows)*. Myelographic contrast material opacifies the meningocele.

Neurenteric Cyst

The neurenteric cyst, which is rare, is composed of both neural and gastrointestinal elements and frequently is attached to both the meninges and gastrointestinal tract. It appears as a homogeneous posterior mediastinal mass and rarely contains air because of communication with abdominal viscera. As with meningocele, it is frequently associated with a vertebral anomaly or scoliosis. As opposed to meningocele, it frequently causes pain and is generally diagnosed at a young age.

Diseases of the Thoracic Spine

Tumors (either benign or malignant), infectious spondylitis, or vertebral fracture with associated hemorrhage can produce a paravertebral mass. Frequently, the abnormality is bilateral and fusiform, allowing it to be distinguished from solitary masses such as a neurogenic tumor. Associated abnormalities of the vertebral bodies or discs assist in diagnosis and should be sought. Preservation of discs in association with vertebral body destruction suggests neoplasm or tuberculosis; disc destruction suggests infection other than tuberculosis.

Extramedullary Hematopoiesis

Extramedullary hematopoiesis can result in paravertebral masses in patients with severe anemia (usually congenital hemolytic anemia or thalassemia). These masses are of unknown origin but perhaps arise from lymph nodes, veins, or an extension of rib marrow. Masses can be multiple and bilateral and are most commonly associated with the lower thoracic spine. They have no specific CT characteristics. With resolution they may appear as fat density.

Fluid Collections

Occasionally, posterior pleural fluid collections can simulate a paravertebral mediastinal mass. Mediastinal extension of a pancreatic pseudocyst through the aortic or esophageal hiatus can occur, but it is rare.

Vascular Abnormalities

Posteriorly located aortic aneurysms can occupy this part of the mediastinum. Also, azygos and hemiazygos vein dilatation will produce abnormalities in this region. Dilated azygos or hemiazygos veins, because they are visible on a number of contiguous slices, are easily distinguished from a focal mass.

☐ DIFFUSE MEDIASTINAL ABNORMALITIES

Mediastinitis

Mediastinal infections (mediastinitis) can be acute or chronic.

Acute Mediastinitis

Acute mediastinitis usually results from esophageal perforation or the spread of infection from adjacent tissue spaces, including the pharynx, lungs, pleura, and lymph nodes. The primary symptoms are substernal chest pain and fever. CT shows mediastinal widening, replacement of normal fat by fluid attenuation, or localized fluid collections. Gas bubbles may be seen (Fig. 4-27).

Granulomatous Mediastinitis

In patients with histoplasmosis, tuberculosis, and sarcoidosis, chronic mediastinal lymph node enlargement and associated fibrosis can result in so-called granulomatous mediastinitis. In these patients, the large nodes and associated fibrous tissue form a mediastinal mass that can compress the superior vena cava, pulmonary arteries or veins, bronchi, and esophagus.

The node enlargement tends to be asymmetrical except in patients with sarcoidosis. Fibrosis can replace normally visible mediastinal fat. Calcification of the nodes can be seen in some patients, indicating the benign nature of the disease process. Compression of the main bronchi (usually the left) or pulmonary arteries (usually the right) can sometimes be recognized.

Sclerosing Mediastinitis

In some patients, similar mediastinal fibrosis is not associated with obvious granulomatous disease. In a few patients, this is associated with fibrosis elsewhere (retroperitoneal fibrosis). Symptoms and radiographic findings are similar to granulomatous mediastinitis, but calcification does not occur.

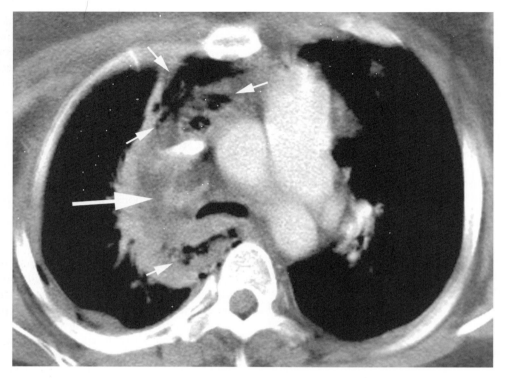

FIGURE 4-27 **Acute mediastinitis caused by esophageal perforation by a car antenna.** There is mediastinal widening, increased attenuation of mediastinal fat as a result of inflammation *(large arrow),* and multiple collections of air *(small arrows).*

Mediastinal Hemorrhage

Mediastinal hemorrhage usually results from trauma such as venous or arterial laceration, from aortic rupture or dissection, or from anti-coagulation (see Chapter 3 and Fig. 3-10). Superior mediastinal widening associated with blurring of normal mediastinal contours is usually present. Mediastinal fluid visible on CT is high in attenuation (>50 H). Blood can dissect extra-pleurally over the lung apex, resulting in a so-called apical cap. In some patients, blood will also be present in the left pleural space. Contrast-enhanced CT may be of value in diagnosing associated aortic aneurysm, dissection, or rupture.

☐ **HEART AND PERICARDIUM**

CT is not commonly used for the evaluation of cardiac abnormalities, but some knowledge of cardiac anatomy on CT is necessary for the proper interpretation of scans and the identification of paracardiac abnormalities or masses and the effect they have on the heart. Only occasionally are incidental cardiac abnormalities detected on CT. CT, however, is excellent for evaluating pericardial abnormalities.

Cardiac Pathology

Although CT can show a number of abnormalities in patients with ischemic heart disease or other cardiac abnormalities, it does not usually play a significant role in the clinical evaluation of patients with cardiac pathology. Echocardiography, magnetic resonance imaging, and angiography are more commonly used.

In patients with an acute myocardial infarction, after the bolus injection of contrast medium, infarcted myocardium can show less opacification than normal myocardium and, to some degree, infarct size can be quantitated. Ventricular thrombus can also be shown in patients with an acute myocardial infarction.

In patients with prior infarct, CT can be valuable in showing ventricular aneurysms and associated thrombus. In patients who have had coronary artery bypass grafts, graft patency can be determined with an accuracy of about 90% with enhanced CT. However, significant stenoses of patent grafts are difficult to see.

Intracardiac abnormalities can be shown with contrast-enhanced CT (Figs. 4-28 and 4-29), but they are rare and usually are evaluated using other techniques. Myocardial wall thickening can be seen in some patients with cardiomyopathy. CT is sensitive in detecting great-vessel (aortic), valve, and annular calcification.

Coronary Artery Calcification

Coronary artery calcification can be identified clearly on CT scans at and below the level of the aortic root. In recent studies, the presence and extent of coronary artery calcification has been correlated with the likelihood of clinically significant coronary artery disease.

The left main coronary artery is about 1 cm in length; it arises from the aorta at about the 4-o'clock position and gives rise to the left anterior descending coronary artery extending anteriorly and inferiorly and the circumflex coronary artery extending posteriorly and inferiorly. Left main coronary calcification is said to be present if calcium is seen proximal to its point of bifurcation into the left anterior descending and circumflex arteries. The right coronary

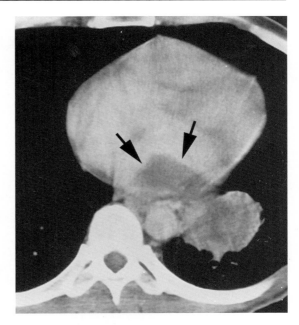

FIGURE 4-29 **Left atrial metastasis.** In a patient with renal cell carcinoma and a left hilar mass, a mass within the opacified left atrium represents a large metastasis *(arrows)*.

artery arises from the anterior aorta (at about the 11-o'clock position) slightly caudal to the left main artery and extends anteriorly and inferiorly in the atrioventricular groove. Left anterior descending artery calcification almost always predominates.

Pericardial Abnormalities

Pericardial Effusion, Thickening, and Fibrosis

Pericardial effusion results in thickening of the normal pericardial stripe. When fluid begins to accumulate, it accumulates first in the dependent portions of the pericardium, typically posterior to the left ventricle (Fig. 4-30). As the effusion increases in size, it is visible lateral and anterior to the right atrium and right ventricle; when large, it appears as a concentric opacity surrounding the heart. Large effusions can also extend into the superior pericardial recess. The presence of tamponade, associated with pericardial effusion, may be more directly related to the speed at which the fluid accumulates and the distensibility of the pericardium than the size of the effusion alone.

Pericardial thickening or fibrosis, usually as a result of inflammation, can produce a similar thickening of the pericardial stripe. With contrast medium infusion, the thickened

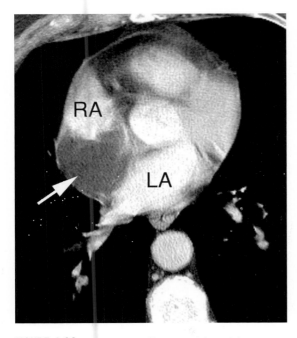

FIGURE 4-28 **Lipomatous infiltration of the atrial septum.** A focal low-attenuation (fatty) mass is visible in the region of the atrial septum *(arrow)*, compressing both the right (RA) and left atria (LA). This abnormality is usually of no consequence, and this patient had no cardiac symptoms.

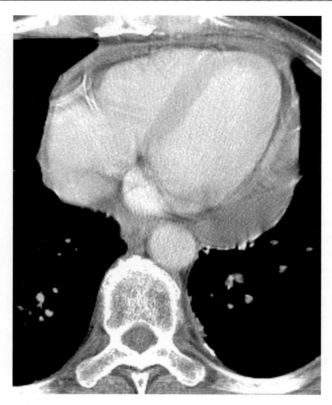

FIGURE 4-30 **Pericardial effusion from metastatic lung cancer.** Fluid accumulates first in the dependent portions of the pericardium, posterior to the left ventricle. In this patient, most fluid collection has accumulated in this region.

pericardium may be seen to enhance, thus distinguishing it from effusion. Also, pericardial thickening may be denser than fluid collections, even without contrast infusion. Thickening may be smooth or focal and nodular. Calcification can occur, particularly as a result of tuberculosis, purulent pericarditis, or hemopericardium.

In the presence of symptoms of constrictive pericarditis, the CT appearance of a normal pericardium rules out the diagnosis, whereas a thickened pericardium allows a presumptive diagnosis of constriction to be made. In the presence of pericardial metastases, CT can show an effusion or nodular masses may be visible, particularly after contrast medium infusion.

☐ PARACARDIAC MASSES

Compression of the atria or right ventricle can be seen in the presence of a paracardiac mass, but left ventricular compression is uncommon because of the thickness of its wall and the relatively high pressure of its contents.

Anterior Cardiophrenic Angle Masses

Although a number of the mediastinal masses already described can occur at the level of the anterior cardiophrenic angle, the differential diagnosis of lesions occurring in this location includes several additional entities. These include pericardial cyst, large epicardial fat pad, Morgagni's hernia, and enlargement of paracardiac lymph nodes (see Fig. 4-2).

Pericardial Cyst

Most commonly, pericardial cysts touch the diaphragm, 60% in the anterior right cardiophrenic angle and 30% in the left cardiophrenic angle; 10% occur higher in the mediastinum. Most patients are asymptomatic. The cysts typically appear as smooth, round, homogeneous masses (Fig. 4-31). They range up to 15 cm in diameter.

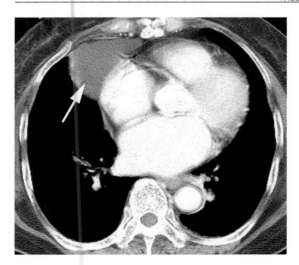

FIGURE 4-31 **Pericardial cyst.** A fluid-attenuation (i.e., 0 H) mass is visible in the right cardiophrenic angle *(arrow)*. This appearance and location are typical of pericardial cyst.

Although they are usually low in attenuation (i.e., near 0 H), their attenuation may be that of soft tissue.

Fat Pad

Deposition of fat in either cardiophrenic angle is not uncommon, particularly in obese patients, and can simulate a mass on plain radiographs. CT, of course, is diagnostic.

Morgagni Hernia

Hernias of abdominal contents through the anteromedial diaphragmatic foramen of Morgagni can result in a cardiophrenic angle mass; 90% of these occur on the right. The hernia usually contains omentum or liver; bowel is less common. When the hernia contains fat, CT can confirm its benign nature but does not allow its differentiation from a fat pad. When it contains liver, CT may allow diagnosis by showing hepatic vessels or bile ducts. If bowel is present in the hernia sac, gas is usually visible.

▪ SUGGESTED READING

AHN JM, LEE KS, GOO JM, et al: Predicting the histology of anterior mediastinal masses: Comparison of chest radiography on CT. J Thorac Imaging 265–271, 1996.

BASHIST B, ELLIS K, GOLD RP: Computed tomography of intrathoracic goiters. AJR Am J Roentgenol 140:455–460, 1983.

BROWN LR, AUGHENBAUGH GL: Masses of the anterior mediastinum: CT and MR imaging. AJR Am J Roentgenol 157:1171–1180, 1991.

CASTELLINO RA, BLANK N, HOPPE RT, et al: Hodgkin disease: Contributions of chest CT in the initial staging evaluation. Radiology 160:603–605, 1986.

CASTELLINO RA, HILTON S, O'BRIEN JP, et al: Non-Hodgkin lymphoma: Contribution of chest CT in the initial staging evaluation. Radiology 199:129–132, 1996.

DALES RE, STARK RM, RAMAN S: Computed tomography to stage lung cancer: Approaching a controversy using meta-analysis. Am Rev Respir Dis 141:1096–1101, 1990.

FREUNDLICH IM, MCGAVRAN MH: Abnormalities of the thymus. J Thorac Imaging 11:58–65, 1996.

GLAZER HS, ARONBERG DJ, SAGEL SS: Pitfalls in CT recognition of mediastinal lymphadenopathy. AJR Am J Roentgenol 144:267–274, 1985.

GLAZER GM, GROSS BH, QUINT LE, et al: Normal mediastinal lymph nodes: Number and size according to American Thoracic Society mapping. AJR Am J Roentgenol 144:261–265, 1985.

GLAZER HS, KAISER LR, ANDERSON DJ, et al: Indeterminate mediastinal invasion in bronchogenic carcinoma: CT evaluation. Radiology 173:37–42, 1989.

GLAZER HS, MOLINA PL, SIEGEL MJ, SAGEL SS: Pictorial essay. Low-attenuation mediastinal masses on CT. AJR Am J Roentgenol 152:1173–1177, 1989.

GLAZER HS, SIEGEL MJ, SAGEL SS: Pictorial essay. High-attenuation mediastinal masses on unenhanced CT. AJR Am J Roentgenol 156:45–50, 1991.

GLAZER HS, WICK MR, ANDERSON DJ, et al: CT of fatty thoracic masses. AJR Am J Roentgenol 159:1181–1187, 1992.

JOLLES H, HENRY DA, ROBERSON JP, et al: Mediastinitis following median sternotomy: CT findings. Radiology 201:463–466, 1996.

KAWASHIMA A, FISHMAN EK, KUHLMAN JE, et al: CT of posterior mediastinal masses. Radiographics 11:1045–1067, 1991.

MCLOUD TC, BOURGOUIN PM, GREENBERG RW, et al: Bronchogenic carcinoma: Analysis of staging in the mediastinum with CT by correlative lymph node mapping and sampling. Radiology 182:319–323, 1992.

MOUNTAIN CF, DRESLER CM: Regional lymph node classification for lung cancer staging. Chest 111:1718–1723, 1997.

MÜLLER NL, WEBB WR, GAMSU G: Paratracheal lymphadenopathy: Radiographic findings and correlation with CT. Radiology 156:761–765, 1985.

MÜLLER NL, WEBB WR, GAMSU G: Subcarinal lymph node enlargement: Radiographic findings and CT correlation. AJR Am J Roentgenol 145:15–19, 1985.

QUINT LE, GLAZER GM, ORRINGER MB, et al: Mediastinal lymph node detection and sizing at CT and autopsy. AJR Am J Roentgenol 147:469–472, 1986.

ROSADO-DE-CHRISTENSON ML, TEMPLETON PA, MORAN CA: Mediastinal germ-cell tumors: Radiologic and pathologic correlation. Radiographics 12:1013–1030, 1992.

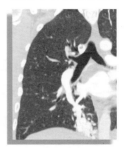

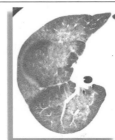

The Pulmonary Hila

W. Richard Webb, M.D.

The pulmonary hila are difficult to evaluate on plain radiographs because they have extremely complex and somewhat variable silhouettes. It is often hard to decide if a hilum is normal or abnormal and, if it is abnormal, what the abnormal finding represents.

CT is helpful in the diagnosis of endobronchial lesions, hilar and parahilar masses, and hilar vascular lesions. The sensitivity and specificity of CT in diagnosing a hilar mass or adenopathy in patients with lung cancer average between 80% and 90% and are greatest when contrast medium enhancement is used.

☐ TECHNIQUE

As with the different parts of the mediastinum described in Chapter 2, it takes about 15 contiguous 5-mm slices to image the hila. The hila are adequately assessed using a routine spiral CT technique, with 5-mm collimation or detector row width infusion of intravenous contrast. Thinner scans may be helpful in identifying subtle bronchial abnormalities, but they are not routinely performed.

Scans are viewed with a mean window level of −600 to −700 H and a window width of 1000 or 1500 H (lung window) for accurate assessment of hilar contours and bronchial anatomy. Scans are also viewed at a mean window value of 0 to 50 H and a window width of 500 H (soft-tissue or mediastinal window) to obtain information about hilar structures, lymph nodes, and masses.

☐ DIAGNOSIS OF HILAR MASS OR ADENOPATHY

A detailed understanding of cross-sectional hilar anatomy is necessary to identify hilar abnormalities on CT. Contrast-enhanced CT simplifies the identification of hilar mass or lymph node enlargement.

Lobar and segmental bronchi (Fig. 5-1) are consistently seen on CT and reliably identify successive hilar levels. Their recognition is key to interpreting the pulmonary hila. In general, hilar anatomy and contours at the same bronchial levels are relatively constant from one patient to the next. The bronchi should be looked at first, whenever you read a CT scan of the hila.

In some locations, normal hilar contours are consistent enough that a diagnosis of hilar adenopathy or mass can be made on the basis of an abnormality in hilar contour alone, seen using a lung window. In other locations, however,

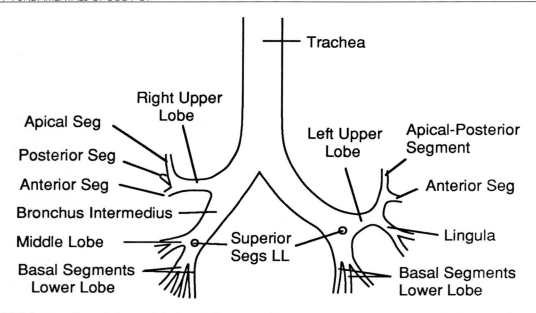

FIGURE 5-1 **Normal bronchial tree.** All the bronchi shown are visible on CT in most patients. Those bronchi that appear horizontal (such as those of the right upper lobe) or nearly vertical are usually seen better than those that have an oblique course relative to the plane of scan (such as right middle lobe or lingular bronchi). LL, lower lobe; Seg, segment.

contours can vary according to the size and position of the hilar pulmonary arteries and veins. In these locations, contrast opacification of the pulmonary vessels is essential for accurate diagnosis. Also, in any location, infusion of a contrast agent can be helpful if you are uncertain about the presence of a mass. It is always wise to perform hilar CT with contrast medium infusion.

A hilar mass or lymph node enlargement may be suggested by a local or generalized alteration in hilar contour; visible mass or lymph node enlargement; bronchial narrowing, obstruction, or displacement; and thickening or obliteration of the walls of bronchi that normally contact lung. As a general rule, any nonenhancing hilar structure larger than 5 mm (in short axis) is usually abnormal, but this is not always the case. Normal soft-tissue collections larger than this, representing fat and normal nodes, are sometimes visible. Also, minimal lymph node enlargement (5–10 mm) is commonly present in patients with inflammatory lung disease (e.g., pneumonia), and such lymph node enlargement should not be of great concern.

Normal and Abnormal Hilar Anatomy

There are two ways to read hilar CT. The first way is to look at each hilum separately, identifying each important structure, and the second is to compare one side with the other at successive scan levels, looking for points of similarity and dissimilarity. In fact, it is wise to do both.

I suggest that as you read the next section, you first learn about right hilar anatomy, skipping what is written about the left hilum. When you finish, and are somewhat oriented, you should start over, reading about both hila, comparing their anatomy, noting what is symmetrical and what is not, and learning how the left hilum differs from the right. Also, you should learn to trace each lobar bronchus from its origin to its segmental branches, because this should be done during interpretation of the CT scan.

Although the hila are not symmetrical structures, they have a number of similarities, and identifying these can be of value. These similarities are emphasized in the following description. To reinforce the normal appearances and their significance, and expected alterations in anatomy occurring because of mass of node enlargement, abnormal findings are discussed at each hilar level described.

Some variation exists among patients in the relative levels of the hila; therefore, there is some variation in the levels at which right and left hilar structures are visible on CT. The right-to-left relations illustrated in Figure 5-1 and described in the following text may or may not be present in individual cases, although variation will usually be minor (1 or 2 cm).

Because recognizing lobar and segmental bronchial anatomy is fundamental to interpreting hilar CT, it is reviewed briefly in Table 5-1. Each of the segments listed is commonly, but not invariably, visible.

Upper Hila

Right Hilum. CT at the level of the distal trachea or carina will show the apical segmental bronchus of the right upper lobe in cross section, surrounded by several vessels of similar size (Fig. 5-2*A* and *B*). On either side, mass or lymphadenopathy is recognized easily. Anything larger than the expected pulmonary vessels is abnormal (Figs. 5-3 and 5-4). Comparing with the opposite side at this level is helpful.

Left Hilum. The apicoposterior segmental bronchus and associated arteries and veins have a similar appearance to the right side at this level (see Fig. 5-2*A* and *B*), as does lymph node enlargement (see Fig. 5-3*A*).

Right Upper Lobe Bronchus and Left Upper Lobe Segments

Right Hilum. Approximately 1 cm distal to the carina, the right upper lobe bronchus is usually visible along its length, with its anterior and posterior segmental branches both generally seen at the same level (Fig. 5-5). The anterior segment, usually lying in or near the scan plane, is commonly seen over a length of 2 to 3 cm. The posterior segment bronchus usually angles slightly cephalad, out of the plane of scan, and may not be seen as well. If it is not seen at the level of the upper lobe bronchus, you should look for it on the next highest level. In some normal subjects, the origin of the apical segment can be seen at this level as a round lucency, usually at the point of bifurcation (or, in this case, trifurcation) of the right upper lobe bronchus.

Anterior to the right upper lobe bronchus, the truncus anterior (pulmonary artery supplying most of the upper lobe) produces an oval opacity of variable size, but often about the same size as the right main bronchus visible at the same level. An upper lobe vein branch (posterior vein), lying in the angle between anterior and posterior segmental branches is present and is visible in almost all patients. The posterior wall of the upper lobe bronchus is usually outlined by lung and appears smooth and 2 to 3 mm in thickness.

Within the anterior right hilum at this level, mass or lymph node enlargement can be identified if a soft-tissue opacity larger than the expected size of the truncus anterior is visible (Fig. 5-6). This, of course, could be confirmed by contrast medium injection. Laterally, in the angle between the anterior and posterior segmental bronchi, anything larger than the expected vein is abnormal (see Fig. 5-6). This vein should not be significantly larger than at the level 1 cm above. Posteriorly, thickening of the wall of the upper lobe bronchus or main bronchus (Fig. 5-7) or a focal soft-tissue opacity behind it will almost always be abnormal. An anomalous pulmonary vein branch may sometimes be seen posterior to the bronchus; it is seen at multiple adjacent levels.

Left Hilum. On the left side, at or near this level, the apicoposterior and anterior segmental bronchi of the left upper lobe are usually visible (see Fig. 5-5). The apicoposterior segment is seen in cross section as a round lucency, whereas the anterior segment is directed anteriorly, roughly in the plane of scan, at about 1 o'clock. In some subjects, the anterior segmental bronchus is seen at a lower level. These bronchi lie lateral to the main branch of the left pulmonary artery, which produces a large convexity in the posterior hilum at this level, and the superior pulmonary vein, which results in an anterior convexity. In many normal subjects, the artery

TABLE 5-1

Lobar and Segmental Bronchial Anatomy

Right Upper Lobe Segments	Left Upper Lobe Segments
Apical	Apicoposterior
Posterior	Anterior
Anterior	Superior lingula
	Inferior lingula

Right Middle Lobe Segments	
Medial	
Lateral	

Right Lower Lobe Segments	Left Lower Lobe Segments
Superior	Superior
Anterior	Anteromedial
Medial	Lateral
Lateral	Posterior
Posterior	

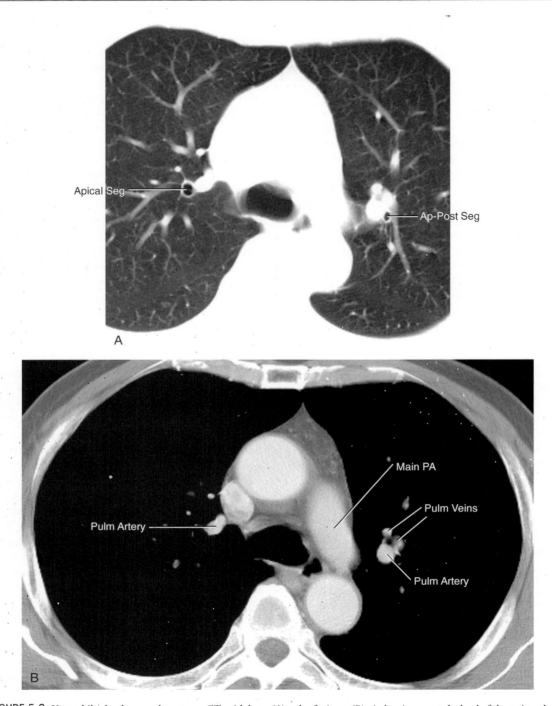

FIGURE 5-2 Upper hilar level: normal anatomy. CT, with lung *(A)* and soft-tissue *(B)* window images at the level of the carina, shows the apical segmental bronchus of the right upper lobe (RUL) in cross section, with several adjacent vessels of similar size. On the left, the apicoposterior segmental bronchus of the left upper lobe (LUL) and associated arteries and veins have a similar appearance. Note that this same patient is also used to illustrate normal anatomy at lower levels, with lung and soft-tissue windows shown together. Generally, the bronchi are identified on the lung window scans, and the vessels are identified on the soft-tissue window scans.

Continued

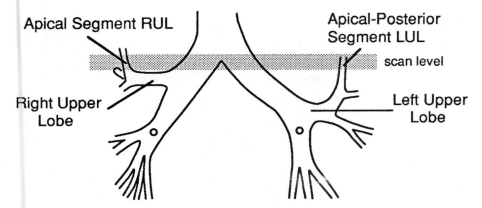

FIGURE 5-2 Cont'd

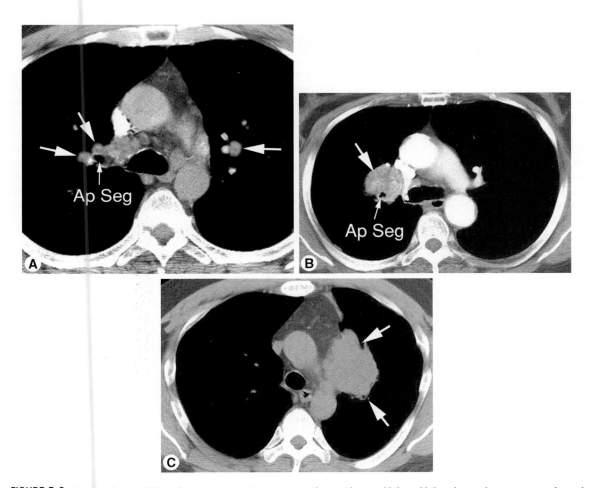

FIGURE 5-3 **Abnormal upper hila in three patients.** *A,* In a patient with sarcoidosis and bilateral hilar adenopathy, a contrast-enhanced scan through the upper hila shows lymph node enlargement *(arrows).* On the right, the apical segmental bronchus (Ap Seg) of the right upper lobe is visible, surrounded by lymph nodes. On the left, an enlarged lymph node is visible lateral to pulmonary vessels. *B,* In a patient with a right upper lobe carcinoma, lymph node enlargement *(arrow)* is visible anterior to the apical segment bronchus (Ap Seg) of the right upper lobe. *C,* In a patient with a right upper lobe carcinoma, tumor *(large arrows)* surrounds the apical segment bronchus (Ap Seg).

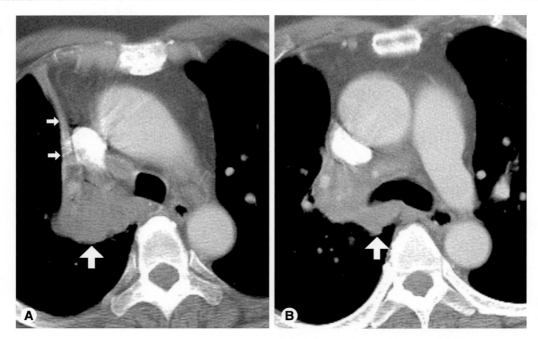

FIGURE 5-4 **Abnormal upper right hilum (bronchogenic carcinoma).** *A,* A large mass *(large arrow)* encompasses the region of the apical segmental bronchus of the right upper lobe. A thin linear opacity *(small arrows)* along the right mediastinum reflects collapse of the right upper lobe. *B,* Below the level shown in *A,* the mass results in obstruction of the right upper lobe bronchus. The mass *(arrow)* is also visible posterior to the right main bronchus.

supplying the anterior segment of the left upper lobe is seen medial to the anterior segment bronchus. Lymphadenopathy can be seen in relation to all these structures and is most easily recognized after contrast infusion (see Fig. 5-6*A* and *B*).

Right Bronchus Intermedius

Below the level of the right upper lobe bronchus the bronchus intermedius is visible as an oval lucency at several adjacent levels (Figs. 5-8 and 5-9). Its posterior wall is sharply outlined by lung. Anterior and lateral to the bronchus the hilar silhouette may vary in appearance, primarily because of variations in the sizes and positions of pulmonary veins. A collection of fat and normal-sized nodes, sometimes measuring more than 10 mm in diameter, is commonly seen at the level of the bifurcation of the right pulmonary artery, anterior and lateral to the bronchus intermedius (see Fig. 5-8). A mass involving the posterior hilum can be readily diagnosed without contrast medium injection, because of thickening of the posterior bronchial wall (see Fig. 5-7); thickening of the posterior wall of the bronchus intermedius is a common finding in patients with right hilar mass, particularly when resulting from lung cancer.

The diagnosis of anterior or lateral hilar masses at this level generally requires contrast administration (Figs. 5-10 to 5-12). Normal soft tissue and nodes (see Fig. 5-8) should not be mistaken for a hilar mass.

Right Middle Lobe Bronchus and Left Upper Lobe/Lingular Bronchus

Right Middle Lobe Bronchus. On the right, at the level of the lower bronchus intermedius, the middle lobe bronchus arises anteriorly and extends anteriorly, laterally, and inferiorly at an angle of about 30 to 45 degrees (Fig. 5-13). Because of its obliquity, only a short segment of its lumen is visible at each level on CT, and this appearance should not be misinterpreted as bronchial obstruction. Often, the superior segmental bronchus of the lower lobe arises posterolaterally at this level (see Fig. 5-13).

At the level of the origin of the middle lobe bronchus, the superior pulmonary veins lie anterior and medial to the bronchus, whereas the descending (interlobar) branch of the right pulmonary artery lies beside and behind it (see Fig. 5-13). Normal lymph nodes (<5 mm in diameter) are commonly visible medial to the artery and lateral to the bronchus. Because of this separation of artery and veins, the lateral hilum at

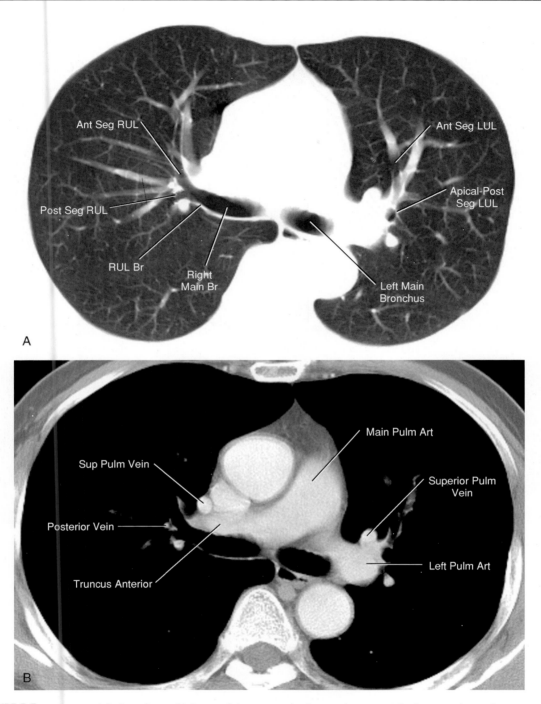

FIGURE 5-5 Right upper lobe bronchus and left upper lobe segments level: normal anatomy. The diagram indicates the approximate plane of scan relative to the bronchial tree. *A and B,* Right hilum: The right upper lobe bronchus (RUL Br) is visible along its length, together with its anterior and posterior segmental branches. The truncus anterior is anterior to the right upper lobe bronchus. An upper lobe vein branch (posterior vein) lies in the angle between the anterior and posterior segmental branches; the superior pulmonary veins result in some lobulation anterior to the truncus anterior. The posterior wall of the upper lobe bronchus appears smooth and 2 to 3 mm in thickness. Left hilum: On the left side, the apicoposterior and anterior segmental bronchi of the left upper lobe are visible. The apicoposterior segment is seen in cross section as a round lucency, whereas the anterior segment is directed anteriorly. These bronchi lie lateral to the main branch of the left pulmonary artery, which produces a convexity in the posterior hilum, and the superior pulmonary vein, which results in an anterior convexity. The artery supplying the anterior segment of the left upper lobe is seen medial to the anterior segment bronchus.

Continued

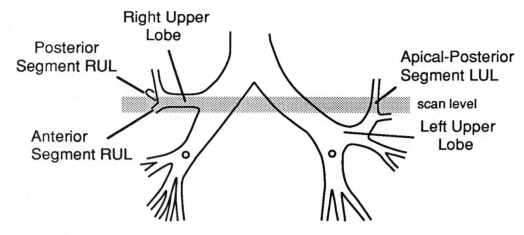

FIGURE 5-5 Cont'd

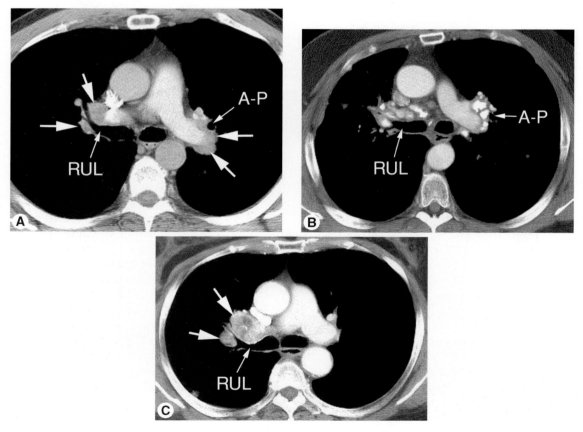

FIGURE 5-6 Hilar adenopathy in three patients. *A,* In the patient with sarcoidosis, as illustrated in Figure 5-3A, there is extensive adenopathy *(arrows)* at the level of the right upper lobe bronchus (RUL) and the apicoposterior segmental bronchus (A-P) of the left upper lobe. On the right, nodes are visible as unopacified structures anteriorly and laterally. The soft-tissue opacity seen in the position of the posterior vein on the right *(small arrow)* is too large to represent a vessel. On the left side, there are enlarged nodes *(arrows)* in both the lateral and posterior hilum, which are distinguishable from the opacified left pulmonary artery. *B,* CT at the level of the right upper lobe bronchus (RUL) and the apicoposterior segmental bronchus (A-P) of the left upper lobe shows extensive lymph node calcification secondary to sarcoidosis. The calcified lymph nodes are similar in location to those shown in *A. C,* Lymph node enlargement *(arrows)* at the level of the right upper lobe bronchus (RUL) in the same patient as shown in Figure 5-3B.

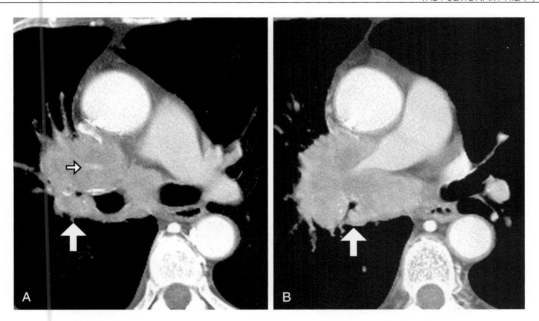

FIGURE 5-7 **Bronchogenic carcinoma with a right hilar mass.** *A,* A large carcinoma causes narrowing of the right upper lobe bronchus and obstruction of the anterior and posterior segmental bronchi. The truncus anterior *(small arrow),* anterior to the bronchus, is markedly narrowed and surrounded by tumor. The posterior walls of the right upper lobe bronchus *(large arrow)* and right main bronchus are thickened. *B,* At a lower level, the bronchus intermedius is narrowed and its posterior wall is thickened *(arrow).* The mass also invades the mediastinum, surrounding and narrowing the right pulmonary artery.

this level (representing the artery) is oval, without prominent lobulations. Any lobulation of significant size suggests hilar adenopathy or mass (Figs. 5-14 to 5-16).

Left Upper Lobe Bronchus. The appearance of the left hilum at the level of the left upper lobe bronchus is quite similar to that of the right hilum at the level of the middle lobe bronchus; however, the left upper lobe bronchus is usually visible about 1 cm above the right middle lobe bronchus (see Fig. 5-9).

The left upper lobe bronchus is usually seen along its axis, extending anteriorly and laterally from its origin, at an angle of 10 to 30 degrees (see Fig. 5-9). The left superior pulmonary veins are anterior and medial to the bronchus at this level, and the descending branch of the left pulmonary artery forms an oval soft-tissue opacity posterior and lateral to it. Normal lymph nodes (<5 mm in diameter) are commonly visible medial to the artery and lateral to the bronchus. Because only the oval artery occupies the lateral hilum, lobulation of the lateral hilum (more than one convexity) indicates mass or lymphadenopathy (see Figs. 5-11 and 5-15). The superior segment bronchus of the left lower lobe can arise at this level.

Although lung contacts and sharply outlines the posterior wall of the bronchus intermedius at several levels, the left posterior bronchial wall is usually outlined only at this level, that is, at the level of the left upper lobe bronchus. In approximately 90% of individuals, lung sharply outlines the posterior wall of the left main or upper lobe bronchus, medial to the descending pulmonary artery (see Fig. 5-9); this is termed the *left retrobronchial stripe.* As on the right, the bronchial wall should measure 2 to 3 mm in thickness. Thickening of this stripe, or a focal soft-tissue opacity behind it, indicates lymph node enlargement or bronchial wall thickening (see Figs. 5-11 and 5-17). In 10% of normal individuals, however, lung does not contact the bronchial wall because the descending pulmonary artery is medially positioned against the aorta. This should not be misinterpreted as abnormal.

Lingular Bronchus. The lingular bronchus is usually visible at a level near the undersurface of the left upper lobe bronchus; its two segments (superior and inferior) can sometimes be seen. The pulmonary artery and veins appear the same as at the level of the left upper lobe bronchus (see Fig. 5-13). As at the level of the left upper lobe bronchus, normal lymph nodes

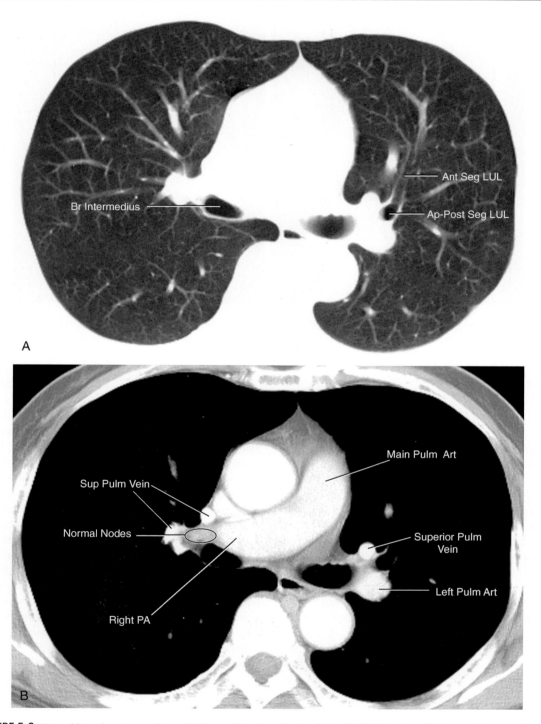

FIGURE 5-8 **Normal bronchus intermedius and left upper lobe bronchus level.** *A* and *B*, The bronchus (Br) intermedius is visible as an oval lucency with its posterior wall sharply outlined by lung. Anterior and lateral to the bronchus, the hilum is made up of the interlobar pulmonary artery (PA) and superior pulmonary veins. Normal lymph nodes and fat are visible in the anterolateral hilum, between the opacified pulmonary artery and veins. On the left, the anterior and the apicoposterior segmental bronchi of the left upper lobe (LUL) are visible. The left superior pulmonary vein is anterior and medial to the bronchi, and the descending branch of the left pulmonary artery forms an oval soft-tissue opacity posterior and lateral to them.

Continued

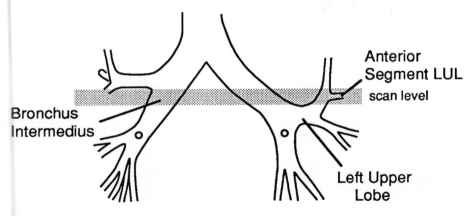

Anterior Segment LUL

scan level

Bronchus Intermedius

Left Upper Lobe

FIGURE 5-8 *Cont'd*

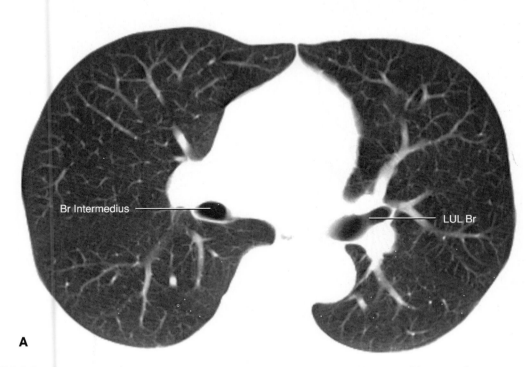

Br Intermedius

LUL Br

A

FIGURE 5-9 *A* and *B,* At a level below Figure 5-8, the bronchus (Br) intermedius is visible as an oval lucency with its posterior wall sharply outlined by lung. The interlobar pulmonary artery (PA) and superior pulmonary veins are anterior and lateral to the bronchus. On the left, the upper lobe (LUL) bronchus is usually seen along its axis, extending anteriorly and laterally from its origin. The left superior pulmonary vein is anterior and medial to the bronchus, and the descending branch of the left pulmonary artery is posterior and lateral to it. The left posterior bronchial wall is outlined by lung at this level. This is termed the *left retrobronchial stripe.*

Continued

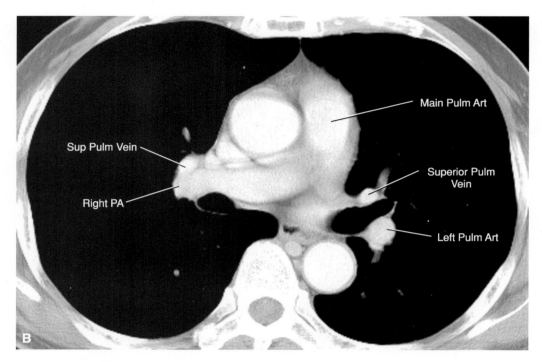

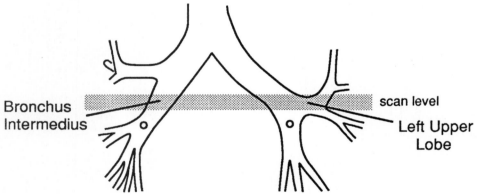

FIGURE 5-9 Cont'd

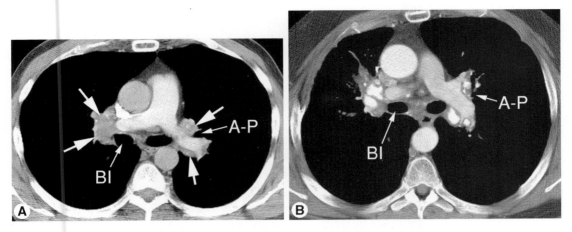

FIGURE 5-10 **Right hilar lymph node enlargement in two patients with sarcoidosis, at the same level as Figure 5-8.** *A,* On the right, a scan at the level of the upper bronchus intermedius (BI) shows enlargement of the normal node group *(arrows)* shown in Figure 5-8*B.* On the left, a scan at the level of the apicoposterior segment bronchus (A-P) shows enlarged lymph nodes *(arrows)* anterior and posterior to the opacified pulmonary artery. This is the same patient as shown in Figures 5-3*A* and 5-6*A.* *B,* In the same patient as shown in Figure 5-6*B,* calcified lymph nodes are visible at the level of the upper bronchus intermedius (BI) and apicoposterior segment bronchus (A-P) of the left upper lobe. Note the locations of the nodes as compared with *A.*

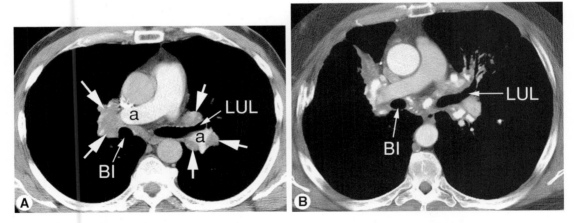

FIGURE 5-11 **Right hilar lymph node enlargement in two patients with sarcoidosis, at the same level as Figure 5-9.** *A,* On the right, a scan at the level of the bronchus intermedius (BI) shows enlargement of the normal node group *(arrows)* shown in Figure 5-8*B,* situated lateral to the pulmonary artery (a). On the left, a scan at the level of the left upper lobe bronchus (LUL) shows enlarged lymph nodes *(arrows)* in the anterior hilum and surrounding the opacified pulmonary artery (a). Enlarged lymph nodes are situated posterior to the left upper lobe bronchus. *B,* A scan at the level of the bronchus intermedius (BI) and left upper lobe bronchus (LUL) shows multiple calcified lymph nodes.

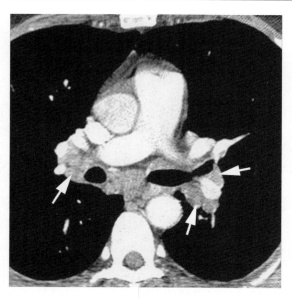

FIGURE 5-12 **Abnormal bronchus intermedius and left upper lobe bronchus level.** In a patient with non–Hodgkin's lymphoma and bilateral hilar adenopathy *(arrows)*, enlarged lymph nodes are clearly distinguished from opacified pulmonary vessels.

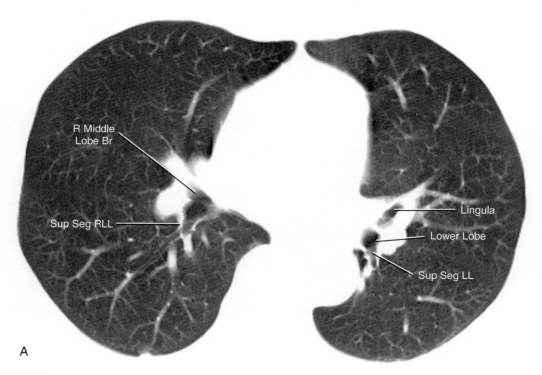

FIGURE 5-13 **Normal right middle lobe and lingular level.** *A* and *B,* Right hilum: The middle lobe bronchus (Br) arises anteriorly and extends anteriorly and laterally at an angle of about 45 degrees. Because it is also angled caudad, only a short segment of its lumen is visible. The superior segmental bronchus of the lower lobe (LL) arises posterolaterally. The superior pulmonary veins lie anterior and medial to the bronchus, whereas the oval descending (interlobar) branch of the right pulmonary artery (RA) lies beside and behind it. The appearance of the right hilum at this level is quite similar to that of the left hilum at the levels of the left upper lobe and lingular bronchi. Left hilum: The lingular bronchus is visible slightly below the level of the upper lobe bronchus. The left lower lobe bronchus and the superior segment branch of the lower lobe are also seen at this level. The descending pulmonary artery appears oval and is located lateral to the bronchi. The appearances of the hila are roughly symmetrical.

Continued

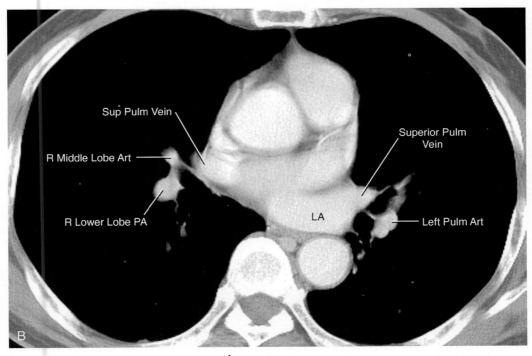

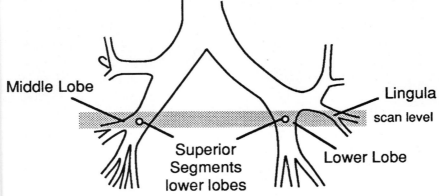

FIGURE 5-13 Cont'd

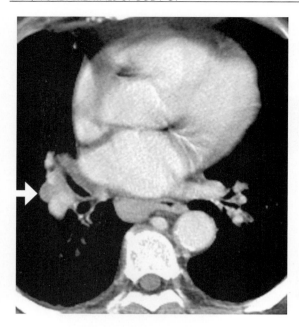

FIGURE 5-14 **Lymphoma with right hilar adenopathy.**
Enlarged lymph nodes *(arrow)* are visible lateral to the
descending right pulmonary artery and middle lobe bronchus.
Lymph node enlargement is also visible in the azygoesophageal
recess.

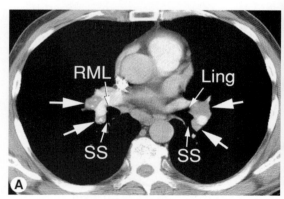

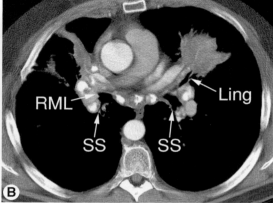

FIGURE 5-15 **Abnormal right middle lobe bronchus level in two patients with sarcoidosis.** *A,* On the right, a scan at the level of the
origin of the right middle lobe bronchus (RML) shows enlargement of nodes *(arrows)* anterior and posterior to the pulmonary artery.
Several of the nodes show calcification. On the left, a scan at the level of the lingular bronchus (Ling) shows enlarged lymph nodes *(arrows)*
anterior and posterior to the opacified pulmonary artery (as on the right side). *B,* As in *A,* a scan at the level of right middle lobe bronchus
(RML) and lingular bronchus (Ling) shows lymph node enlargement (and calcification) anterior and posterior to the pulmonary artery.
SS, superior segment bronchus of the lower lobe.

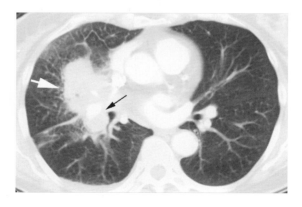

FIGURE 5-16 **Right hilar mass (bronchogenic carcinoma).**
The right middle lobe bronchus is invisible *(small black arrow)* and
obstructed. A large right hilar mass *(large white arrow)* is present.

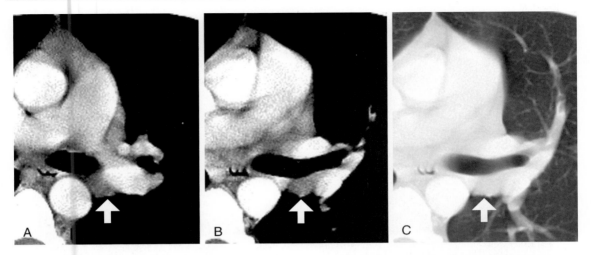

FIGURE 5-17 **Left hilar adenopathy (left upper lobe bronchus level).** *A,* Lymph node enlargement *(arrow)* is visible in the posterior hilum, behind the left upper lobe bronchus, and between the aorta and left pulmonary artery. *B* and *C,* The enlarged lymph node *(arrows)* lies posterior to the bronchus (i.e., in the region of the retrobronchial stripe) and prevents lung from outlining its posterior wall.

are commonly visible medial to the artery. At this level, significant lobulation of the lateral hilar contour indicates mass or adenopathy (see Fig. 5-15). As can the right upper lobe bronchus, the lingular bronchus can appear as the mirror image of the right middle lobe.

Lower Lobe Bronchi (Basal Segments)

Right and Left Hilum. At this level, the hila are relatively symmetrical, and comparing one side to the other can be helpful. The main lower lobe bronchial trunk on each side (Fig. 5-18), which eventually gives rise to the basal

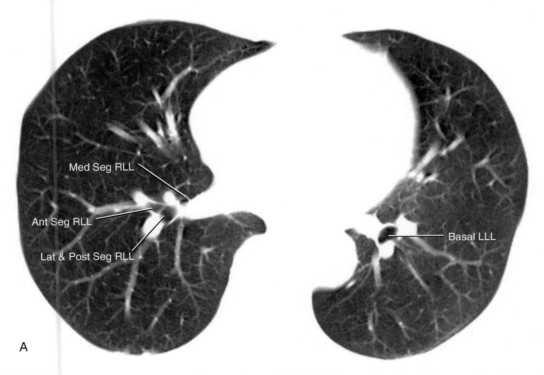

FIGURE 5-18 **Normal lower lobe bronchi (basal segments).** *A* and *B,* On the right, anterior and medial segmental bronchi are visible, whereas a common trunk is yet to divide into the lateral and posterior branches. The basal segmental bronchi arise in a variable fashion. The inferior pulmonary veins are posterior and medial, and pulmonary artery branches accompany the bronchi. On the left, a single undivided basal lower lobe bronchial trunk is seen.

Continued

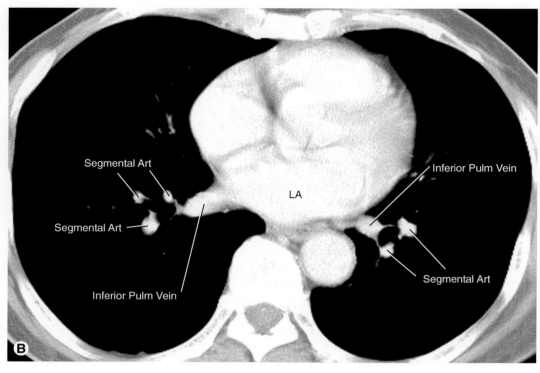

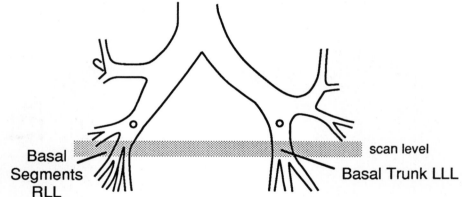

FIGURE 5-18 Cont'd

Continued

segmental bronchi, branches in a variable fashion. It is common for the lower lobe bronchial trunk on the right to divide into two basal bronchial branches or trunks at a level above the origins of the basal segmental bronchi.

At the level of the lower lobe bronchial trunk, on either side, the anterior bronchial wall is usually outlined by lung, with pulmonary artery branches being lateral to the bronchus and veins being posterior and medial to the bronchus (see Fig. 5-18*A* and *B*). Enlarged

lymph nodes can be identified anterior to the bronchus at this level.

The basal segmental branches of the lower lobe bronchi vary in appearance depending on their courses (see Fig. 5-18). On the right, the four segmental branches (medial, anterior, lateral, and posterior) are usually visible; on the left, there are three basal segments (anteromedial, lateral, and posterior). These segments are much better seen with thin slices.

The segmental bronchi are accompanied by pulmonary artery branches that are slightly

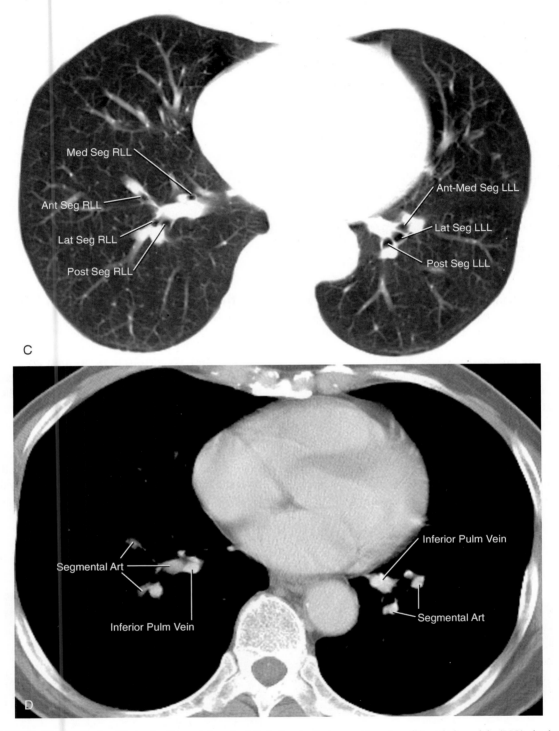

FIGURE 5-18 **Cont'd** *C* and *D,* At a level 7 mm below *A* and *B,* the four basal segmental branches of the right lower lobe (RLL), the three segmental branches of the left lower lobe (LLL), and their associated vessels are all visible. LA, left atrium.

Continued

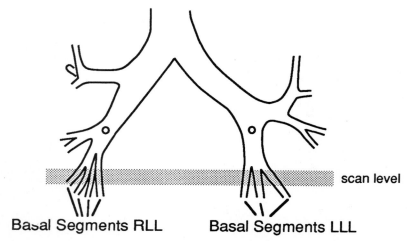

Basal Segments RLL   scan level   **Basal Segments LLL**

FIGURE 5-18 Cont'd

larger than the bronchi; the bronchi and arteries are nearly perpendicular to the scan plane, and thus are seen in cross section (see Fig. 5-18). The inferior pulmonary veins pass behind and medial to the bronchi to enter the left atrium and, unlike the arteries, tend to be seen along their axis. Hilar masses or lymph node enlargement can be diagnosed on the basis of contour abnormalities or asymmetries between the hila. Soft-tissue densities that seem too large to be the pulmonary artery or vein branches should be regarded with suspicion (Figs. 5-19 to 5-21). The largest nodes seen at this level tend to be anterior.

☐ BRONCHIAL ABNORMALITIES

The excellent contrast and spatial resolution of CT allow for good assessment of bronchial lesions, and CT is often performed to guide bronchoscopy in patients who have a suspected hilar or bronchial abnormality. Accurate indicators of bronchial pathology are: (1) bronchial wall thickening, (2) an endobronchial mass, and (3) narrowing of the bronchial lumen.

Bronchial wall thickening is most easily assessed on CT in regions where the hilar bronchi lie adjacent to lung: the posterior walls of the right main and both upper lobe bronchi and

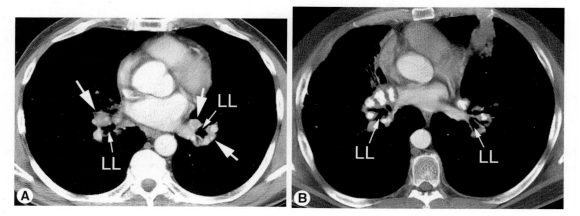

FIGURE 5-19 **Abnormal lower lobe bronchi level in two patients with sarcoidosis.** *A* and *B,* At the level of the lower lobe segments (LL), abnormal lymph nodes *(arrows)* are visible anteriorly and adjacent to the vascular branches.

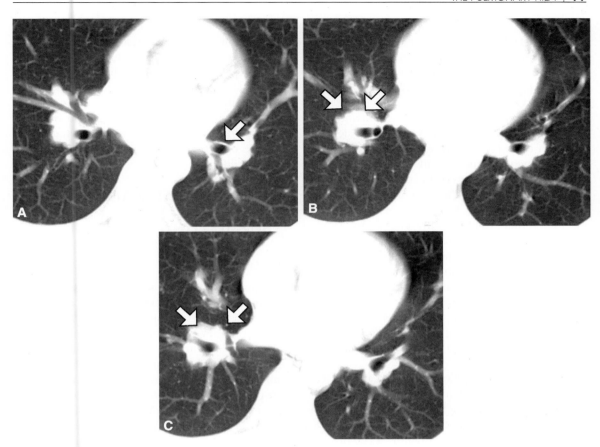

FIGURE 5-20 Right hilar adenopathy, lower lobe bronchi, and basal segments. *A,* Lobulation of the right hilum at the level of the right middle lobe bronchus indicates lymph node enlargement. Note that lung contacts the anterior wall of the left lower lobe bronchial trunk *(arrow),* with arteries and veins being lateral, posterior, and medial to the bronchus. This appearance is normal. *B,* The right lower lobe bronchial trunk has divided into two branches. Soft tissue anterior to these branches represents lymph node enlargement *(arrows).* On the left, the lower lobe bronchial trunk remains outlined by lung anteriorly. *C,* At the level of the basal segments, the right and left sides appear asymmetrical. The right bronchial segments are surrounded by soft tissue. Nodes *(arrows)* are anterior to the bronchi.

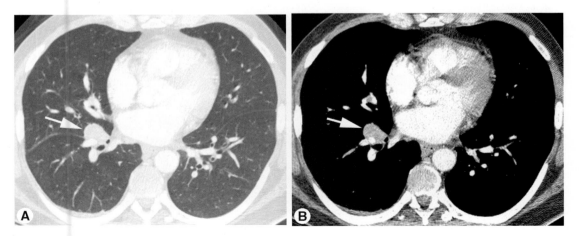

FIGURE 5-21 Right hilar adenopathy, lower lobe bronchial trunk. *A* and *B,* In a patient with non–Hodgkin's lymphoma, an enlarged lymph node *(arrow)* is visible anterior to the right lower lobe bronchial branches.

the posterior wall of the bronchus intermedius. Smooth bronchial wall thickening can be caused by inflammation or tumor infiltration (see Figs. 5-7 and 5-22), whereas a localized or lobulated thickening usually indicates tumor or lymph node enlargement (see Fig. 5-17).

Bronchial narrowing and endobronchial lesions that may be extremely difficult to detect on plain radiographs can be diagnosed reliably on CT. However, it may be difficult to distinguish endobronchial tumor from compression by an extrinsic mass (see Fig. 5-7). Abrupt changes in bronchial caliber on CT usually indicate circumferential tumor infiltration or an endobronchial mass (Figs. 5-23 and 5-24); but it is important to look at adjacent scans to confirm that the apparent bronchial narrowing does not reflect an oblique bronchial course, with the bronchus leaving the plane of scan (as with the right middle lobe bronchus). Bronchial abnormalities that are primarily mucosal can be missed using CT because of their minimal thickness.

In general, scans viewed with a lung window setting are best for identifying normal bronchi and detecting bronchial abnormalities, but they often overestimate the degree of bronchial narrowing. Also, volume averaging at the upper or lower edges of a normal bronchus can mimic the presence of bronchial obstruction. Soft-tissue (mediastinal) window settings more accurately assess bronchial lumen diameter in the presence of an abnormality (and show mass lesions), but they somewhat overestimate luminal diameter. If a bronchial lesion is suspected, both window settings should be used. Thin scans, particularly with multidetector CT, can be of great value in identifying bronchial abnormalities.

☐ DIFFERENTIAL DIAGNOSIS OF HILAR AND BRONCHIAL ABNORMALITIES

Lung Cancer

The most common cause of hilar mass or lymph node enlargement is bronchogenic carcinoma. The hilar mass can appear irregular because of local infiltration of the lung parenchyma. In patients with tumors arising centrally (usually squamous cell carcinoma or small-cell carcinoma), bronchial abnormalities (narrowing, obstruction) visible on CT are common. In such patients, an endobronchial lesion is commonly visible at bronchoscopy, correlating with the CT abnormality. If the bronchial abnormality involves the tracheal carina, resection may

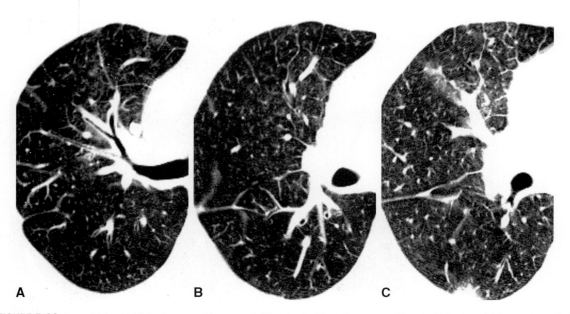

FIGURE 5-22 Bronchial wall thickening caused by tumor infiltration by Kaposi's sarcoma. There is thickening of the posterior wall of the right upper lobe bronchus *(A)* and bronchus intermedius *(B and C)*. Interlobular septal thickening is visible in the right lung, as is typical of lymphangitic spread of carcinoma.

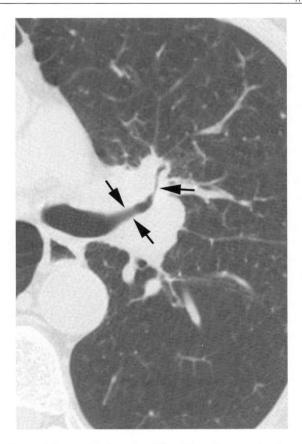

FIGURE 5-23 **Bronchogenic carcinoma, left upper lobe bronchus.** There is irregular narrowing *(arrows)* of the left upper lobe bronchus and the anterior segmental bronchus. The wall of the anterior segmental bronchus is thickened.

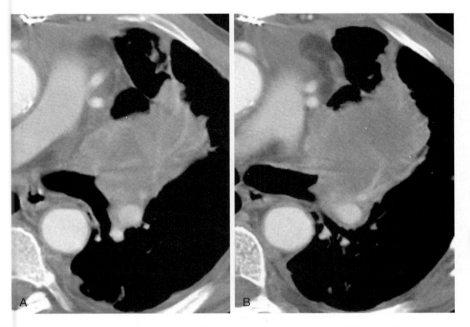

FIGURE 5-24 **Bronchogenic carcinoma with left upper lobe bronchus obstruction.** *A* and *B,* There is abrupt termination of the left upper lobe bronchus, associated with distal collapse and consolidation of the left upper lobe. This appearance strongly suggests bronchogenic carcinoma.

be impossible; bronchoscopy rather than CT, however, is most accurate for making this determination.

When the carcinoma arises in the peripheral lung, and the hila are abnormal because of lymph node metastases, the hilar mass or masses may be smoother and more sharply defined than when the hilar mass represents the primary tumor. However, this distinction is not always made easily. Patients with a central mass and bronchial obstruction often show peripheral parenchymal abnormalities. In patients with hilar node metastases, a bronchial abnormality seen at CT usually reflects external compression by the enlarged hilar nodes, but bronchial invasion also may be present. Hilar node metastases are present at surgery in 15% to 40% of patients with lung cancer.

In patients with bronchogenic carcinoma, enlarged hilar nodes visible on CT may not be caused by node metastasis. Hyperplastic nodal enlargement often occurs in patients with lung cancer, particularly when there is bronchial obstruction and distal pneumonia or atelectasis. Conversely, a normal-sized hilar node can harbor microscopic metastases. In the lung cancer staging system, ipsilateral hilar lymph node metastases are termed *N1*. Contralateral hilar lymph node metastases are *N3*.

Other Primary Bronchial Tumors

Other primary bronchial tumors can be associated with a hilar mass. The most common of these is carcinoid tumor. This malignant tumor arises from the main, lobar, or segmental bronchi in 80% to 90% of cases. It tends to grow slowly and to be invasive locally. A well-defined endobronchial mass is typical, but a large, exobronchial, hilar mass is sometimes seen as well. Carcinoid tumors are highly vascular and usually enhance densely after contrast medium infusion. Carcinoid tumors occasionally calcify.

Adenoid cystic carcinoma (cylindroma) can result in a CT appearance similar to carcinoid, but dense enhancement is not typical. It arises in the trachea (see Fig. 4-23) more commonly than does carcinoid.

Benign bronchial tumors, such as hamartoma, fibroma, chondroma, or lipoma, usually appear focal and endobronchial on CT (Fig. 5-25), rather than infiltrative, and they are not commonly associated with an extrinsic mass. Obstruction is the primary finding on CT.

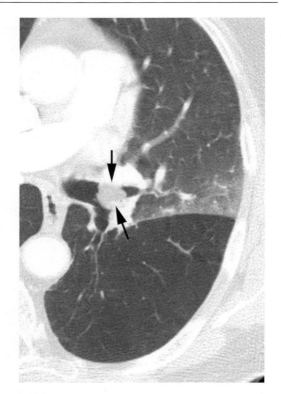

FIGURE 5-25 **Endobronchial lipoma.** A rounded, polypoid mass *(arrows)* is visible within the left upper lobe bronchus. There is no associated bronchial wall thickening, extrinsic mass, or lymph node enlargement. Increased density in the upper lobe reflects associated atelectasis.

Lymphoma

Hilar adenopathy is present in 25% of patients with Hodgkin's lymphoma and 10% of patients with non–Hodgkin's lymphoma. Hilar involvement is usually asymmetrical. Multiple nodes in the hilum or mediastinum are usually involved. Endobronchial lesions can also be seen, or bronchi may be compressed by enlarged nodes, but this is much less common than with lung cancer. There are no specific features of the hilar abnormality seen in patients with lymphoma that allow a definite diagnosis.

Metastases

Metastases to hilar lymph nodes from an extrathoracic primary tumor are not uncommon. Hilar node metastases may be unilateral or bilateral. Endobronchial metastases can also be seen (Fig. 5-26) without there being hilar node metastases; these may appear to be focal and endo-

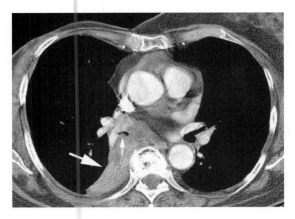

FIGURE 5-26 Endobronchial metastasis from breast carcinoma. In a patient with a right mastectomy, a focal lesion narrowing the lower lobe bronchus *(small arrow)* is associated with right lower lobe atelectasis *(large arrow)*. This represented an endobronchial metastasis.

bronchial or infiltrative. Head and neck carcinomas, thyroid carcinoma, genitourinary tumors (particularly renal cell and testicular carcinoma), melanoma, and breast carcinomas are most commonly responsible for hilar or endobronchial metastases.

Inflammatory Disease

Unilateral or bilateral hilar lymphadenopathy and bronchial narrowing can be seen in a number of infectious or inflammatory conditions. Primary tuberculosis usually causes unilateral hilar adenopathy. Fungal infections, most notably histoplasmosis and coccidioidomycosis, cause unilateral or bilateral adenopathy. Sarcoidosis causes bilateral and symmetrical adenopathy in most patients (see Fig. 5-11). Silicosis and coal-worker's pneumoconiosis are also commonly associated with bilateral hilar lymph node enlargement.

In patients with prior tuberculosis, histoplasmosis, sarcoidosis, or silicosis, calcified hilar nodes are commonly seen (see Fig. 5-11). Egg-shell (peripheral) calcification of lymph nodes is most commonly seen with silicosis, sarcoidosis, or tuberculosis. Calcified nodes can erode into a bronchus causing obstruction, that is, so-called broncholithiasis.

Mucus

Blobs of mucus may simulate one or more endobronchial lesions on CT; these are usually located along the posterior bronchial wall. If this diagnosis is suggested, for instance, if you see a focal bronchial lesion when you do not expect one, a repeat scan can be obtained after having the patient cough. The abnormality will disappear. Large mucus plugs can also mimic hilar masses or be seen as a bronchial abnormality on CT.

□ PULMONARY VASCULAR DISEASE

CT is useful in differentiating pulmonary vascular disease from hilar adenopathy. Pulmonary hypertension with dilatation of the pulmonary arteries is relatively common and can simulate a hilar mass on plain radiographs (Fig. 5-27). CT can accurately define the size of the pulmonary arteries in patients with arterial dilatation. If the main pulmonary artery is larger than the ascending aorta, pulmonary hypertension is likely present. Rarely, in patients with chronic pulmonary hypertension, pulmonary artery calcification can be seen as a result of atherosclerosis.

Encasement or compression of one of the main pulmonary arteries by tumor in patients with a bronchogenic carcinoma can be diagnosed with CT and can be of value in assessing the extent of surgery that will be required for resection. For example, tumor surrounding the left pulmonary artery generally indicates that

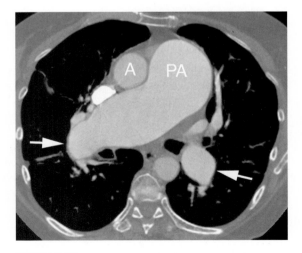

FIGURE 5-27 Pulmonary artery enlargement in pulmonary hypertension. The main pulmonary artery (PA) is larger than the ascending aorta (A), which is a good sign of pulmonary hypertension. Enlargement of the hilar arteries *(arrows)* is also seen.

pneumonectomy rather than lobectomy is required. However, caution must be exercised; narrowing of the pulmonary artery can reflect compression rather than encasement. Adequate assessment requires the use of intravenous contrast. Chapter 3 discusses the CT diagnosis of pulmonary embolism.

MASS VERSUS ATELECTASIS

In patients with a hilar mass and bronchial obstruction, collapse or consolidation of distal lung can obscure the margins of the mass, making it difficult to diagnose. On plain radiographs, the mass can sometimes be detected because of alterations in the shape of the collapsed or consolidated lobe or lobes (i.e., Golden's S sign). Similarly, alterations in the shape of a collapsed lobe can be seen on CT in the presence of a mass.

If contrast is injected, the collapsed lobe usually can be seen to enhance to a greater degree than the mass causing collapse (Fig. 5-28).

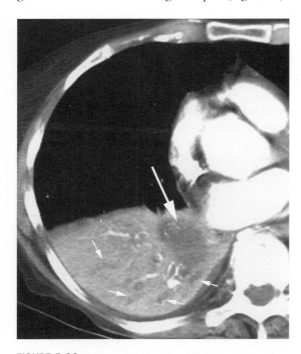

FIGURE 5-28 Hilar mass with atelectasis. In a patient with right hilar carcinoma, associated with right lower lobe atelectasis, the hilar mass can be distinguished from collapsed lung after contrast infusion. The mass *(large arrow)* appears less dense than opacified and enhanced lung. Low-attenuation, mucus-filled bronchi *(small arrows)* are visible within consolidated lung. These are associated with bronchial obstruction and are termed *mucous bronchograms.*

Of additional value in distinguishing mass and lung consolidation are air bronchograms. These indicate the presence of lung consolidation and are not usually visible with the mass itself. In some patients, low-attenuation, fluid-filled bronchi (i.e., *mucous bronchograms*) are seen within the collapsed lung instead of air bronchograms.

SUGGESTED READING

GLAZER GM, GROSS BH, AISEN AM, et al: Imaging of the pulmonary hilum: A prospective comparative study in patients with lung cancer. AJR Am J Roentgenol 145:245–248, 1985.

MÜLLER NL, WEBB WR: Radiographic imaging of the pulmonary hila. Invest Radiol 20:661–671, 1985.

NAIDICH DP, KHOURI NF, SCOTT WJ, et al: Computed tomography of the pulmonary hila: I. Normal anatomy. J Comput Assist Tomogr 5:459–467, 1981.

NAIDICH DP, KHOURI NF, STITIK FP, et al: Computed tomography of the pulmonary hila: II. Abnormal anatomy. J Comput Assist Tomogr 5:468–475, 1981.

NG CS, WELLS AU, PADLEY SP: A CT sign of chronic pulmonary arterial hypertension: The ratio of main pulmonary artery to aortic diameter. J Thorac Imaging 14:270–278, 1999.

PARK CK, WEBB WR, KLEIN JS: Inferior hilar window. Radiology 178:163–168, 1991.

REMY-JARDIN M, DUYCK P, REMY J, et al: Hilar lymph nodes: Identification with spiral CT and histologic correlation. Radiology 196:387–394, 1995.

REMY-JARDIN M, REMY J, ARTAUD D, et al: Volume rendering of the tracheobronchial tree: Clinical evaluation of bronchographic images. Radiology 208:761–770, 1998.

SONE S, HIGASHIHARA T, MORIMOTO S, et al: CT anatomy of hilar lymphadenopathy. AJR Am J Roentgenol 140:887–892, 1983.

WEBB WR, GAMSU G: Computed tomography of the left retrobronchial stripe. J Comput Assist Tomogr 7:65–69, 1983.

WEBB WR, GAMSU G, GLAZER G: Computed tomography of the abnormal pulmonary hilum. J Comput Assist Tomogr 5:485–490, 1981.

WEBB WR, GLAZER G, GAMSU G: Computed tomography of the normal pulmonary hilum. J Comput Assist Tomogr 5:476–484, 1981.

WEBB WR, HIRJI M, GAMSU G: Posterior wall of the bronchus intermedius: Radiographic-CT correlation. AJR Am J Roentgenol 142:907–911, 1984.

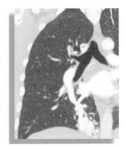

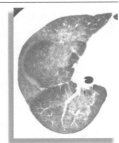

6

Lung Disease

W. Richard Webb, M.D.

On CT, normal lung varies in appearance depending on the window settings used. With a window mean of −600 to −700 H and a width of 1000 to 1500 H, the lungs appear dark, but not as black as the air visible in the trachea or bronchi. This slight difference in attenuation between lung parenchyma and air should be sought in choosing an appropriate window setting. If the lungs are viewed with too high a window mean, soft-tissue structures in the lung (vessels, bronchi, or lung nodules) are difficult to see or are underestimated as to their size, and any areas of lucency, such as bullae, may be missed. The lungs, after all, are not simply bags of air, and they should not appear to be. If too low a window mean is used, the size of soft-tissue structures in the lung will be overestimated.

☐ NORMAL ANATOMY

Intrapulmonary Fissures and Lobar Anatomy

Major Fissures

Because they are thin and oblique relative to the plane of the scan, the normal major fissures are not usually visible on CT obtained with 5-mm collimation. However, the position of each major fissure can be inferred from the location of the relatively avascular region of lung 1 to 2 cm in thickness (representing the lung on each side of the fissure), which contains no large vessels (Fig. 6-1). Sometimes, an ill-defined band of density is seen in the middle of the avascular area; this band represents volume averaging of the fissure with adjacent lung. In 10% to 20% of patients, the major fissures are visible as a thin line. On thin slices or high-resolution CT (HRCT), the major fissures are almost always recognizable as thin white lines. The major fissures are incomplete in many patients (i.e., they do not completely separate the lobes).

Within the lower thorax, the major fissures angle anterolaterally from the mediastinum, contacting the anterior third of the hemidiaphragms. They separate the lower lobes posteriorly from the upper lobe on the left and the middle and upper lobes on the right. In the upper thorax, the major fissures angle posterolaterally. Above the aortic arch, they contact the posterior chest wall.

Minor Fissure

The minor fissure is usually hard to see because it parallels the plane of scan. However, its approximate position can be determined by noting

105

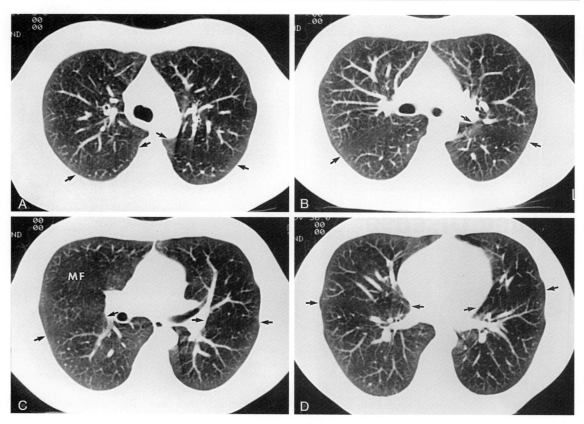

FIGURE 6-1 **Normal fissures.** *A,* At the level of the aortic arch, an avascular band *(arrows)* within the posterior lungs marks the locations of the major fissures. They angle posterolaterly. *B,* Several centimeters lower, the major fissures *(arrows)* are more anteriorly positioned. The upper lobes are anterior to the fissures. *C,* The major fissures *(arrows)* remain visible. The location of the minor fissure is indicated by the rounded region (MF), which contains no large vessels. *D,* Near the diaphragm, the major fissures angle anterolaterly *(arrows).* The middle lobe is located anterior to the right major fissure.

a lucent, avascular region in the anterior right lung, corresponding to lung on each side of the fissure (see Fig. 6-1*C*). This avascular plane is visible on CT in most patients. In some patients, the minor fissure mimics the appearance of the major fissure but is seen anterior to it. On thin-section CT or HRCT, the minor fissure often can be seen as a white line of varying sharpness and thickness, depending on its orientation.

Because the minor fissure often angles caudally, the lower, middle, and upper lobe may all be seen on a single scan (Fig. 6-2). If the minor fissure is concave caudad, it can sometimes be seen in two locations or can appear ring shaped (see Fig. 6-2), with the middle lobe between the fissure lines or in the center of the ring and the upper lobe anterior to the most anterior part of the fissure.

Accessory Fissures

In patients with an azygos lobe, the four layers of the *mesoazygos,* or azygos fissure, are invariably visible above the level of the intrapulmonary azygos vein. The azygos fissure is C shaped and convex laterally, beginning anteriorly at the right brachiocephalic vein and ending posteriorly at the right anterolateral surface of the vertebral body (see Fig. 6-8 and also Fig. 3-16). Other accessory fissures, most commonly the inferior accessory fissure, are occasionally seen on CT. They are not generally of diagnostic significance.

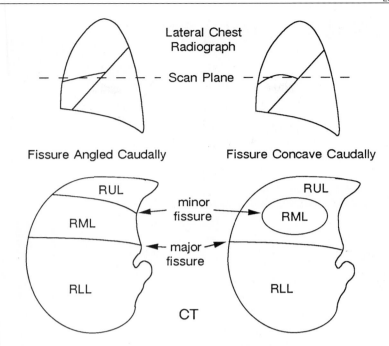

FIGURE 6-2 **Possible appearances of minor fissure.** Depending on the orientation of the minor fissure, its appearance and the relations of the lobes of the right lung can vary. If the minor fissure angles downward, both the middle and upper lobes can be seen on a single scan. If the minor fissure is concave caudad, it may appear ring shaped. RLL, right lower lobe; RML, right middle lobe; RUL, right upper lobe.

☐ CONGENITAL LESIONS

Pulmonary Agenesis and Aplasia

Pulmonary agenesis consists of complete absence of lung, bronchi, and vascular supply. With pulmonary aplasia, a rudimentary bronchus is present, ending in a blind pouch, but lung parenchyma and pulmonary vessels are absent (Fig. 6-3).

☐ BRONCHIAL ANOMALIES

Tracheal Bronchus

Tracheal bronchus represents the origin of all or part (usually the apical segment) of the right upper lobe bronchus from the trachea (Fig. 6-4); its incidence is less than 1%. A left tracheal bronchus is much less common. Tracheal bronchus is common in cloven-hoofed animals such as the pig, sheep, goat, camel, and giraffe; it may be associated with recurrent infection (in humans).

Bronchial Isomerism

Bronchial isomerism refers to bilateral symmetry of the bronchi. It may be isolated or associated with a variety of anomalies.

Bronchial Atresia

Bronchial atresia is characterized by local narrowing or obliteration of a lobar, segmental, or subsegmental bronchus. It is most common in the left upper lobe, followed by the right upper and right middle lobes. Mucus commonly accumulates in dilated bronchi distal to the obstruction, resulting in a tubular, branching, or ovoid mucus plug. Air trapping in the lobe or segment distal to the obstruction occurs because of collateral ventilation. Obstructed distal lung often appears hyperlucent and hypovascular.

☐ BRONCHOGENIC CYST

The appearance of mediastinal bronchogenic cyst has been described. Pulmonary bronchogenic

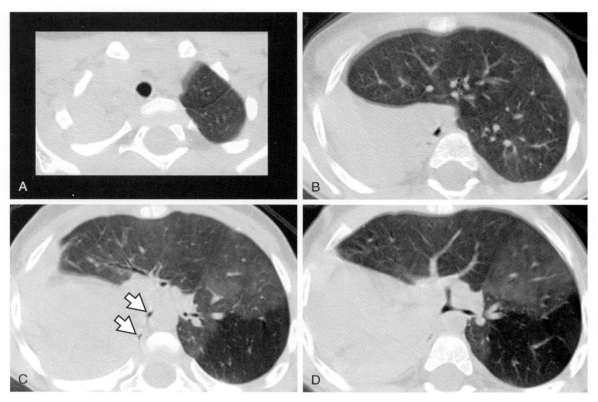

FIGURE 6-3 **Pulmonary aplasia in a child.** *A–D,* The right lung is completely absent with mediastinal shift to the right and herniation of the left lung across the midline. The presence of rudimentary bronchi on the right *(arrows, C)* indicates that this represents aplasia rather than agenesis.

cysts are typically well defined, round or oval, and of fluid or soft-tissue attenuation; previously infected cysts can contain air or an air–fluid level. When a cyst contains air, its wall appears very thin, although consolidation of surrounding lung may be present.

☐ ARTERIOVENOUS FISTULA

Pulmonary arteriovenous fistulas can be single (65%) or multiple (35%) and are often associated with Osler-Weber-Rendu syndrome (65%). On CT, an arteriovenous fistula can appear in either

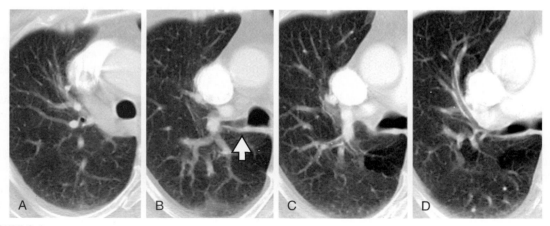

FIGURE 6-4 **Tracheal bronchus.** Four images *(A–D)* at contiguous levels in a patient with tracheal bronchus. The tracheal bronchus *(arrow, B)* arises from the lateral tracheal wall *(B)* above the level of the right upper lobe bronchus *(D).* The tracheal bronchus supplies the apical segment of the right upper lobe. Note that the azygos arch is visible above the tracheal bronchus.

of two forms: (1) a single dilated vascular sac, visible as a smooth, sharply defined, round or oval nodule (most common); or (2) a tangle of dilated tortuous vessels seen as a lobulated or serpiginous mass. In each type, the feeding pulmonary artery branch and draining pulmonary vein are dilated and should be easily seen on CT (Fig. 6-5). In most cases, the fistula is immediately subpleural in location. These findings should be sufficient to make a specific diagnosis on scans without contrast infusion. Spiral CT without contrast infusion is more accurate than angiography in the diagnosis of arteriovenous fistulas and in showing their vascular architecture.

Although contrast medium is not usually needed for diagnosis, an arteriovenous fistula shows rapid and dense opacification after bolus contrast injection, followed by rapid washout of the contrast (see Fig. 6-5). As would be expected, opacification occurs just after opacification of the right ventricle. Solid tumors can opacify after contrast medium injection, but

rapid and dense opacification and rapid washout of contrast medium is not seen with tumors.

☐ SEQUESTRATION

Pulmonary sequestrations can appear cystic or solid on CT. From 70% to 90% are located posteromedially on the left; all have anomalous systemic arterial supply from the thoracic or abdominal aorta. There is no bronchial or pulmonary artery supply to the lesion. In many cases of sequestration, the feeding systemic artery is visible on contrast-enhanced CT (Figs. 6-6 and 6-7).

Intralobar Sequestration

Intralobar sequestration is usually diagnosed in adults, and recurrent or chronic infection is common. Venous drainage is usually by means of the pulmonary veins, although systemic (azygos) vein drainage may also be seen. Intralobar sequestration typically contains air but can be

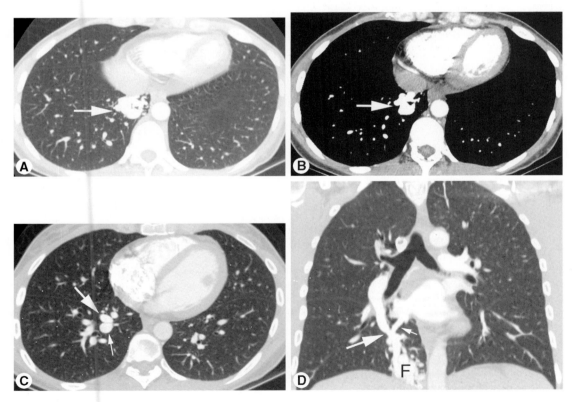

FIGURE 6-5 Arteriovenous fistula. *A,* Contrast-enhanced multidetector CT with 1.25-mm slice thickness (lung window) shows a lobulated and serpiginous mass at the right lung base typical of an arteriovenous fistula *(arrow)*. *B,* With a soft-tissue window setting, dense enhancement is visible *(arrow)*. *C,* At a more cephalad level, the feeding artery *(large arrow)* and draining vein *(small arrow)* are visible. *D,* A coronal reformation shows the feeding artery *(large arrow)*, draining vein *(small arrow)*, and subpleural fistula (F).

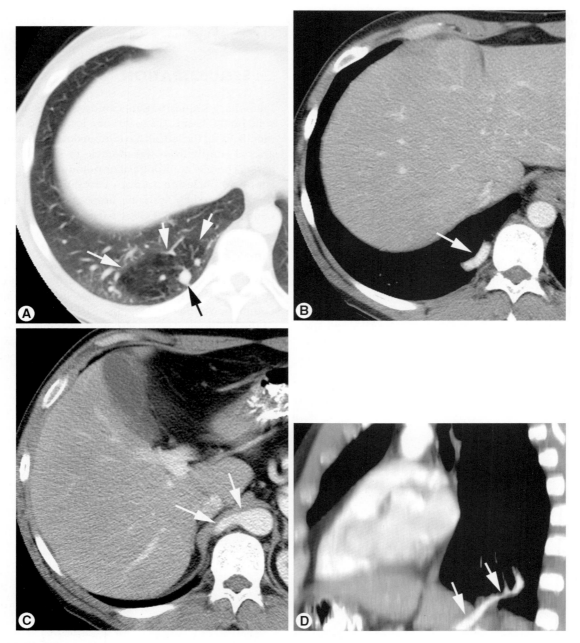

FIGURE 6-6 **Intralobar sequestration appearing as hyperlucent lung.** *A,* Contrast-enhanced CT (lung window) in a patient with intralobar sequestration shows an area of lucent lung *(white arrows)* at the right base. An abnormal vessel *(black arrow)* is visible within the area of lucency. *B,* Soft-tissue window at a lower level shows the abnormal vessel *(arrow). C,* A scan near the lung base shows that the abnormal vessel arises from the aorta *(arrows). D,* Sagittal reformation shows the abnormal vessel *(arrows),* originating in the abdomen, supplying the posterior lower lobe.

quite variable in appearance. On CT, intralobar sequestration can appear as follows:

1. A region of hyperlucent lung (see Fig. 6-6A)
2. A cystic or multicystic structure (sometimes with air–fluid levels)
3. Consolidated or collapsed lung (see Fig. 6-7)
4. A combination of these findings

Areas of lucent lung in association with, or representing part of, an intralobar sequestration are common (see Fig. 6-6A); these areas are

1. Hypoplasia of the lung with abnormal segmental or lobar anatomy
2. Hypoplasia of the ipsilateral pulmonary artery
3. Anomalous pulmonary venous return (the *scimitar vein*) from the right upper lobe or the entire right lung, usually to the vena cava or right atrium
4. Anomalous systemic arterial supply to a portion of the hypoplastic lung, usually the lower lobe

On CT, the hypoplastic lung is recognizable because of dextroposition of the heart and mediastinal shift to the right (Fig. 6-8). The hypoplastic lung may also show abnormal bronchial anatomy, deficient bronchial divisions, or mirror image bronchial or pulmonary artery branching. When the anomalous (scimitar) vein is present, it is clearly visible on CT. Hypoplasia of the pulmonary artery is usually recognizable by the decreased size of vessels in the hypoplastic lung. This entity may be associated with congenital heart disease.

☐ PULMONARY VEIN ANOMALIES AND VEIN VARIX

Anomalous Pulmonary Venous Return

An anomalous pulmonary vein branch is present in about 0.5% of the population and is usually asymptomatic. The anomalous vein may drain into various vascular structures. On the right, the most common are the superior vena cava, azygos vein, inferior vena cava, and right atrium. On the left, drainage may be via left brachiocephalic vein, persistent left superior vena cava, or coronary sinus (Fig. 6-9). Drainage may also be below the diaphragm. These can be seen as an isolated anomaly or in association with congenital heart disease.

Pulmonary Vein Varix

A dilated central pulmonary vein, or vein varix, can be congenital or result from increased left atrial pressure (often with mitral stenosis). It is most common on the right side, corresponding to the inferior pulmonary vein branch in most cases. The dilated segment of vein opacifies after contrast infusion. In some cases, a vein varix may be associated with anomalous pulmonary venous return.

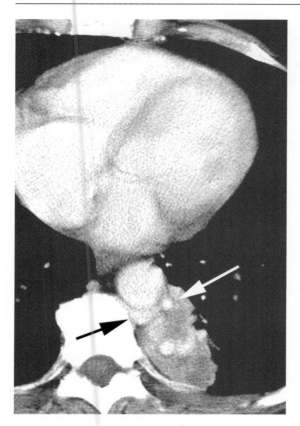

FIGURE 6-7 **Intralobar sequestration appearing as consolidated lung.** Contrast-enhanced CT (lung window) in a patient with an intralobar sequestration shows an area of consolidation adjacent to the aorta in the left lower lobe. An anomalous artery *(white arrow)* arises from the descending aorta and supplies the sequestration. The draining vein *(black arrow)* communicates with the hemiazygos vein.

usually caused by air trapping. Normal bronchi are not seen in the sequestration; and if the sequestration is aerated, the vascular branching pattern within it may appear abnormal.

Extralobar Sequestration

Extralobar sequestration is usually diagnosed in infants or children, and infection is rare. It almost always appears as a solid mass and rarely contains air. Venous drainage is usually through systemic veins.

☐ HYPOGENETIC LUNG (SCIMITAR) SYNDROME

Hypogenetic lung (scimitar) syndrome, a rare anomaly almost always occurring on the right side, is characterized by four features that coexist to varying degrees:

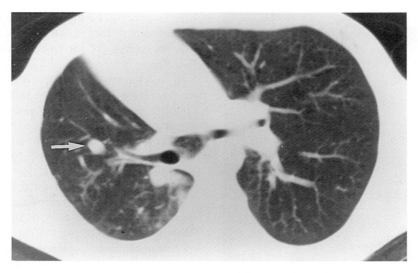

FIGURE 6-8 **Hypogenetic lung syndrome.** The right lung is reduced in volume, and the mediastinum is shifted toward the right. The scimitar vein *(arrow)* is visible within the right lung.

☐ THE SOLITARY PULMONARY NODULE AND FOCAL LUNG LESIONS

CT is often used to evaluate a solitary nodule or focal lesion detected on chest radiographs. It is of value in several ways, including: (1) confirming the presence of a parenchymal lesion, (2) determining its morphology, (3) detecting the presence of calcium or fat, (4) determining if the lesion opacifies after contrast infusion, and (5) planning biopsy.

Morphology of Some Focal Lesions and Lung Nodules

HRCT scans are valuable in defining the morphology of focal pulmonary parenchymal lesions. With single-detector CT, scanning through the nodule with 1-mm collimation and a pitch of 1 is recommended; with multidetector CT, scans obtained using 1.25-mm detectors are sufficient. A high-resolution reconstruction algorithm should be used. Lung cancers and several other focal lesions can have characteristic appearances on CT.

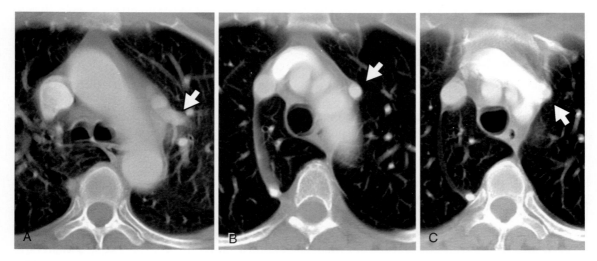

FIGURE 6-9 **Anomalous pulmonary vein drainage.** A pulmonary vein branch *(arrow, A)* enters the left mediastinum, draining through an anomalous left vertical vein *(arrow, B)*, which drains *(arrow, C)* into the left brachiocephalic vein. An azygos lobe is also present.

Lung Cancer

A definite diagnosis of lung cancer cannot be made on CT. However, CT findings that strongly suggest malignancy in a patient with a solitary nodule include the following:

1. An irregular or spiculated edge, usually caused by fibrosis surrounding the tumor (90% of nodules with a spiculated edge are malignant; Fig. 6-10)
2. A lobulated contour (Fig. 6-11)
3. Air bronchograms (see Fig. 6-10), cystic or "bubbly" air-containing regions within the nodule (seen in 65% of cancers but only 5% of benign lesions)
4. Cavitation (see Fig. 6-11), with a nodular cavity wall or a wall exceeding 15 mm in greatest thickness (90% are cancers)
5. A diameter exceeding 2 cm (95% are cancers)

A spiculated edge and the presence of air bronchograms or cystic regions are particularly common with adenocarcinomas and bronchioloalveolar carcinoma. Lobulation also suggests the diagnosis of carcinoma but may be seen with other lesions as well, particularly hamartomas.

Both primary lung carcinomas and metastases can cavitate. Typically, a cavitary carcinoma has a thick, irregular, and nodular wall (see Fig. 6-11), but some metastatic tumors, particu-

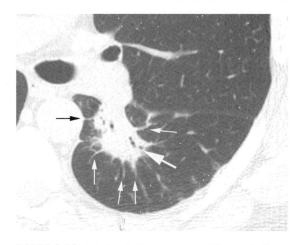

FIGURE 6-10 **Spiculated adenocarcinoma.** High-resolution CT in a patient with a left lower lobe nodule shows a spiculated mass *(small white arrows)*, suggestive of carcinoma. When a linear opacity contacts the pleural surface *(black arrow)*, the resulting opacity is termed a *pleural tail*. Note that the nodule contains several air bronchograms *(large white arrow)*.

larly those of squamous cell origin, can be relatively thin walled. A cavitary nodule with a thin wall (<5 mm) is likely (90%) benign.

Some cancers, particularly bronchioloalveolar carcinoma, may also present with a nodule of ground-glass opacity, opacity that does not obscure vessels, or the "halo sign" (see later). Such tumors tend to have a better prognosis than solid (homogenously dense) tumors.

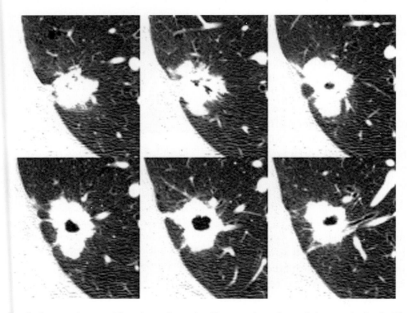

FIGURE 6-11 **Spiculated adenocarcinoma with an irregular cavity.** Six scans through a nodule were obtained with spiral technique and 1-mm collimation. The nodule has a lobulated and spiculated margin and contains a thick-walled cavity. Pleural tails are also visible.

Hamartoma

HRCT can be valuable in diagnosing pulmonary hamartomas. Hamartomas appear smooth and rounded or lobulated in contour. Using CT with thin sections, about two thirds of hamartomas can be correctly diagnosed because of visible fat (60%; Fig. 6-12*A*), either focal or diffuse (see Fig. 6-12), fat and calcification (30%; see Fig. 6-12), or diffuse calcification (10%). Usually, fat is easily seen on the scans; CT numbers range between −40 and −120 H. Calcification may have a "popcorn" appearance because of calcification of nodules of cartilage (see Fig. 6-12*B*).

Rounded Atelectasis

Rounded atelectasis represents focal, collapsed, and often folded lung. It almost always occurs in association with pleural thickening or effusion. It is frequently seen in clinical practice.

Rounded atelectasis is most common in the posterior, paravertebral regions and may be bilateral in patients with bilateral pleural disease. Areas of rounded atelectasis are usually several centimeters in diameter. Bending or bowing of adjacent bronchi and arteries toward the edge of the area of round atelectasis, because of volume loss or folding of lung, is characteristic (Fig. 6-13) and has been likened to a "comet tail." Air bronchograms can sometimes be seen within the mass. Rounded atelectasis opacifies densely after contrast infusion.

Four findings must be present to make a confident diagnosis of rounded atelectasis on CT; if these are present, follow-up is usually sufficient (see Fig. 6-13). If one of these findings is lacking, you should be cautious in making the diagnosis, and biopsy may be necessary. These four findings are:

1. Ipsilateral pleural thickening or effusion
2. Significant contact between the lung lesion and the abnormal pleural surface
3. The "comet tail" sign
4. Volume loss in the lobe in which the opacity is seen

Rounded atelectasis is most commonly associated with pleural effusion. It is also commonly associated with asbestos-related pleural thickening, occurring adjacent to regions of thickened pleura; but often it has an atypical appearance. Areas of atelectasis or focal fibrosis in patients exposed to asbestos can be irregular,

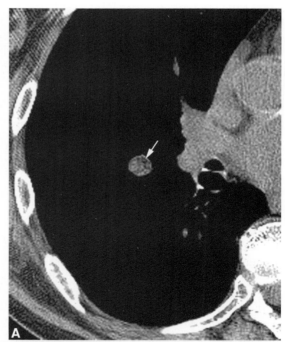

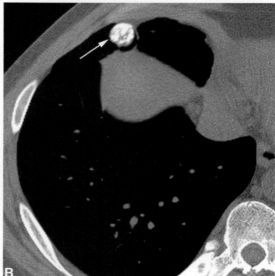

FIGURE 6-12 **Hamartoma, common appearances in two patients.** *A,* High-resolution CT with soft-tissue (mediastinal) window settings in a patient with a small lung nodule detected on plain films. The nodule is round and sharply defined. It contains areas of low attenuation *(arrow),* indicating the presence of fat. This appearance is diagnostic of hamartoma. *B,* In another patient with hamartoma *(arrow),* a rounded and sharply defined nodule shows "popcorn" calcification. This appearance is seen in some patients with hamartoma.

may not have extensive pleural contact, and may not be associated with the "comet tail" sign. Biopsy is often warranted in this setting.

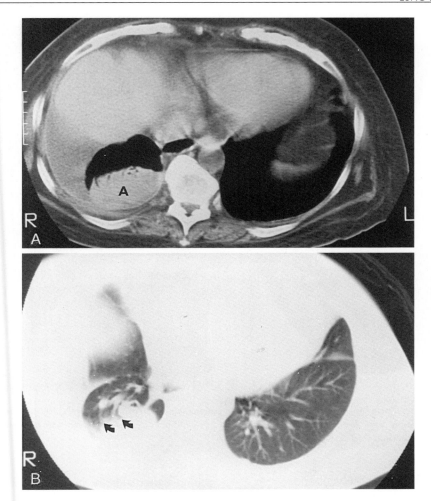

FIGURE 6-13 **Rounded atelectasis.** *A,* Adjacent to an area of pleural thickening and effusion, the atelectatic lung (A) shows air bronchograms curving into its edge. The lesion shows extensive pleural contact. *B,* At a lung window setting, the curved vessels and bronchi *(arrows)* entering the atelectatic lung are visible, and there is posterior displacement of the major fissure, indicating volume loss.

Pulmonary Infarction and Septic Embolism

Infarcts can result in a focal pulmonary opacity. Septic emboli are usually multiple. In either instance, nodules typically are: (1) peripheral or abut a pleural surface; (2) round, wedge shaped, or truncated; and (3) seen to have a pulmonary artery branch leading to them.

Using contrast-enhanced CT, associated clot may be identified in the proximal pulmonary artery in patients with pulmonary infarction. In patients with septic embolism, cavitation of lung nodules is common.

The "Halo" Sign and Invasive Aspergillosis

The "halo" sign is said to be present if a soft-tissue attenuation nodule is surrounded by a less dense rim or halo of ground-glass opacity (Fig. 6-14). In immunosuppressed patients, particularly those with treated leukemia and low white blood cell counts, this appearance is typical of invasive aspergillosis. Although suggestive of invasive aspergillosis in the proper clinical setting, the halo sign is nonspecific and can be seen with other infections (tuberculosis, legionellosis, nocardiosis, and cytomegalovirus infection), some tumors (particularly bronchioloalveolar carcinoma, lymphoma, and Kaposi's sarcoma), and in patients with infarction and Wegener's granulomatosis. Although the histologic appearance of the halo varies with the entity, it often represents hemorrhage (aspergillosis, Kaposi's sarcoma, infarction, Wegener's granulomatosis) or inhomogeneous inflammation (infections) or infiltration of lung (carcinoma).

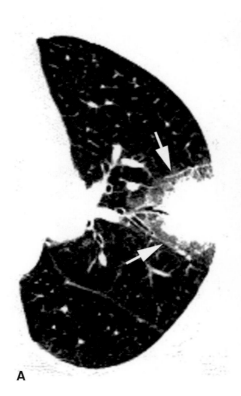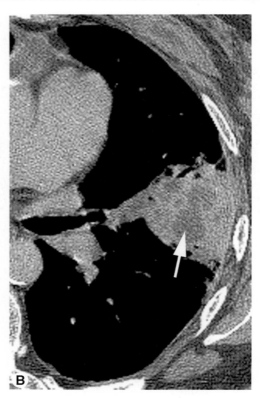

FIGURE 6-14 **Invasive aspergillosis with the halo sign.** *A,* In an immunosuppressed patient with leukemia, an ill-defined lung mass is surrounded by a less-dense "halo" *(arrows)*. This finding is highly suggestive of this diagnosis in a patient with the appropriate history. *B,* Soft-tissue window at the same level shows central necrosis *(arrow)*.

The Air-Crescent Sign and Mycetoma

The presence of a lung mass capped by a crescent of air is termed the *air-crescent sign* (Fig. 6-15). It usually indicates the presence of a mass within a cavity. The air-crescent sign is most typical of mycetoma, but it may also be seen in the later stages of invasive aspergillosis, clot or neoplasm within a cavity, and echinococcal cyst.

In patients with a preexisting pulmonary cyst or cavity, a mycetoma or fungus ball can form as a result of saprophytic infection, usually by *Aspergillus*. On CT, a round or oval mass (the fungus ball) can be seen within the cavity, in a dependent location, and is typically mobile. The mass is capped by a crescent of air within the cavity. Thickening of the cavity wall is common. In patients with a developing mycetoma, the fungus ball can contain multiple air collections. The same appearance can represent semi-invasive aspergillosis, in which the fungus also invades the wall of the cyst or cavity. Hemorrhage and hemoptysis are common associations. With invasive aspergillosis, septic infarction of

lung can result in an air-crescent sign as the patient recovers (see Fig. 6-15).

Lung Abscess

A lung abscess can occur with a variety of bacterial, fungal, and parasitic infections. The hallmark of lung abscess is necrosis or cavitation within an area of pneumonia or dense consolidation; the necrotic region can appear quite irregular (see Fig. 6-14). Necrosis is commonly visible on contrast-enhanced CT as one or more areas of low attenuation within opacified lung. Cavitation is said to be present if air is visible within the lesion, and often CT is obtained to confirm this diagnosis when the plain radiograph is suggestive. An air–fluid level or levels are commonly present (Fig. 6-16). CT can also be helpful in distinguishing a lung abscess from an empyema. Chapter 7 contrasts the CT appearances of lung abscess and empyema.

Granulomatous Lesions and "Satellite Nodules"

Granulomas usually appear rounded and well defined. They may contain calcium. Inflamma-

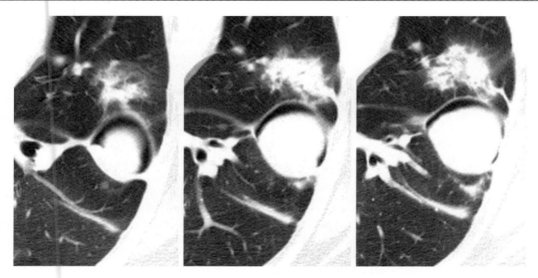

FIGURE 6-15 **Invasive aspergillosis with an air-crescent sign.** A crescent of air outlines a mass within a cavity. In invasive aspergillosis, the mass represents a ball of infarcted lung and the cavity represents the space the lung used to occupy. This is distinct from aspergilloma, in which an air-crescent sign reflects fungus within a preexisting cavity. Focal consolidation is visible anterior to the cavitary lesion, because of acute infection.

tory and particularly granulomatous lesions may be associated with small *satellite nodules*— that is, small nodules grouped together or seen surrounding a larger nodule or cavity (Fig. 6-17). In patients with sarcoidosis, this appearance has been referred to as the *galaxy sign*. These are seen in only 1% to 2% of carcinomas.

Lipoid Pneumonia
Chronic aspiration of lipid (animal, vegetable, or mineral) can lead to lipoid pneumonia, with fat and variable amounts of fibrosis resulting in focal consolidations or masses. In some patients, most typically those with mineral oil aspiration, CT shows low-attenuation (-50 to -140 H) consolidation indicative of its lipid content. When fibrosis predominates, the masses are of soft-tissue attenuation. Lipoid pneumonia differs from hamartoma, which may also contain fat, in that masses are larger, less well defined, and usually appear more irregular.

Linear Opacities (Scars or Atelectasis)
Sometimes, patients with a solitary nodule visible on chest radiographs show something on CT that is best categorized as a linear opacity. This may represent scarring from prior infection or

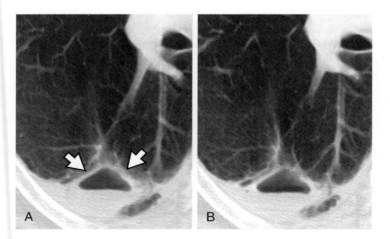

FIGURE 6-16 **Lung abscess.** *A* and *B,* A thin-walled lung abscess *(arrows)* is visible in the posterior lung, containing an air–fluid level.

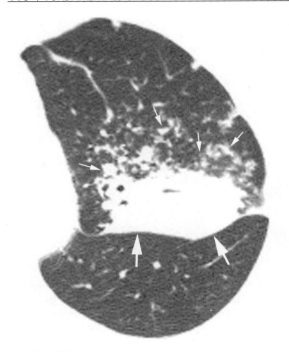

FIGURE 6-17 **Satellite nodules in sarcoidosis.** High-resolution CT in a patient with an ill-defined sarcoidosis and a left upper lobe mass, marginated posteriorly by the major fissure *(large arrows).* On high-resolution CT, the mass is surrounded by a number of smaller "satellite" nodules *(small arrows).* This appearance is most typical of a granulomatous process. It has also been referred to as the "galaxy sign."

infarction or a region of focal atelectasis. Although the cause cannot be determined, these opacities can be distinguished from cancers, which appear round or mass-like. Although their appearance indicates they are likely benign, follow-up may be appropriate.

Pleural (Fissural) Lesions

Occasionally, a pleural abnormality located in a fissure (e.g., a plaque, loculated effusion, or localized fibrous tumor of the pleura) may be misinterpreted as a lung nodule. Looking for the fissures on CT, and obtaining HRCT, will sometimes allow you to avoid this mistake. Correlating the CT with the chest radiographs also can prove valuable.

CT Diagnosis of Nodule Calcification

CT can be used to detect calcification in a lung nodule, indicating that the nodule is benign and that resection is not necessary. About 25% to 35% of benign nodules appearing uncalcified on radiographs show calcification on thin slices.

Calcification of lung nodules can sometimes be seen using CT with conventional technique (5-mm collimation). However, thin collimation (1–2 mm) and HRCT technique should be used to make this diagnosis. Calcium easily diagnosable on thin-slice CT is often invisible with thicker collimation. Soft-tissue window settings are best for detecting calcium.

When using CT to detect "benign" calcification, you must be sure that the calcification is benign in appearance (Fig. 6-18*A*); that is, it must be: (1) diffuse calcification (see Fig. 6-18*B*), typical of a granuloma; (2) dense, central (i.e., bull's-eye) calcification within the nodule, most typical of histoplasmosis (see Fig. 6-18*C*), (3) central and "popcorn" calcification, typical of hamartoma (see Fig. 6-12*B*); or (4) concentric rings of calcification (see Fig. 6-18*D*), typical of histoplasmosis. Nodules that show visible calcification will generally have measured CT numbers exceeding 100 to 200 H.

About 5% to 10% of carcinomas contain some calcium, either as a result of tumor calcification or because the carcinoma has engulfed a preexisting granuloma. Calcification in tumors is typically punctate or stippled, or is eccentric within the nodule (Fig. 6-19). Although these patterns of calcification may also be seen in benign lesions, when interpreting CT, they should be considered to be indeterminate or potentially associated with malignancy (see Fig. 6-19*A*).

Nodule Opacification

Lung cancers have a greater tendency to enhance after contrast infusion than do many benign lesions. Contrast enhancement greater than 15 H is sensitive in detecting cancers, but some benign lesions, such as benign tumors and active granulomatous lesions, also can enhance.

Because the degree of enhancement depends on the amount and rapidity of contrast medium infusion, it is important to use a consistent technique. In one study, 420 mg iodine/kg (usually 75–125 mL) was injected at a rate of 2 mL/second, with HRCT scans through the nodule obtained before the infusion and at 1-minute intervals for 4 minutes after the start of the injection. When enhancement of 15 HU or more is used to distinguish malignant from benign lesions, sensitivity is 98%, but specificity is only 73%.

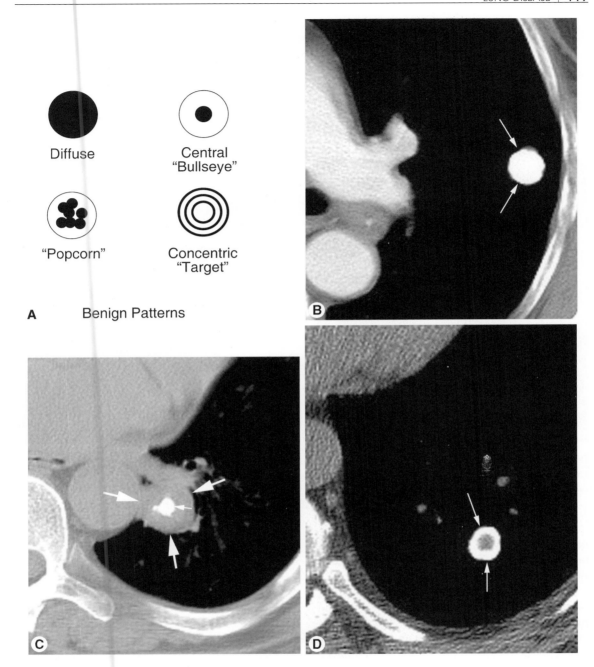

FIGURE 6-18 **Benign patterns of calcification.** *A,* Patterns of calcification typically associated with benign nodules. *B,* Diffuse nodule calcification *(arrows)* in tuberculoma. *C,* A left lower lobe nodule *(large arrows)* shows dense central (bull's-eye) calcification *(small arrow)*. *D,* A concentric ring of calcification *(arrows)* outlines a lung nodule.

Nodule Growth

The growth rate of a nodule, the time required for a doubling of volume (doubling time), may be used to determine its likelihood of being malignant. A pulmonary nodule that doubles in volume in less than 1 month or more than 16 months is usually benign. However, the overlap-ping growth rates of benign and malignant lesions make it difficult to use doubling time as an absolute indicator. In my opinion, you should be suspicious of malignancy if any growth occurs, no matter how slow; some lung cancers have a doubling time exceeding 1,000 days. It is generally agreed that a solitary pulmonary

Eccentric

Stippled

A Indeterminant Patterns

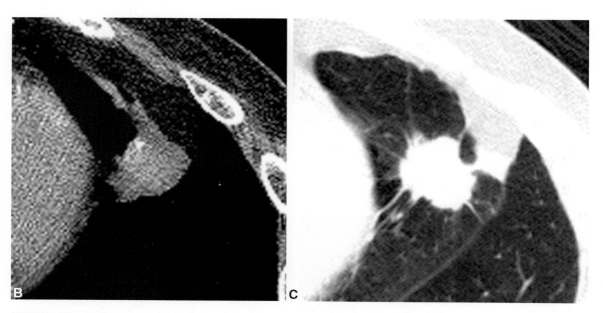

FIGURE 6-19 **Indeterminate calcification.** *A,* Patterns of calcification that may be seen in either benign or malignant nodules. *B* and *C,* High-resolution CT in a patient with an adenocarcinoma in the lingula shows a spiculated nodule with eccentric calcification. Eccentric calcification can be seen in carcinomas.

nodule that does not grow over a 2-year period is benign and does not require resection. However, this is not always true.

CT is commonly used to follow a newly diagnosed lung nodule to determine its doubling time. Follow-up CT at an initial interval of 3 months, then increasing to 6 months, is commonly used. However, the growth of nodules a few millimeters in diameter is difficult to assess using CT, and longer follow-up periods (e.g., 1 year) are likely appropriate in such cases. Because a 26% increase in nodule diameter equals a doubling of volume, for a 3-mm nodule, a volume doubling is equivalent to a diameter increase of less than 1 mm. This change is difficult to detect on CT.

Notably, on occasion, a lung cancer shows a transient decrease in size on follow-up. A single follow-up scan showing a nodule to be decreased in size is not sufficient to call it benign.

A second scan showing continued decrease in size or resolution is a good practice.

CT Lung Cancer Screening

CT may be used to screen patients at high risk for lung cancer. Using CT, more lung cancers (4:1), smaller lung cancers, and more early-stage (stage 1) cancers (6:1) are detected compared with using chest radiographs. However, false positives are common (up to 70% of screened patients show at least one lung nodule), limiting its usefulness. Furthermore, the value of screening in reducing lung cancer mortality has not been proven. Consequently, CT lung cancer screening is controversial; several studies are underway to determine its value and the costs involved.

CT lung cancer screening is ideally performed using multidetector CT, thin detector rows (1.25–2.5 mm), and a low-dose technique (obtained by reducing the milliampere setting). Because of the small size of nodules detected, follow-up scans (at 3- to 6-month intervals) are usually required to assess the significance of detected nodules.

Use of CT to Guide Biopsy of a Lung Nodule

If CT does not allow a specific diagnosis to be made in a patient with a solitary nodule, and no calcification is visible, further evaluation is often appropriate. This may involve positron emission tomography scanning, which has a high sensitivity (97%) and specificity (80%) in diagnosing cancer, or biopsy of the nodule.

Bronchoscopy is most accurate in diagnosing central masses that have an endobronchial component, whereas needle biopsy is best for peripheral lung lesions. For lesions in the central half of the lung, if an endobronchial abnormality is seen on CT or a *bronchus sign* (bronchial narrowing or obstruction at the site of a nodule, or a bronchus within the mass lesion) is visible, bronchoscopy directed to the proper site is most appropriate. If there is no evidence of an abnormal bronchus at CT, needle biopsy should probably be performed first.

CT can be helpful in planning a needle aspiration biopsy, even if CT is not used for the biopsy itself. First, CT can indicate the depth of the lesion and the needle can be marked accordingly. This is of particular value if only single-plane fluoroscopy is available for the biopsy procedure. Second, CT can help in planning the biopsy approach. If bullae lie in the path of the needle, or the needle must cross a fissure to reach the lesion, the risk for pneumothorax is increased, and a different approach might be chosen.

Thoracoscopic biopsy or resection of peripheral lung nodules can be assisted by CT-guided localization techniques. These may involve injection of methylene blue or placement of hooked wires in the nodule.

☐ MULTIPLE LUNG NODULES AND PULMONARY METASTASES

CT is much more sensitive than plain radiographs in detecting lung nodules. Nodules as small as a few millimeters can be detected easily using CT (Figs. 6-20 and 6-21).

Nodules can mimic the appearance of vessels seen in cross section. However, small nodules are usually visible on only one or two adjacent scans, whereas longitudinally oriented vessels can be followed on a number of scans and can be traced to their point of origin or seen to branch. Contrast injection is not usually of value in making this distinction, except in the case of large central nodules, in contiguity with the hilar vessels.

The differential diagnosis of multiple large (>1 cm) pulmonary nodules includes metastases; lymphoma; bronchogenic carcinoma with synchronous primary tumors; bacterial, fungal, and sometimes viral infections (Fig. 6-22); granulomatous diseases; sarcoidosis; Wegener's granulomatosis; rheumatoid lung disease; amyloidosis; and septic emboli. In most cases, the CT appearance of large nodules is nonspecific. The differential diagnosis of multiple small nodules (<1 cm) is discussed in the section on HRCT and Diffuse Infiltrative Lung Disease.

Metastases

Pulmonary metastases resulting from tumor embolization are typically diffuse or have a predilection for the peripheral, subpleural lung (see Figs. 6-20 and 6-21). Normal subpleural lymphoid aggregates and granulomas can also result in the presence of small peripheral nodules and are common in clinical practice. Because small nodules are often too small to evaluate using

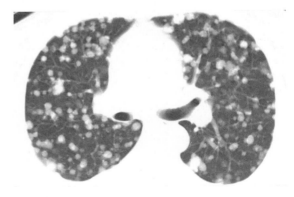

FIGURE 6-20 **Pulmonary metastases.** CT shows multiple nodules with a diffuse distribution. Despite their small size, nodules are sharply defined. This pattern of nodules is termed *random*.

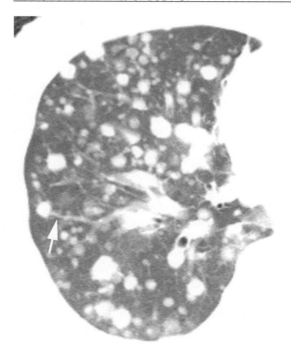

FIGURE 6-21 **Pulmonary metastases with the feeding vessel sign.** Multiple well-defined nodules represent metastases from a renal cell carcinoma. Involvement of the peripheral lung is typical. A few of these nodules *(arrow)* appear to be related to a pulmonary vessel, the so-called feeding vessel sign.

percutaneous biopsy, follow-up CT at 1 to 3 months is often used to assess their significance. Metastases increase in size.

In obtaining follow-up CT to assess a small lung nodule(s) for change in size, it is important to obtain scans at exactly the same levels and with the same window settings as in the original study. A small nodule can be missed if the patient breathes differently for two supposedly contiguous scans (the nodule may fall at a level between the two "adjacent" scans), or it can appear to be smaller if it is slightly out of the scan plane; the use of spiral CT during a single breath hold helps to avoid these problems. Identifying the pattern of branching vessels within the lung, in the region of the nodule, is an easy way of knowing exactly what level you are viewing. If the same vessels are visible on both the original and follow-up scans, and the nodule looks different, then the nodule is different. If a different branching pattern is visible, an apparent difference in nodule size may not be real. If follow-up scans are viewed at window settings different from the original study, a nodule may appear to be a different size. As stated earlier, low window mean settings make a nodule appear larger.

Pulmonary metastases are typically round and well defined (see Fig. 6-20). Some metastases with surrounding hemorrhage can be ill defined or associated with the halo sign. Cavitation and calcification can be seen with some metastatic

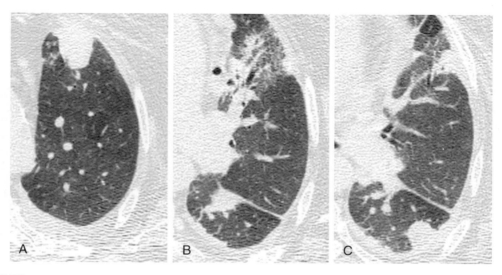

FIGURE 6-22 **Nocardiosis with multiple nodules.** Multiple ill-defined nodules reflect nocardia pneumonia in an immunosuppressed patient.

tumors. Pulmonary metastases may be seen to have a connection with a pulmonary artery branch, reflecting their embolic nature (i.e., "the feeding vessel sign"; see Fig. 6-21). However, this finding can be present with other causes of pulmonary nodules, such as Wegener's granulomatosis and bland or septic emboli.

Bronchioloalveolar Carcinoma

Approximately 50% of patients with bronchioloalveolar carcinoma present with diffuse or patchy lung consolidation or multiple lung nodules (Fig. 6-23). The presence of visible opacified arteries within the areas of consolidation on contrast-enhanced CT (i.e., "the CT angiogram sign") has been reported to be suggestive of this tumor, but it can also be seen with other causes of consolidation, such as pneumonia. In patients with bronchioloalveolar carcinoma, the tumor can secrete large amounts of low-attenuation fluid or mucus, which is partially responsible for lung consolidation and the pres-

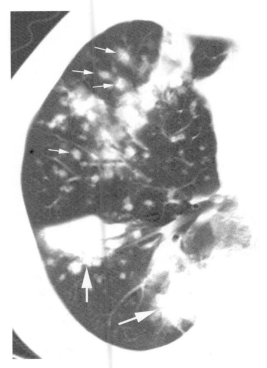

FIGURE 6-23 **Bronchioloalveolar carcinoma with consolidation and multiple nodules.** Focal areas of consolidation *(large arrows)* are visible in the right lung. Multiple nodules *(small arrows)* are also visible; these nodules are usually centrilobular in location and reflect endobronchial spread of tumor.

ence of the CT angiogram sign. Bronchorrhea (excessive sputum production) can also result.

Lymphoma

Pulmonary parenchymal involvement is seen in 10% of patients with Hodgkin's disease at the time of presentation. Direct extension from hilar nodes, focal discrete areas of consolidation, or masslike lesions can be seen. Air bronchograms or areas of cavitation may be visible within the abnormal regions. In patients with untreated Hodgkin's disease, lung involvement usually does not occur in the absence of radiographically demonstrable mediastinal (and usually ipsilateral hilar) adenopathy.

In patients with non-Hodgkin's lymphoma, pulmonary disease can occur in the absence of lymph node enlargement. This is common in patients with acquired immunodeficiency syndrome. Large, ill-defined nodules can be seen.

☐ BRONCHIECTASIS AND BRONCHIAL ABNORMALITIES

HRCT or spiral CT obtained with thin (3 mm) collimation or detector width should be obtained to diagnosis bronchiectasis. In normal patients, a bronchus and its adjacent pulmonary artery branch are usually about the same size. In patients with bronchiectasis, the pulmonary artery branch and adjacent dilated, ring-shaped bronchus give their combined shadow the appearance of a signet ring (Fig. 6-24). The *signet ring sign* is characteristic of bronchiectasis. By definition, the signet ring sign is present if the internal diameter of a bronchus exceeds the diameter of the adjacent artery; this appearance is occasionally seen in healthy subjects. In patients with bronchiectasis, bronchial wall thickening is also usually present. Bronchiectasis is usually classified as cylindrical, varicose, and cystic, but these designations are of little clinical significance.

Mucus plugs associated with bronchiectasis, cystic fibrosis, allergic bronchopulmonary aspergillosis (Fig. 6-25), bronchial obstruction, or congenital bronchial atresia can sometimes produce nodular opacities that are difficult to diagnose on chest radiographs. On CT, their relation to the bronchial tree, their often branching shape, and their associated bronchiectasis are diagnostic.

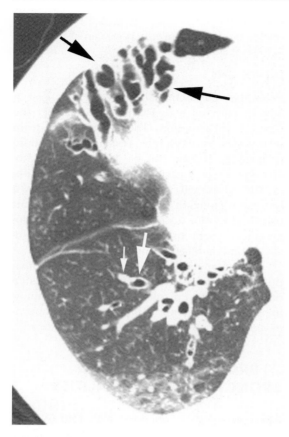

FIGURE 6-24 **Bronchiectasis.** High-resolution CT shows multifocal bronchiectasis. Thick-walled and irregularly dilated bronchi are visible in the middle lobe *(black arrows).* Their appearance would be classified as cylindrical or varicose. In the right lower lobe, several bronchi *(large white arrow)* appear larger than the adjacent pulmonary artery *(small white arrow).* This occurrence is termed the signet-ring sign.

Most patients with bronchiectasis have nonspecific findings, with abnormalities being most severe peripherally and in the lower lobes. Several diseases show other appearances. Cystic fibrosis usually shows bilateral bronchiectasis involving the upper lobes and being most severe in the central (parahilar) lung regions. Allergic bronchopulmonary aspergillosis also shows central bronchiectasis; mucous plugs are common and are often high in attenuation because of calcification (see Fig. 6-25). Tuberculosis shows upper lobe bronchiectasis, which is often asymmetric.

In patients with bronchiolitis obliterans (i.e., constrictive bronchiolitis or the Swyer–James syndrome), in addition to findings of bronchiectasis, areas of pulmonary hyperlucency can also be seen on CT, as a result of decreased perfusion within areas of lung that are poorly ventilated. This occurrence gives the lung a patchy inhomogeneous appearance and is termed *mosaic perfusion.* It is best shown on HRCT (Fig. 6-26). Typically, vessels within the relatively lucent regions appear smaller than in relatively dense lung regions.

☐ ATELECTASIS: TYPES AND PATTERNS

Atelectasis most commonly occurs because of bronchial obstruction (obstructive atelectasis), pleural effusion or other pleural processes that allow the lung to collapse (passive or relaxation atelectasis), or lung fibrosis (cicatrization atelectasis). These can have different appearances. General signs of volume loss on CT are the same as those on chest radiographs. Mediastinal shift (particularly of the anterior mediastinum), elevation of the diaphragm, and displacement of fissures are well seen on CT.

Obstructive Atelectasis

Obstructive atelectasis often occurs because of a tumor, and the bronchi should be examined closely. For the most part, the CT findings of obstructive atelectasis are what would be expected from our experience with plain films. Typically, the affected lobe is partially or completely consolidated (Fig. 6-27). Air bronchograms may be visible (see Fig. 6-27), but typically they are not. Mucus-bronchograms (low-density fluid or mucus within obstructed bronchi) can sometimes be seen on CT. The air- or mucus-filled bronchi can be dilated in the presence of atelectasis, simulating bronchiectasis. If contrast medium infusion is used, opacified vessels are often visible within the consolidated lobe. If little volume loss if present, the term *obstructive pneumonia* is often used instead (Fig. 6-28).

On CT, atelectasis can be diagnosed when displacement of fissures is seen. As on plain films, typical patterns of collapse can be identified (Figs. 6-29 and 6-30).

Right Upper Lobe Collapse

The major fissure rotates anteriorly and medially as the upper lobe progressively flattens against the mediastinum (see Figs. 6-27 and 6-29). The

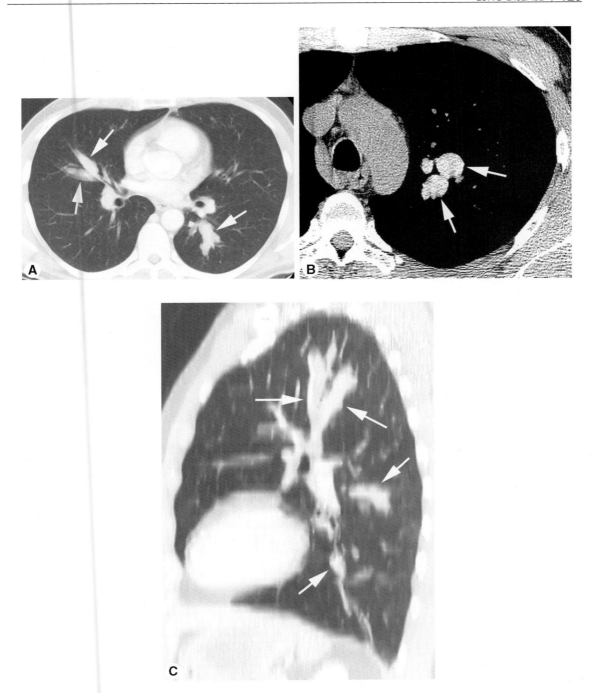

FIGURE 6-25 **Mucous plugging with allergic bronchopulmonary aspergillosis (ABPA).** *A,* CT with lung windows shows branching opacities *(arrows)* suggestive of mucous plugs. *B,* The mucous plugs *(arrows)* appear higher in attenuation than soft tissue using a mediastinal window. This strongly suggests ABPA. *C,* Sagittal reformation shows the mucous plugs *(arrows)* and some branching.

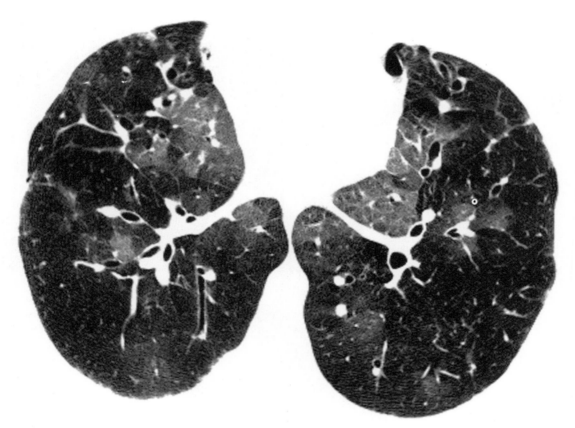

FIGURE 6-26 **Bronchiolitis obliterans with mosaic perfusion.** In a patient with bronchiolitis obliterans resulting from a bone marrow transplantation and graft-versus-host reaction, the lung has a patchy appearance on a high-resolution CT. Differences in lung density reflect differences in lung perfusion secondary to abnormal ventilation related to airway obstruction. Note that vessels look larger in the dense lung regions than in the lucent lung regions; this is an important clue to the presence of mosaic perfusion.

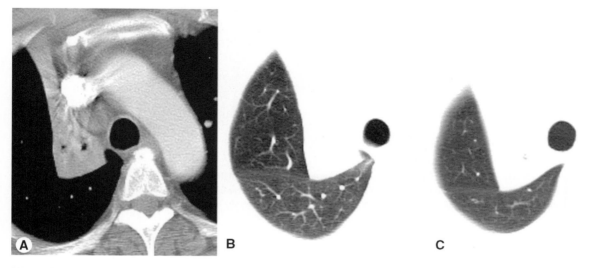

FIGURE 6-27 **Right upper lobe collapse.** In a patient with carcinoma obstructing the right upper lobe bronchus, both air bronchograms and opacified vessels are visible *(A).* The collapsed upper lobe has a triangular shape *(B* and *C).* The middle lobe borders the lateral aspect of the collapsed lobe, whereas the lower lobe is posterior to it.

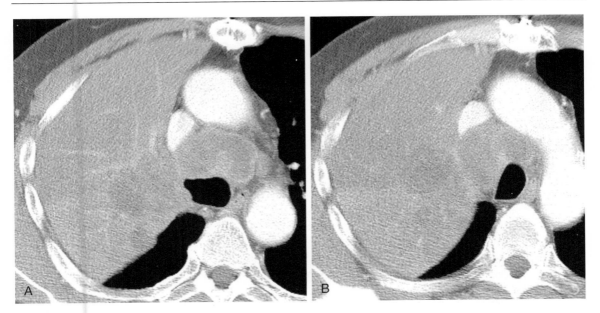

FIGURE 6-28 **Lung carcinoma with obstructive pneumonia.** *A* and *B,* The right upper lobe is consolidated, but no volume loss is present. No air bronchograms are seen, but opacified vessels are visible. Large, low-density, necrotic mediastinal lymph nodes are also present.

fissure can be bowed anteriorly. In the presence of a hilar mass, an appearance similar to Golden's S sign, as seen on plain radiographs, is visible. In some patients, the lobe assumes a triangular shape (see Fig. 6-27).

Left Upper Lobe Collapse

As on the right, the major fissure rotates anteromedially. However, above the hilum, the superior segment of the lower lobe may displace part of the upper lobe away from the mediastinum, giving the posterior margin of the collapsed lobe a V shape (see Fig. 6-29). A similar appearance is sometimes seen on the right.

Middle Lobe Collapse

As the middle lobe loses volume, the minor fissure, which normally is difficult to see because it lies in the plane of scan, rotates downward and medially and becomes visible on CT. The collapsed lobe assumes a triangular shape, with one side of the triangle abutting the mediastinum (see Fig. 6-30). The upper lobe can be seen anterolaterally, bordering the collapsed lobe, with the lower lobe bordering it posterolaterally. These aerated lobes usually separate the collapsed middle lobe from the lateral chest wall.

Lower Lobe Collapse

On either side, the major fissure rotates posteromedially (see Fig. 6-30). The collapsed lobe contacts the posterior mediastinum and posteromedial chest wall and maintains contact with the medial diaphragm.

Passive Atelectasis

In the presence of pleural effusion, the lung tends to retract or collapse toward the hilum, and fluid entering the fissures allows the lobes to separate. With the injection of contrast, the lung opacifies and is clearly distinguishable from surrounding fluid. Air bronchograms may be seen within the collapsed lobes. Rounded atelectasis is a form of passive atelectasis.

Cicatrization Atelectasis

Cicatrization atelectasis occurs in the presence of pulmonary fibrosis and may be associated with tuberculosis, radiation, or chronic bronchiectasis. In this condition, there is no evidence of bronchial obstruction. Rather, air bronchograms and bronchial dilatation (bronchiectasis) are usually visible within the area of collapse. The volume loss is often severe.

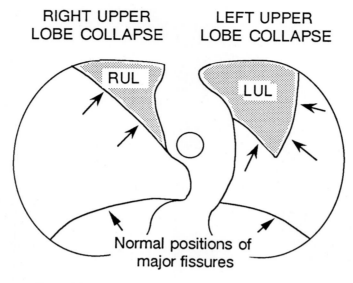

FIGURE 6-29 **Typical patterns of upper lobe collapse.** LUL, left upper lobe; RUL, right upper lobe.

☐ **DIFFUSE INFILTRATIVE LUNG DISEASE**

The term *diffuse infiltrative lung disease* is used to describe a variety of conditions, both air-space and interstitial, manifested by a generalized parenchymal abnormality. Included in this category are such disparate diseases as diffuse pneumonia, pulmonary edema, and chronic interstitial diseases.

CT is not generally used to evaluate patients with acute diffuse lung consolidation or acute interstitial disease visible on chest radiographs (although the use of CT for pulmonary embolism diagnosis has led to an increase in imaging acute lung disease), because, in most cases, the diagnosis of such diseases is clinical. Common causes would be acute pneumonia, pulmonary edema, and acute respiratory distress syndrome.

In some patients with an acute abnormality, however, CT may be done to look for associated findings such as pleural effusion, bronchial obstruction or associated mass, adenopathy, or cavitation, which might be valuable in diagnosis.

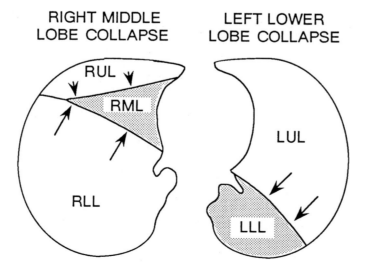

FIGURE 6-30 **Typical patterns of middle and lower lobe collapse.** LLL, left lower lobe; LUL, left upper lobe; RLL, right lower lobe; RML, right middle lobe; RUL, right upper lobe.

CT, particularly HRCT, has been reported to be of some value in the diagnosis of acute lung disease in immunosuppressed patients, especially those with the acquired immunodeficiency syndrome.

High-Resolution CT Diagnosis of Diffuse Lung Disease

HRCT is commonly used to evaluate diffuse infiltrative lung diseases, particularly when chronic or progressive, and when the diagnosis is in question. Generally, HRCT is used: (1) to detect lung disease in patients with symptoms of respiratory distress or abnormal pulmonary function tests who have normal chest radiograph results (approximately 10–15% of patients with infiltrative lung disease have normal chest radiograph results); (2) to characterize lung disease as to its morphologic pattern (e.g., Is there honeycombing?), and perhaps make a specific diagnosis; (3) to assess disease activity; and (4) to localize areas of abnormality in patients who are having a lung biopsy. Compared with plain radiographs, HRCT is more sensitive (94% vs. 80%), more specific (96% vs. 82%), and more accurate in making a diagnosis (by >10%).

HRCT scans are usually obtained at 1- to 2-cm intervals, because this technique is intended to "sample" lung anatomy at different levels. Scans are usually obtained during full inspiration in the supine position. Prone scans are commonly obtained to avoid misdiagnosis when posterior atelectasis develops with the patient lying supine. Some dependent lung collapse is often seen on HRCT, and having scans in both positions allows us to differentiate this finding from true pathologic processes. Post-expiratory scans at three to five levels are often obtained to detect air trapping associated with airways disease.

High-Resolution Findings in Healthy Subjects

Secondary pulmonary lobules are polygonal in shape and usually measure 1 to 3 cm in diameter. They are marginated by interlobular septa, containing veins and lymphatics (Fig. 6-31). In the center of the lobule are pulmonary artery and bronchiolar branches. On HRCT, normal interlobular septa are sometimes visible as very thin, straight lines of uniform thickness, 1 to 2 cm in length; but usually, only a few well-defined septa are visible in healthy subjects. A linear, branching, or dotlike density seen within the secondary lobule, or within a centimeter of the pleural surface, represents the centrilobular artery branch. The centrilobular bronchiole is not normally visible. The visible artery in the center of the lobule does not extend to the pleural surface in the absence of atelectasis. In healthy subjects, the pleural surfaces, fissures, and margins of central vessels and bronchi appear smooth and sharply defined.

Abnormal High-Resolution Findings

Thickened Interlobular Septa

Thickening of interlobular septa can be seen in patients with a variety of interstitial lung diseases (Fig. 6-32). Within the central lung, thickened septa can outline lobules that appear

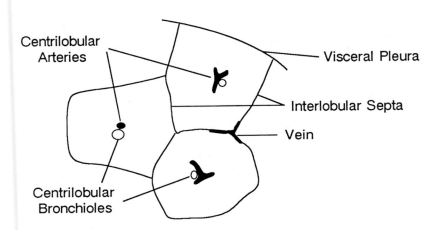

FIGURE 6-31 Normal pulmonary lobules.

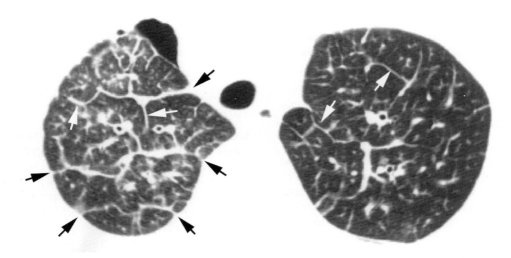

FIGURE 6-32 **Thickening of interlobular septa.** In a patient with lymphangitic spread of breast carcinoma, high-resolution CT shows evidence of septal thickening *(arrows)* characteristic of this disease. Although the septal thickening is bilateral, it is most severe on the right side. A small right pneumothorax is also present.

hexagonal or polygonal and contain a visible central arterial branch. In the peripheral lung, thickened septa often extend to the pleural surface. Septal thickening can appear smooth, nodular, or irregular in different diseases.

Often, thickened septa in the peripheral lung reflect generalized interstitial thickening and are also associated with the following: (1) thickening of fissures caused by subpleural interstitial thickening, (2) prominent centrilobular structures caused by thickening of the sheath of connective tissue that surrounds them, and (3) thickening of the interstitium surrounding central vessels and bronchi (i.e., peribronchial cuffing).

Common causes of interlobular septal thickening as the predominant HRCT finding include:

1. Lymphangitic spread of carcinoma (smooth or nodular septal thickening; see Fig. 6-32)
2. Interstitial pulmonary edema (smooth)
3. Alveolar proteinosis (smooth, in association with ground-glass opacity)
4. Sarcoidosis (nodular when granulomas present; irregular in fibrotic or end-stage disease)

Pulmonary Fibrosis

Fibrosis results in an irregular reticular pattern on HRCT. *Intralobular interstitial thickening* is a common finding in early fibrosis and appears

as a fine reticulation. Fibrosis associated with areas of lung destruction and the disorganization of lung architecture is termed *honeycombing.* Honeycombing results in a coarser reticular pattern or cystic appearance on HRCT, which is characteristic (Fig. 6-33). Cystic spaces are several millimeters to several centimeters in diameter; are often peripheral and subpleural; are characterized by thick, clearly definable walls; and tend to occur in groups or layers, with adjacent cysts sharing walls. *Traction bronchiectasis,* dilatation of bronchi in regions of fibrosis, is another common finding. Also, intralobular bronchioles may be visible on HRCT in patients with honeycombing because of a combination of traction bronchiolectasis and thickening of the peribronchiolar interstitium. *Conglomerate masses* of fibrous tissue can be seen in the upper lobes of patients with sarcoidosis or silicosis.

Common causes of fibrosis and honeycombing as the predominant HRCT finding include the following:

1. Idiopathic pulmonary fibrosis (IPF; 60–70% of cases)
2. Collagen vascular diseases, particularly rheumatoid arthritis and scleroderma
3. Drug-related fibrosis
4. Asbestosis, in association with pleural thickening
5. End-stage hypersensitivity pneumonitis

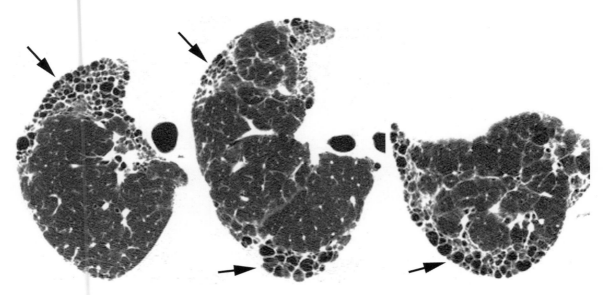

FIGURE 6-33 **Pulmonary fibrosis and honeycombing in rheumatoid arthritis.** High-resolution CT of the right lung at three levels shows characteristic small, thick-walled cysts (honeycomb cysts), which are most evident peripherally *(arrows)*. This appearance is diagnostic of fibrosis.

6. End-stage sarcoidosis (a small percentage of patients)

Nodules

Small nodules (a few millimeters to 1 cm in diameter) can be detected on HRCT in patients with granulomatous diseases such as sarcoidosis and miliary tuberculosis, in patients with meta-static tumor, and in patients with small airways disease. Three distributions of lung nodules can be identified on HRCT (Fig. 6-34); recognition of one of these three is invaluable in differential diagnosis.

Perilymphatic nodules predominate in relation to the following areas: (1) the pleural surfaces (particularly the fissures), (2) large vessels and bronchi, (3) interlobular septa, and (4) the centrilobular regions. They are typically patchy in distribution. They are most common in sarcoidosis (see Figs. 6-34 and 6-35), silicosis, and lymphangitic carcinoma.

Random nodules also involve the pleural surfaces but have a diffuse and uniform distribution, with a random distribution in relation to lung structures. They are most typical of miliary tuberculosis and hematogenous metastases (see Fig. 6-20).

Centrilobular nodules usually spare the pleural surfaces and are centrilobular in distribution (Fig. 6-36). They tend to occur in relation

to small vessels, with the most peripheral nodules being 5 to 10 mm from the pleural surface. They usually reflect diseases occurring in relation to small airways and are common with endobronchial spread of infection (e.g., tuberculosis, bacterial bronchopneumonia), endobronchial spread of tumor (e.g., bronchioloalveolar carcinoma), hypersensitivity pneumonitis, bronchiolitis obliterans organizing pneumonia, and diseases causing or associated with bronchiectasis.

Centrilobular nodules may be associated with a finding termed *tree-in-bud,* which is what it looks like (Fig. 6-37). Tree-in-bud reflects mucus or pus in dilated centrilobular bronchioles. The presence of this finding indicates airways disease, almost always caused by infection, such as caused by endobronchial spread of tuberculosis or *Mycobacterium avium/ M. intracellulare* complex, bacterial bronchopneumonia, cystic fibrosis, or bronchiectasis.

In attempting to make the diagnosis of one of these three patterns of multiple nodules, it is easiest to first determine the presence or absence of nodules in relation to the pleural surfaces and particularly along the fissures. If pleural nodules are absent, the distribution is centrilobular; if they are present, then the distribution of lung nodules determines the pattern present. Nodules with a patchy distribution and occurring in relation to the specific structures

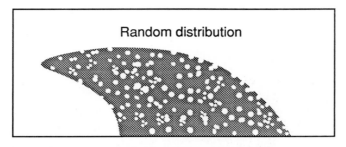

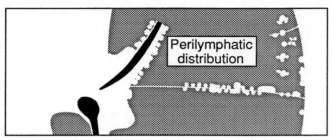

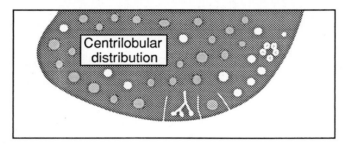

FIGURE 6-34 Distributions of lung nodules.

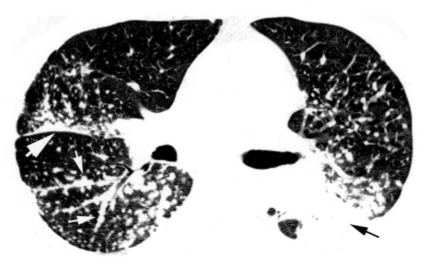

FIGURE 6-35 **Perilymphatic nodules (sarcoidosis).** Multiple nodules are visible adjacent to the major fissure *(large white arrow)* and central bronchi and vessels *(small white arrows).* This pattern is characteristic of sarcoidosis. Note the patchy distribution, with some lung regions being involved, whereas others appear normal. A conglomerate mass associated with satellite nodules is visible on the left *(black arrow).*

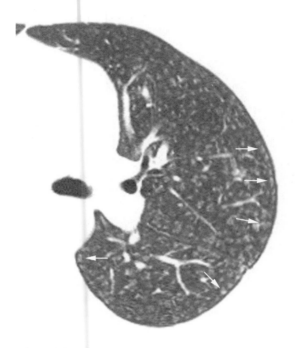

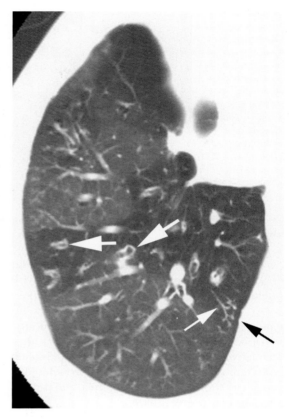

FIGURE 6-36 **Centrilobular nodules in a patient with hypersensitivity pneumonitis.** Small, ill-defined nodules of ground-glass opacity are visible. The most peripheral nodules *(arrows)* are about 5 mm from the fissure or the pleural surfaces. The pleural surfaces are spared.

FIGURE 6-37 **Tree-in-bud associated with cystic fibrosis.** A nodular branching opacity in the posterior right lower lobe *(small arrows)* represents a dilated, pus-filled bronchiole. Bronchial wall thickening and bronchiectasis is also present *(large arrows)*. Areas of low-attenuation lung represent mosaic perfusion.

listed earlier indicate a perilymphatic distribution; a diffuse and uniform distribution indicates a random pattern. This method can be used to correctly categorize more than 95% of the cases you will see.

Consolidation

HRCT findings of air space consolidation are similar to those seen on plain radiographs, with obscuration of pulmonary vessels and air bronchograms being the most characteristic findings (Fig. 6-38). Centrilobular nodules (as described earlier), measuring 0.5 to 1 cm in diameter, can also be seen on HRCT in patients with air space diseases (e.g., bronchioloalveolar carcinoma [see Fig. 6-23] or endobronchial spread of tuberculosis).

The differential diagnosis of consolidation is primarily based on the duration of symptoms present. Consolidation associated with acute symptoms usually represents pneumonia (see Fig. 6-38), severe edema or hemorrhage, or acute respiratory distress syndrome. In patients with consolidation and chronic (i.e., >4-6 weeks) symptoms, common causes of lung consolidation include bronchiolitis obliterans

obstructing pneumonia (see Fig. 6-44), bronchioloalveolar carcinoma (see Fig. 6-23), and chronic eosinophilic pneumonia.

Ground-Glass Opacity

In some patients with minimal interstitial disease, alveolar wall thickening, or minimal air space consolidation, a hazy increase in lung density can be observed on HRCT (Fig. 6-39); this is termed *ground-glass opacity*. Ground-glass opacity is differentiated from consolidation in that areas of increased opacity do not obscure underlying pulmonary vessels.

Ground-glass opacity is nonspecific and can be seen with a variety of diseases. As in patients with consolidation, the differential diagnosis of ground-glass opacity is primarily based on the duration of symptoms. Ground-glass opacity associated with acute symptoms usually represents an atypical pneumonia (*Pneumocystis*

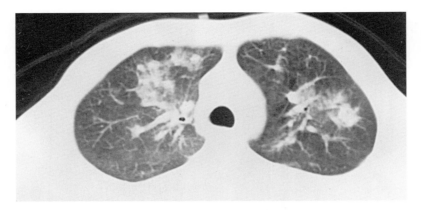

FIGURE 6-38 Patchy consolidation from pneumonia. Patchy consolidation is visible bilaterally in a patient with fever and acute shortness of breath.

carinii or viral pneumonia), edema (see Fig. 6-39), hemorrhage, or acute hypersensitivity pneumonitis. In patients with chronic (i.e., >4–6 weeks) symptoms, common causes include subacute hypersensitivity pneumonitis, nonspecific interstitial pneumonia (NSIP), desquamative interstitial pneumonia, bronchiolitis obliterans obstructing pneumonia, bronchioloalveolar carcinoma, lipoid pneumonia, and pulmonary alveolar proteinosis.

In all patients with acute symptoms, ground-glass opacity indicates active disease. In 60% to 80% of patients with more chronic symptoms, this appearance correlates with some type of active lung disease. If ground-glass opacity is seen only in lung regions that also show findings of fibrosis (e.g., honeycombing or traction bronchiectasis), it is likely that the ground-glass opacity represents fibrosis rather than active disease. This is typical in patient with usual interstitial pneumonia (UIP) and IPF.

Lung Cysts

Lung cysts are thin-walled, air-filled spaces within the lung parenchyma. Cysts are seen in honeycombing, cystic bronchiectasis, bullous emphysema, and pneumonias resulting in pneumatocele formation (e.g., Pneumocystis pneumonia). Several rare lung diseases result in lung cysts as a primary manifestation of the

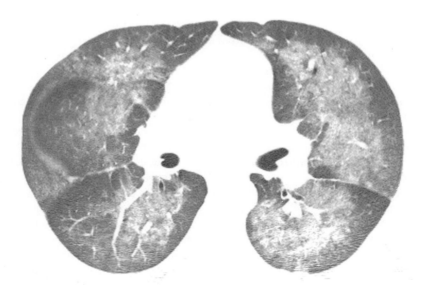

FIGURE 6-39 Ground-glass opacity. Perihilar ground-glass opacity in this patient reflects pulmonary edema and hemorrhage related to an acute reaction to cocaine use. Note the appearances of the major and minor fissures (compare with Fig. 6-2).

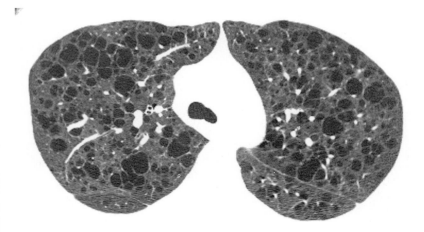

FIGURE 6-40 **Lung cysts in lymphangiomyomatosis (LAM).** Diffuse, thin-walled, rounded lung cysts are visible in a young woman. This appearance is typical of LAM.

disease. These include Langerhans histiocytosis, lymphangiomyomatosis (Fig. 6-40), and lympho-cytic interstitial pneumonia, particularly in asso-ciation with Sjögren's syndrome.

High-Resolution CT Appearances in Specific Diseases: The Top 10

Although more than 200 diseases can result in a diffuse pulmonary abnormality, knowledge of relatively few allows you to correctly diagnose most cases you will see. More than 90% of patients with diffuse lung disease have one of about only 10 possible diseases.

Metastatic Carcinoma

Although lymphangitic and hematogenous sp-read of carcinoma produce somewhat different patterns, overlap is common, and many patients will show some features of both.

In a patient with the appropriate history of malignancy and progressive dyspnea, the HRCT appearance of lymphangitic spread is diagnos-tic. Often, the plain radiograph will be normal or equivocal in this setting. *Lymphangitic spread of carcinoma* is characterized by

1. Interlobular septal thickening, smooth or nodular (see Fig. 6-32 and also Fig. 5-22)
2. Peribronchial interstitial thickening (peri-bronchial cuffing)
3. Thickening of fissures (smooth or nodular)
4. A patchy or unilateral distribution (in many cases)
5. Lymph node enlargement (in some cases)

Hematogenous spread of tumor can be characterized by

1. A random distribution of small nodules, sometimes with a peripheral predominance (see Figs. 6-20 and 6-21)
2. Involvement of fissures and the pleural sur-faces
3. A bilateral distribution
4. Presence of large nodules

Idiopathic Pulmonary Fibrosis and Usual Interstitial Pneumonia

IPF accounts for two thirds of cases of diffuse pulmonary fibrosis with honeycombing. Histo-logically, IPF is manifested by the histologic pattern of UIP. Progressive dyspnea is present. The prognosis is poor. Patients with this disorder typically demonstrate the following characteristics:

1. Intralobular interstitial thickening
2. Honeycombing (Fig. 6-41)
3. Traction bronchiectasis and bronchiolectasis
4. A predominance in subpleural, posterior, and basal lung regions
5. Ground-glass opacity (can be present in some patients; it usually is associated with traction bronchiectasis or honeycombing and indicates lung fibrosis)

Nonspecific Interstitial Pneumonia

NSIP is a recently described histologic abnormal-ity commonly associated with collagen vascular disease. It is less common than UIP and IPF. NSIP

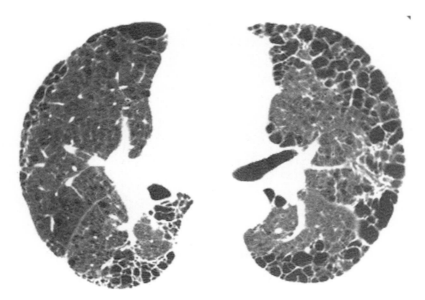

FIGURE 6-41 **Idiopathic pulmonary fibrosis (IPF) and usual interstitial pneumonia (UIP).** There is extensive subpleural honeycombing typical of UIP and IPF.

has a variable appearance, but often has the following characteristics:

1. Ground-glass opacity (Fig. 6-42)
2. A predominance in posterior and basal lung regions, but often sparing the immediate subpleural lung (see Fig. 6-42)
3. Reticulation, traction bronchiectasis, and bronchiolectasis may be present
4. Honeycombing is rare

Collagen Vascular Disease

Rheumatoid lung disease, scleroderma, and other collagen diseases may result in findings of UIP or NSIP (see Figs. 6-33 and 6-42). Bronchiolitis obliterans obstructing pneumonia may also be seen.

Sarcoidosis

Sarcoidosis can have a highly diagnostic appearance in some patients. Patients may be

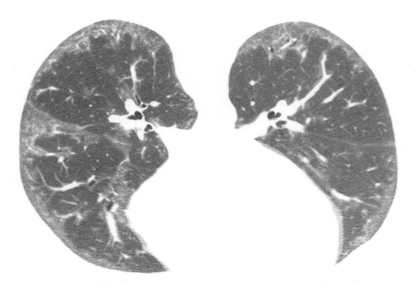

FIGURE 6-42 **Nonspecific interstitial pneumonia (NSIP) in a patient with scleroderma.** High-resolution CT in the prone position shows peripheral, subpleural ground-glass opacity. This appearance is typical of NSIP.

relatively asymptomatic. HRCT findings in patients with active and end-stage disease differ. Typical findings in patients with active sarcoid are:

1. Perilymphatic nodules, 1 to 10 mm (particularly subpleural and peribronchial; see Figs. 6-17 and 6-35); calcification can occur
2. A patchy distribution, often asymmetric
3. Upper lobe predominance
4. Hilar and mediastinal node enlargement (helpful in diagnosis but not always present); calcification can be present
5. Ground-glass opacity (uncommon), reflecting the presence of small granulomas

HRCT findings in patients with end-stage sarcoidosis and fibrosis include:

1. Irregular septal thickening
2. Architectural distortion
3. Parahilar conglomerate masses containing crowded, ectatic bronchi, often involving the upper lobes
4. Honeycombing (a small percentage)
5. Hilar and mediastinal node enlargement (not always present)

Silicosis and Coal Workers' Pneumoconiosis

Findings for silicosis and coal workers' pneumoconiosis can be similar to those of sarcoidosis, but significant differences are recognizable. Findings include:

1. Perilymphatic nodules, 1 to 10 mm (particularly centrilobular and subpleural), with calcification in some
2. Symmetric distribution
3. Posterior lung predominance
4. Upper lobe predominance
5. Conglomerate masses of nodules or fibrosis in the upper lobes
6. Hilar and mediastinal node enlargement; egg-shell calcification may be present

Tuberculosis

Tuberculosis has different appearances depending on the form of disease. The features of primary tuberculosis resemble those of pneumonia, and HRCT is not commonly used for diagnosis. In patients with disseminated tuberculosis, HRCT findings depend on the mode of spread; for example,

Endobronchial Spread
1. Centrilobular nodules
2. Tree-in-bud
3. Focal areas of consolidation
4. Bronchial wall thickening or bronchiectasis
5. Usually patchy or focal

Miliary Spread
1. Random nodules, 1 to 5 mm (see Fig. 6-34)
2. Usually diffuse

Pulmonary Alveolar Proteinosis

Pulmonary alveolar proteinosis is characterized by filling of the alveolar spaces by a lipid-rich proteinaceous material. A majority of cases are idiopathic, but some are associated with exposure to dusts (particularly silica), hematologic or lymphatic malignancies, or chemotherapy. Nocardial or mycobacterial superinfection may occur. HRCT findings can be diagnostic and include: (1) patchy or geographic ground-glass opacity; and (2) smooth, interlobular septal thickening in regions of ground-glass opacity. This combination is termed "*crazy paving.*"

Hypersensitivity Pneumonitis

Hypersensitivity pneumonitis is an allergic lung disease resulting from exposure to one of a number of organic dusts (e.g., farmer's lung). In the acute and subacute stages, interstitial and alveolar infiltrates and ill-defined peribronchiolar granulomas are present. In the chronic stage, fibrosis and honeycombing occur. In the subacute stage, HRCT typically shows the following characteristics:

1. Patchy or geographic ground-glass opacity (Fig. 6-43)
2. Poorly defined centrilobular nodules of ground-glass opacity (see Fig. 6-36)
3. Mosaic perfusion caused by bronchiolar abnormalities
4. Air trapping (commonly present on expiratory scans)

Bronchiolitis Obliterans Organizing Pneumonia

Bronchiolitis obliterans organizing pneumonia can be idiopathic or result from infections, toxic exposures, drug reactions, or autoimmune diseases. It typically results in progressive dyspnea and low-grade fever. Organizing pneumonia is the predominant histologic feature, and the idiopathic form of this disease is also called

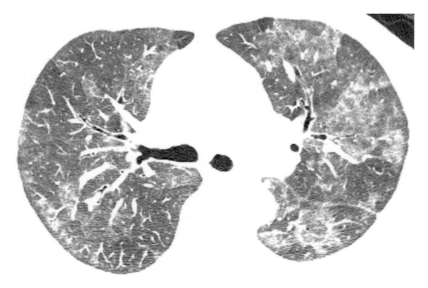

FIGURE 6-43 **Ground-glass opacity in hypersensitivity pneumonitis.** Multiple patchy areas of increased lung attenuation are typical of ground-glass opacity. Note that vessels remain visible within the abnormal lung regions. Ill-defined centrilobular nodules of ground-glass opacity are also visible. This appearance is typical of hypersensitivity pneumonitis.

cryptogenic organizing pneumonia. HRCT features are nonspecific and include:

1. Patchy or nodular consolidation
2. Patchy or nodular ground-glass opacity (Fig. 6-44)
3. A peripheral or peribronchial distribution

Chronic Eosinophilic Pneumonia

Chronic eosinophilic pneumonia is idiopathic and is characterized by filling of alveoli by a mixed inflammatory infiltrate consisting primarily of eosinophils. Blood eosinophilia is usually present. Patients present with fever, cough, and shortness of breath; symptoms are of a month in duration. HRCT features are nonspecific and are similar to those of bronchiolitis obliterans obstructing pneumonia, including (1) patchy consolidation or, less often, ground-glass opacity; and (2) a peripheral distribution.

Histiocytosis

Histiocytosis (Langerhans histiocytosis or eosinophilic granuloma) is associated with centrilob-

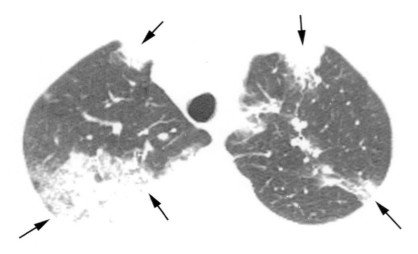

FIGURE 6-44 **Bronchiolitis obliterans organizing pneumonia.** Patchy areas of consolidation are noted in the peripheral lung *(arrows).* This appearance in a patient with chronic symptoms is typical.

ular nodules early in the disease and cystic lesions late in the disease. Nodules and cysts can coexist. It occurs in both men and women and has the following features:

1. Centrilobular nodules, which may be cavitary
2. Thin-walled, irregularly shaped lung cysts
3. Normal-appearing intervening lung
4. Upper lobe predominance
5. Sparing of costophrenic angles

Lymphangiomyomatosis

HRCT demonstrates thin-walled cysts, with intervening lung appearing normal. When seen in a patient with a characteristic history (i.e., dyspnea, spontaneous pneumothorax, and chylous pleural effusions), the findings are diagnostic. Lymphangiomyomatosis occurs only in women of child-bearing age, but an identical abnormality can occur in patients with tuberous sclerosis, almost entirely in women. Its features include:

1. Thin-walled, usually rounded lung cysts (see Fig. 6-40)
2. Normal-appearing intervening lung
3. A diffuse distribution, without sparing of the lung bases
4. Lymph node enlargement or pleural effusion

☐ EMPHYSEMA

On routine CT, emphysema can sometimes be diagnosed if areas of low attenuation are visible; a paucity of vessels, or draping of vessels around bullae, may also be seen. However, emphysema is most accurately depicted using HRCT. On HRCT, emphysema results in areas of low attenuation that can be easily contrasted with surrounding normal lung parenchyma. Emphysema is usually distinguishable from honeycombing or cystic lung disease because, in most cases, the lucent areas lack visible walls (Fig. 6-45). Emphysema can be diagnosed using HRCT in symptomatic patients when chest radiographs and pulmonary function tests are normal. On HRCT, emphysema may be classified as centrilobular, panlobular, paraseptal, and bullous.

Centrilobular emphysema is most common, is usually associated with smoking, and is typically most severe in the upper lobes (see Fig. 6-45). Sometimes it appears "centrilobular" on HRCT, but the presence of "spotty" lucency is diagnostic.

Panlobular emphysema is much less common and is often related to α_1-antitrypsin deficiency. It is diffuse or most severe at the lung bases and is manifested by an overall decrease in lung attenuation and in the size of pulmonary vessels (Fig. 6-46). Early panlobular emphysema can be quite subtle.

Paraseptal emphysema is common. It involves the subpleural lung adjacent to the chest wall and mediastinum. Emphysematous spaces several centimeters in diameter are typical, and their walls are seen easily (Fig. 6-47). It can occur as an isolated abnormality in young patients or be associated with centrilobular emphysema.

Bullous emphysema is said to be present when bullae predominate. It is most often associated with paraseptal emphysema. Large bullae can be seen, particularly in young men. Bullae sometimes contain fluid, as well as air, which may indicate infection.

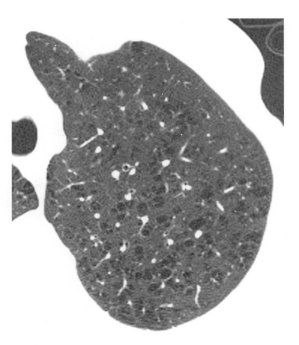

FIGURE 6-45 **Centrilobular emphysema.** On high-resolution CT, multiple spotty areas of cystic lucency without visible walls are typical of centrilobular emphysema.

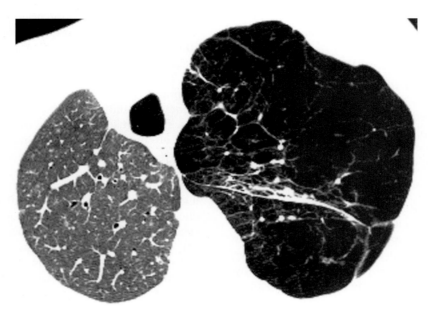

FIGURE 6-46 Panlobular emphysema. Panlobular emphysema in a patient with a right lung transplant. The native left lung, involved by emphysema, is too lucent and vessels are abnormally small.

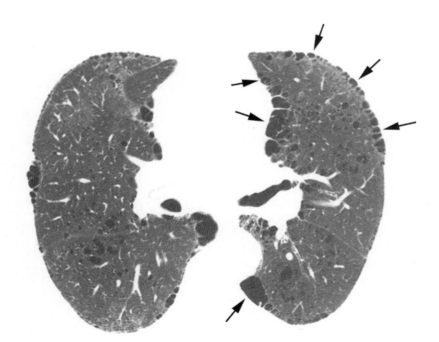

FIGURE 6-47 Paraseptal emphysema. Subpleural lucency *(arrows)* is typical of paraseptal emphysema. Centrilobular emphysema is also present. It is similar in appearance to honeycombing, but typically occurs in a single layer, predominates in the upper lobes, and is not associated with findings of fibrosis.

■ SUGGESTED READING

ABERLE DR, HANSELL DM, BROWN K, TASHKIN DP: Lymphangiomyomatosis: CT, chest radiographic, and functional correlations. Radiology 176: 381–387, 1990.

AKIRA M, YAMAMOTO S, YOKOYAMA K, et al: Asbestosis: High-resolution CT-pathologic correlation. Radiology 176:389–394, 1990.

American Thoracic Society/European Respiratory Society International Multidisciplinary Consensus Classification of the Idiopathic Interstitial Pneumonias. Am J Respir Crit Care Med 165:277–304, 2002.

AQUINO SL, GAMSU G, WEBB WR, KEE SL: Tree-in-bud pattern: Frequency and significance on thin section CT. J Comput Assist Tomogr 20:594–599, 1996.

AUSTIN JH, MÜLLER NL, FRIEDMAN PJ, et al: Glossary of terms for CT of the lungs: recommendations of the Nomenclature Committee of the Fleischner Society. Radiology 200:327–331, 1996.

BALAKRISHNAN J, MEZIANE MA, SIEGELMAN SS, FISHMAN EK: Pulmonary infarction: CT appearance with pathologic correlation. J Comput Assist Tomogr 13:941–945, 1989.

BRAUNER MW, GRENIER P, MOMPOINT D, et al: Pulmonary sarcoidosis: Evaluation with high-resolution CT. Radiology 172:467–471, 1989.

CARTIER Y, KAVANAGH PV, JOHKOH T, et al: Bronchiectasis: Accuracy of high-resolution CT in the differentiation of specific diseases. AJR Am J Roentgenol 173:47–52, 1999.

DAVIS SD: CT evaluation for pulmonary metastases in patients with extrathoracic malignancy. Radiology 180:1–12, 1991.

ENGELER CE, TASHJIAN JH, TRENKNER SW, WALSH JW: Ground-glass opacity of the lung parenchyma: A guide to analysis with high-resolution CT. AJR Am J Roentgenol 160:249–251, 1993.

FOSTER WL, GIMENEZ EI, ROUBIDOUX MA, et al: The emphysemas: Radiologic-pathologic correlations. Radiographics 13:311–328, 1993.

GRUDEN JF, WEBB WR, NAIDICH DP, McGUINNESS G: Multinodular disease: Anatomic localization at thin-section CT—multireader evaluation of a simple algorithm. Radiology 210:711–720, 1999.

GRUDEN JF, WEBB WR, WARNOCK M: Centrilobular opacities in the lung on high-resolution CT: diagnostic considerations and pathologic correlation. AJR Am J Roentgenol 162:569–574, 1994.

IKEZOE J, MURAYAMA S, GODWIN JD, et al: Bronchopulmonary sequestration: CT assessment. Radiology 176:375–379, 1990.

JOHKOH T, MÜLLER NL, CARTIER Y, et al: Idiopathic interstitial pneumonias: Diagnostic accuracy of thin-section CT in 129 patients. Radiology 211:555–560, 1999.

KUHLMAN JE, REYES BL, HRUBAN RH, et al: Abnormal air-filled spaces in the lung. Radiographics 13: 47–75, 1993.

LEUNG AN, MILLER RR, MÜLLER NL: Parenchymal opacification in chronic infiltrative lung diseases: CT-pathologic correlation. Radiology 188:209–214, 1993.

LEWIS ER, CASKEY CI, FISHMAN EK: Lymphoma of the lung: CT findings in 31 patients. AJR Am J Roentgenol 156:711–714, 1991.

MAHONEY MC, SHIPLEY RT, COCORAN HL, DICKSON BA: CT demonstration of calcification in carcinoma of the lung. AJR Am J Roentgenol 154:255–258, 1990.

McGUINNESS G, NAIDICH DP, LEITMAN BS, McCAULEY DI: Bronchiectasis: CT evaluation. AJR Am J Roentgenol 160:253–259, 1993.

McHUGH K, BLAQUIERE RM: CT features of rounded atelectasis. AJR Am J Roentgenol 153:257–260, 1989.

MOORE AD, GODWIN JD, MÜLLER NL, et al: Pulmonary histiocytosis X: Comparison of radiographic and CT findings. Radiology 172:249–254, 1989.

MÜLLER NL, COLBY TV: Idiopathic interstitial pneumonias: High-resolution CT and histologic findings. Radiographics 17:1016–1022, 1997.

MÜLLER NL, MILLER RR: Computed tomography of chronic diffuse infiltrative lung disease: I. Am Rev Respir Dis 142:1206–1215, 1990.

MÜLLER NL, MILLER RR: Computed tomography of chronic diffuse infiltrative lung disease: II. Am Rev Respir Dis 142:1440–1448, 1990.

MÜLLER NL, MILLER RR: Diseases of the bronchioles: CT and histopathologic findings. Radiology 196: 3–12, 1995.

NAIDICH DP: High-resolution computed tomography of cystic lung disease. Semin Roentgenol 26: 151–174, 1991.

NAIDICH DP, ETTINGER N, LEITMAN BS, McCAULEY DI: CT of lobar collapse. Semin Roentgenol 19:222–235, 1984.

PARK JS, LEE KS, KIM JS, et al: Nonspecific interstitial pneumonia with fibrosis: Radiographic and CT findings in seven patients. Radiology 195: 645–648, 1995.

PATEL RA, SELLAMI D, GOTWAY MB, et al: Hypersensitivity pneumonitis: Patterns on high-resolution CT. J Comput Assist Tomogr 24:965–970, 2000.

PRIMACK SL, HARTMAN TE, LEE KS, MÜLLER NL: Pulmonary nodules and the CT halo sign. Radiology 190:513–515, 1994.

PRIMACK SL, MÜLLER NL: Radiologic manifestations of the systemic autoimmune diseases. Clin Chest Med 19:573–586, 1998.

PROTO AV, BALL JB: Computed tomography of the major and minor fissures. AJR Am J Roentgenol 140:439–448, 1983.

REMY J, REMY-JARDIN M, GIRAUD F, WATTINNE L: Angioarchitecture of pulmonary arteriovenous malformations: Clinical utility of three-dimensional helical CT. Radiology 191:657–664, 1994.

SIEGELMAN SS, KHOURI NF, SCOTT WW, et al: Pulmonary hamartoma: CT findings. Radiology 160:313–317, 1986.

STERN EJ, FRANK MS: CT of the lung in patients with pulmonary emphysema: Diagnosis, quantification, and correlation with pathologic and physiologic findings. AJR Am J Roentgenol 162:791–798, 1994.

SWENSEN SJ, VIGGIANO RW, MIDTHUN DE, et al: Lung nodule enhancement at CT: Multicenter study. Radiology 214:73–80, 2000.

TEMPLETON PA, ZERHOUNI EA: High-resolution computed tomography of focal lung disease. Semin Roentgenol 26:143–150, 1991.

TRAILL ZC, MASKELL GF, GLEESON FV: High-resolution CT findings of pulmonary sarcoidosis. AJR Am J Roentgenol 168:1557–1560, 1997.

WEBB WR: Radiologic evaluation of the solitary pulmonary nodule. AJR Am J Roentgenol 154:701–708, 1990.

WEBB WR: High-resolution computed tomography of the lung: Normal and abnormal anatomy. Semin Roentgenol 26:110–117, 1991.

WEBB WR: High-resolution computed tomography of obstructive lung disease. Radiol Clin North Am 32:745–757, 1994.

ZWIREWICH CV, VEDAL S, MILLER RR, MÜLLER NL: Solitary pulmonary nodule: High-resolution CT and radiologic-pathologic correlation. Radiology 179:469–476, 1991.

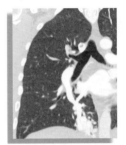

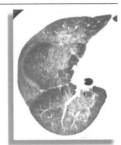

7

Pleura, Chest Wall, and Diaphragm

W. Richard Webb, M.D.

CT plays an important role in the diagnosis of pleural and chest wall abnormalities. The cross-sectional format and excellent density resolution of CT often provide anatomic information that cannot be obtained using conventional radiographs.

☐ TECHNICAL CONSIDERATIONS

In general, the pleura and chest wall are well evaluated using routine thoracic CT techniques. High-resolution CT (HRCT) techniques can demonstrate the anatomy of the lung/pleura/chest wall interface better than can conventional CT; this is occasionally of value. CT after contrast infusion is helpful in showing pleural thickening and in allowing its differentiation from pleural fluid. Soft-tissue window settings are most suitable for evaluating pleural abnormalities, the chest wall, and the diaphragm.

One must keep in mind that the diaphragm and posterior pleural space extend well below the lung bases, and scans inferior to the diaphragmatic domes must be obtained to evaluate these structures completely. Scanning with the patient in the prone position may be of assistance in evaluating pleural diseases; free pleural effusions shift to the dependent portion of the pleural space when the patient is moved from the supine position to the prone or decubitus position, whereas loculated effusions or fibrosis shows little or no change. Also, the movement of an effusion helps reveal underlying pulmonary parenchymal or pleural lesions that are otherwise obscured.

☐ PLEURA

Anatomy

Because of the oblique orientation of the lateral ribs, usually only a short segment of each rib is visible on a single CT scan; each progressively more anterior rib represents the one arising at a higher thoracic level (Fig. 7-1). Thus, at any given level, the fifth rib, for example, is anterior to the sixth, and the fourth is anterior to the fifth. At the level of the lung apex, the first rib can be identified by its anterior position and by its articulation with the manubrium immediately below the level of the clavicle.

In many patients, a bony spur projects inferiorly from the undersurface of the first rib at its junction with the manubrium. In cross section, this bony spur can appear to be surrounded by lung and can mimic a lung nodule.

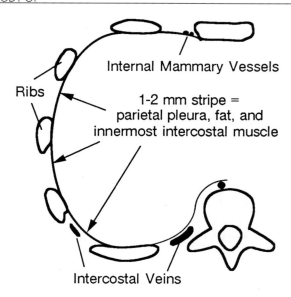

FIGURE 7-1 **Normal pleura.** A 1- to 2-mm line of opacity at the pleural surface primarily represents the innermost intercostal muscle, combined with the two pleural layers and the endothoracic fascia. In the paravertebral region, this stripe is much thinner or invisible.

This appearance is usually bilateral and symmetric, providing a clue as to its true nature. As would be expected, it often appears calcified.

Costal Pleura

On CT or HRCT in normal subjects, a 1- to 2-mm thick opaque stripe is commonly seen in the intercostal spaces, between adjacent rib segments (see Fig. 7-1). This stripe primarily represents the innermost intercostal muscle. In the paravertebral regions, the innermost intercostal muscle is absent, and a much thinner line (or no line at all) is visible at the pleural surface. The visceral and parietal pleura lie internal to ribs and innermost intercostal muscles and are separated from them by a layer of extrapleural fat, but they are not normally visible on CT.

Intrapulmonary Fissures

Intrapulmonary fissures were described in Chapter 6 (see Fig. 6-1). Normal collections of fat extending into the inferior aspects of the major fissures at the diaphragmatic surface can simulate fissural pleural thickening or effusion. These will be low in attenuation at mediastinal window settings.

Inferior Pulmonary Ligament

On each side, below the inferior pulmonary vein, the parietal and visceral pleural layers join, forming a fold that extends inferiorly along the mediastinal surface of the lung and ends at the level of the diaphragm. This fold, the *inferior pulmonary ligament,* anchors the lower lobe. On CT images viewed at lung window settings, it appears as, or is related to, a small, triangular opacity 1 cm or less in size with its apex pointing laterally into the lung and its base against the mediastinum. On each side, it usually lies adjacent to the esophagus (Fig. 7-2). Pleural effusion or pneumothoraces can be limited and marginated by the inferior pulmonary ligament.

A similar opacity can be seen on the right, lateral to the inferior vena cava (and thus anterior to the inferior pulmonary ligament), extending inferiorly to the diaphragm, and then laterally for several centimeters along the diaphragmatic surface (see Fig. 7-2). This represents the right phrenic nerve and its pleural reflection. Its only significance is that it is commonly seen and is just as commonly confusing.

Pleural Abnormalities

Pleural Thickening and Look-Alikes

Pleural thickening is visible on CT as a soft-tissue curvilinear stripe, passing internal to the ribs and innermost intercostal muscles. Anytime the pleura is visible on CT, it is thickened. Thickened pleura enhances and is best seen after contrast infusion.

In the presence of pleural thickening, the extrapleural fat layer is often thickened as well,

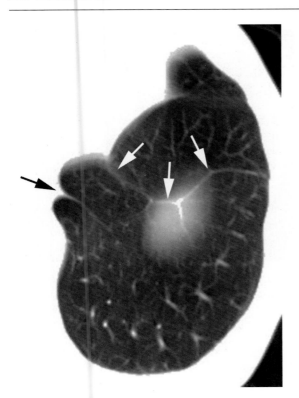

FIGURE 7-2 **Inferior pulmonary ligament and phrenic nerve.**
A small, triangular opacity *(black arrow)* arising adjacent to the
esophagus represents the left inferior pulmonary ligament.
Longer linear densities near the surface of the diaphragm *(white
arrows)* represent pleural reflections adjacent to the phrenic
nerves.

and the visible pleura is often seen to be separated from the ribs and intercostal muscles by this fat layer. In the paravertebral regions or adjacent to the mediastinum, a distinct opaque stripe is visible in the presence of pleural thickening.

A small *pleural effusion* can mimic the appearance of pleural thickening; however, effusion is usually dependent in location and crescentic. Thickened pleura can often be distinguished from small pleural fluid collections by contrast medium infusion; thickened pleura enhances, whereas fluid does not.

Normal *extrapleural fat pads,* a few millimeters in thickness, can sometimes be seen internal to ribs, particularly in the lower posterolateral thorax, and may not be easily distinguishable from pleural thickening or fluid. However, normal fat pads appear low in attenuation and are often symmetric, whereas pleural abnormalities generally are not. Identifying these fat pads as low in attenuation is easiest on HRCT.

The *subcostalis muscles* are sometimes visible posteriorly in the lower thorax, as a 1- to 2-mm-thick stripe internal to one or more ribs. In contrast to pleural thickening, these muscles are smooth, uniform in thickness, and symmetric bilaterally.

Segments of *intercostal veins* are commonly visible in the paravertebral regions and can mimic focal pleural thickening. Continuity of these opacities with the azygos or hemiazygos veins can sometimes allow them to be identified correctly.

Pleural Effusion

Pleural fluid collections are generally crescentic, elliptical, or lenticular in shape (Fig. 7-3; see also Fig. 7-6). A crescentic and dependent fluid collection is likely free, rather than loculated, but a definite diagnosis of free pleural fluid requires that a shift in effusion be demonstrated in association with a shift in patient position (see Fig. 7-3). Large effusions often extend into the major fissures, displacing the lower lobes medially and posteriorly. Elliptical or crescentic effusions and effusions that are nondependent are likely loculated.

Characterization of Pleural Fluid: Exudates and Transudates

Most effusions appear to be near to water in attenuation. CT numbers cannot be used to predict the specific gravity of the fluid or its cause. One exception, however, is acute or subacute hemothorax. Hemothorax may be dense (>50H) or may appear inhomogeneous, with some areas, particularly dependent regions, having an attenuation value greater than that of water. A fluid–fluid level (a hematocrit effect) or dependent clot may be seen with hemothorax (Fig. 7-4). Hemothorax is defined as a pleural effusion having a hematocrit equal to 50% of the blood hematocrit. It may be traumatic or related to other causes of bleeding.

In patients with effusion, the presence of pleural thickening on contrast-enhanced CT (Figs. 7-5 and 7-6) indicates that the effusion is an *exudate* (a high-protein effusion associated with pleural disease) rather than a *transudate* (a low-protein effusion associated with alteration in systemic factors governing formation of pleural fluid) (Table 7-1). By definition, the pleura is considered thickened if it is visible on contrast-enhanced (or unenhanced) CT. Transudates are never associated with pleural thickening

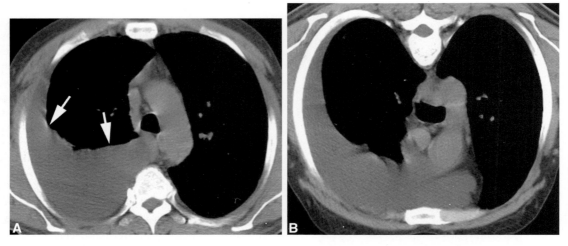

FIGURE 7-3 **Free pleural effusion with gravitational shift.** *A,* A large crescentic fluid collection *(arrows)* is visible posteriorly on the right. *B,* With the patient in the prone position, the fluid shifts to the anterior thorax. This indicates it is free rather than located. No pleural thickening is seen.

(except in the rare case of a patient with preexisting pleural disease who subsequently experiences development of an unrelated transudate).

In contrast, the absence of pleural thickening on contrast–enhanced CT is less helpful; in this case, the effusion can be an exudate or a transudate (see Fig. 7-6). Only about 60% of exudates are associated with visible pleural thickening. However, the absence of pleural thickening on a contrast–enhanced scan rules out empyema; empyema is always associated with parietal pleural thickening on contrast-enhanced CT.

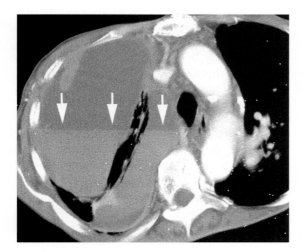

FIGURE 7-4 **Hemothorax.** A large right pleural effusion shows a distinct fluid–fluid level or hematocrit effect, with dense blood or clot layering posteriorly *(arrows).*

Diagnosis of Paradiaphragmatic Fluid Collections

The visceral pleura covers the surface of the lung, and its inferior extent is defined by the inferior extent of lung in the costophrenic angles. The parietal pleura is contiguous with the chest wall and diaphragm and extends well below the level of the lung bases, in the costophrenic angles. Thus, pleural fluid collections in the costophrenic angles can be seen below the lung base and can mimic collections of fluid in the peritoneal cavity.

The parallel curvilinear configuration of the pleural and peritoneal cavities at the level of the perihepatic and perisplenic recesses allows fluid in either cavity to appear as an arcuate or semilunar opacity displacing liver or spleen away from the adjacent chest wall. The relation of the fluid collection to the ipsilateral diaphragmatic crus (see later) helps to determine its location. Pleural fluid collections in the posterior costophrenic angle lie posterior to the diaphragm and cause lateral displacement of the crus. Peritoneal fluid collections are anterior to the diaphragm and lateral to the crus, displacing it medially.

Pleural fluid can also be distinguished from ascites by the clarity of the interface of the fluid with the liver and spleen (Fig. 7-7). With pleural fluid, the interface is hazy, whereas with ascites, it is sharp. In patients with both pleural and peritoneal fluid, the diaphragm often can be seen as a uniform, curvilinear structure of mus-

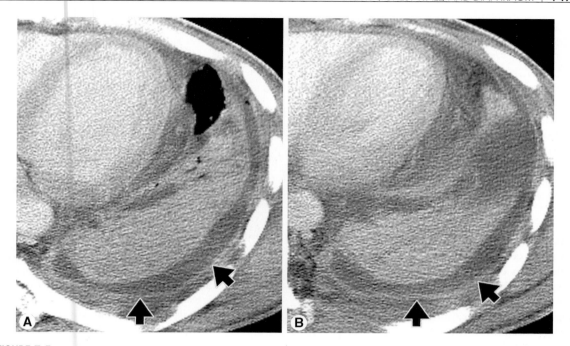

FIGURE 7-5 **Pleural effusion with pleural thickening.** In this patient with empyema, the parietal pleura is thickened (i.e., it is visible; *arrows*). The left lower lobe is consolidated. No visceral pleural thickening is visible.

cle attenuation with relatively low-attenuation fluid both anteriorly and posteriorly or medially and laterally (see Fig. 7-7). Fluid seen posterior to the liver is within the pleural space; the peritoneal space does not extend into this region (this is the "bare area" of the liver).

A large pleural effusion will allow the lower lobe to float anteriorly and lose volume. The posterior edge of the lower lobe, when surrounded by fluid both anteriorly and posteriorly, can appear to represent the diaphragm (a pseudodiaphragm), with pleural fluid posteriorly

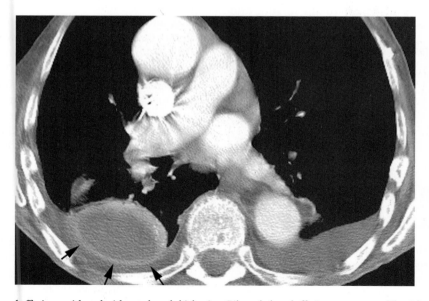

FIGURE 7-6 **Pleural effusions, with and without pleural thickening.** Bilateral pleural effusions are present. The right pleural effusion is lenticular in shape and is associated with pleural thickening *(arrows)* and the split-pleura sign. It represents an empyema. The left pleural effusion is not associated with pleural thickening. It is transudative.

TABLE 7-1

Common Causes of Exudates and Transudates

Exudates	Transudates
Parapneumonic effusion	Congestive heart failure
Empyema	Liver disease
Malignancy	Renal disease
Collagen vascular disease	Overhydration
Pulmonary embolism	Low serum protein
Abdominal disease	
Hemothorax	
Chylothorax	

and ascites anteriorly (Fig. 7-8). Sequential scans at more cephalad levels, however, generally will allow the correct interpretation to be made. Typically, the arcuate opacity of the atelectatic lower lobe becomes thicker superiorly, is contiguous with the remainder of the lower lobe, and often contains air bronchograms.

Fissural Fluid

A focal or loculated collection of pleural fluid in a major or minor fissure can have a confusing appearance on CT scans and can be misinterpreted as representing a parenchymal mass. However, careful analysis of contiguous images usually will confirm the relation of the mass to the plane of the fissure. If the abnormality also is of fluid attenuation, the diagnosis becomes more likely. The edges of the fluid collection may be seen to taper, conforming to the fissure and

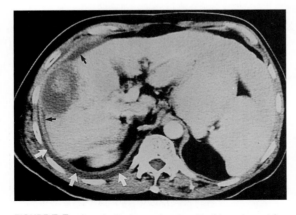

FIGURE 7-7 Pleural effusion and ascites. In this patient with a liver abscess, both pleural effusion and ascites are present. The effusion *(white arrows)* is posterior to the diaphragm. The ascites *(black arrows)* is medial to the diaphragm, and a sharp interface with the liver is evident. Note that the diaphragm is visible as a white stripe with fluid on each side. No ascites is visible posterior to the liver.

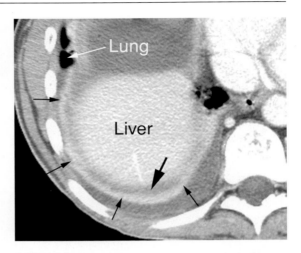

FIGURE 7-8 Subpulmonic effusion and a pseudodiaphragm mimicking ascites. In a patient with a large right pleural effusion, the collapsed posterior lower lobe *(small black arrows)* simulates the diaphragm. Fluid *(large black arrow)* separating this opacity from the liver is in the region of the "bare area" of the liver. Ascites does not occur in this location. Aerated lower lobe *(white arrow)* is seen in association with the anterior aspect of the pseudodiaphragm.

forming a "beak" (Fig. 7-9). Correlation of CT scans with the plain radiographs can be helpful, particularly for fluid localized in the minor fissure.

Parapneumonic Effusions

Pleural fluid can accumulate in patients with pneumonia, even when the pleural space is uninfected. This is termed a *parapneumonic effusion,* and it results from increased permeability of the visceral pleura associated with the inflammation. The effusion is usually an exudate. Distinguishing pleural effusion from adjacent consolidated lung may be difficult unless contrast medium is injected, resulting in lung opacification; the pleural fluid remains low in attenuation. Parietal pleural thickening is present in about half of patients, whereas visceral pleural thickening is seen in one fourth of patients. Because loculation is not present, the effusion is crescentic and dependent (Fig. 7-10).

Empyema

Empyema is diagnosed if pleural fluid contains infectious organisms on smear or culture. Classically, an empyema is associated with the "split-pleura" sign. This sign is said to be present when the thickened visceral and parietal pleural layers are split apart by and surround the empyema (Figs. 7-11 and 7-12; see also Fig. 7-6); these

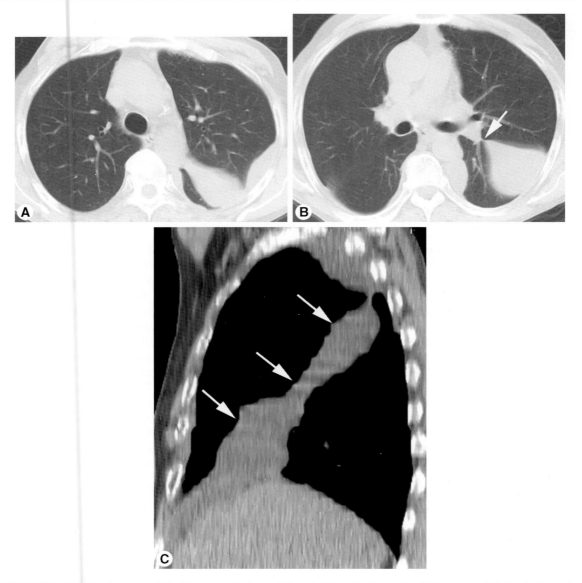

FIGURE 7-9 **Fluid in a fissure.** *A–C,* In this patient, fluid extends into the left major fissure. The fluid tapers medially in relation to the fissure *(arrow, B),* forming a "beak." Sagittal reformation *(C)* shows the fissural fluid *(arrows)* to best advantage.

pleural layers are generally of similar thickness. However, this sign is not always present. Although empyema is always associated with parietal pleural thickening on contrast–enhanced CT, visceral pleural thickening (and thus the split-pleura sign) is only present in half (see Fig. 7-5). Multiple loculations may be present (see Fig. 7-12*B*).

Empyemas can be free or loculated and crescentic (see Figs. 7-4 and 7-11), rounded, elliptical, or lenticular (see Figs. 7-5, 7-6, 7-11, and 7-12). In patients having a dependent and crescentic effusion, associated with pleural thickening, simple parapneumonic effusion and

empyema cannot be distinguished. Loculated effusions are typically elliptical or lenticular and often nondependent; loculation is not usually present in parapneumonic effusion.

The presence of air within the empyema almost always is caused by recent thoracentesis but may also indicate bronchopleural fistula (Fig. 7-13) or a gas-forming organism. In the absence of thoracentesis as a cause for the gas, this finding is usually an indication for tube drainage.

Extension of an empyema to involve the chest wall is termed *empyema necessitatis.* Two thirds of cases result from tuberculosis, but other responsible organisms include *Actinomyces* and

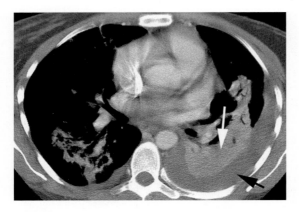

FIGURE 7-10 **Parapneumonic pleural effusion.** A patient with left lower lobe pneumonia *(white arrow)* also shows a left pleural effusion *(black arrow).* The effusion is dependent and crescentic in appearance; it is not associated with pleural thickening.

Nocardia. CT findings include low-attenuation fluid collections within the chest wall.

Differentiation of Empyema from Lung Abscess

Distinguishing empyema from lung abscess is sometimes important in patients who are clinically infected; empyema is often treated using tube drainage, whereas lung abscess generally is not. CT can be helpful in making this distinction, particularly when contrast medium is infused.

The outer edge of an empyema is sharply demarcated from adjacent lung, and on contrast–enhanced scans, the empyema wall appears regular in thickness. When a bronchopleural fistula is present and air is contained within the empyema cavity, or when air is introduced into the empyema at thoracentesis, its inner margin usually appears smooth.

In contrast, lung abscesses are irregularly shaped and often contain multiple areas of low-attenuation necrosis or collections of air and fluid. On contrast–enhanced scans, the abscess wall generally will opacify relative to fluid in the abscess cavity. The inner surfaces of an abscess are often irregular and ragged, and their outer edges may be poorly defined because of adjacent pulmonary parenchymal consolidation.

At their point of contact with the chest wall, empyemas can show acute or obtuse angles (see Fig. 7-11), whereas abscesses typically have acute angles. Empyemas also tend to compress and displace lung and vessels, acting as a space-occupying mass, whereas lung abscesses destroy lung without displacing it (usually).

Organizing Empyema (Pleural Peel)

In patients with chronic empyema, especially tuberculous in origin, ingrowth of fibroblasts can result in pleural fibrosis and the development of chronic pleural thickening. CT may show a thickened pleural peel (Fig. 7-14). The presence of decreased volume of the affected hemithorax is an important finding (see Fig. 7-14). Calcification, which typically is focal in its early stages (Fig. 7-15), may become extensive (Fig. 7-16). Frequently, a thickened layer of extrapleural fat is also visible, separating the parietal pleura and the ribs (this layer is considerably thicker than the fat pads, which can be seen normally). Treatment requires pleural stripping.

Dense pleural thickening, even with calcification, does not indicate that the pleural disease is inactive. Loculated fluid collections resulting from active infection (see Fig. 7-16) may be seen on CT within the thickened pleura.

Thoracostomy Tubes

Infected pleural fluid collections often become loculated and can be difficult to drain. CT is

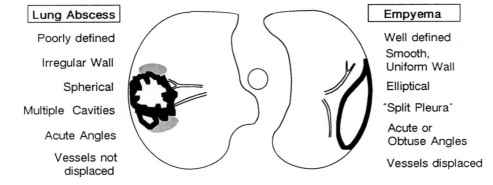

Lung Abscess	Empyema
Poorly defined	Well defined
Irregular Wall	Smooth, Uniform Wall
Spherical	Elliptical
Multiple Cavities	"Split Pleura"
Acute Angles	Acute or Obtuse Angles
Vessels not displaced	Vessels displaced

FIGURE 7-11 **Empyema versus lung abscess.**

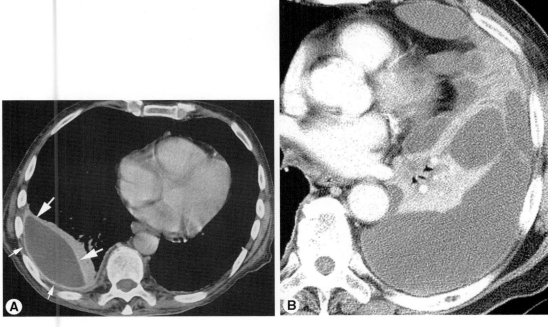

FIGURE 7-12 Empyema in two patients. *A,* A classic empyema is lenticular and well defined. After contrast injection, the thickened visceral *(large white arrows)* and parietal pleura *(small white arrows)* and the split-pleura sign are visible. *B,* An empyema is associated with a large left pleural effusion, pleural thickening, and multiple loculations.

sometimes indicated to evaluate thoracostomy tube position when the tube is functioning poorly. Malpositioned chest tubes can lie within a fissure, within a loculated fluid collection (whereas other collections remain undrained), or outside the empyema.

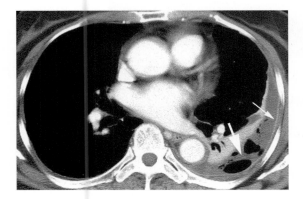

FIGURE 7-13 Empyema and bronchopleural fistula. A crescentic left pleural effusion is associated with pleural thickening *(small arrow).* Multiple collections of air *(large arrow)* in the left effusion are caused by a bronchopleural fistula. The presence of multiple discrete air bubbles indicates the presence of a multiseptated pleural effusion.

Asbestos-Related Pleural Disease

Asbestos-related pleural thickening has a typical appearance on CT. Early pleural thickening is discontinuous, with the intervening pleura appearing normal; focal areas of pleural thickening are termed *pleural plaques* (Fig. 7-17). The pleural disease is typically bilateral. Calcification is common. Diffuse pleural thickening, which is probably the result of prior asbestos-related benign pleural effusion, can also be seen (Fig. 7-18). In patients with asbestos-related pleural disease, the pleural thickening, plaques, or calcification typically involve the parietal pleura, but this is difficult to recognize on CT unless the presence of pleural fluid separates the visceral and parietal pleural layers.

The diaphragmatic pleura is commonly involved in patients with asbestos-related pleural disease. However, the diaphragm lies roughly in the plane of the scan, and the detection of uncalcified pleural plaques on the diaphragmatic surface can be difficult. In some patients, diaphragmatic pleural plaques are visible deep in the posterior costophrenic angle, below the lung base; in this location, the pleural disease

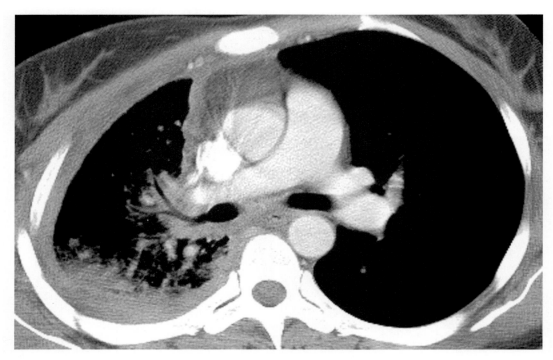

FIGURE 7-14 **Pleural peel.** A patient with prior empyema shows extensive smooth thickening of the right pleura. Note that the hemithorax is reduced in volume. This is typical of pleural fibrosis.

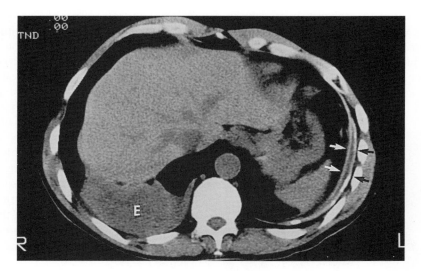

FIGURE 7-15 **Acute and chronic empyemas.** On the right side, a fluid collection (E) posterior to the liver is in the pleural space; it represents an acute empyema. On the left, pleural thickening *(arrows)* with areas of calcification reflects a healed tuberculous empyema. The split-pleura sign is present.

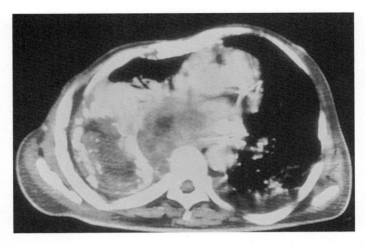

FIGURE 7-16 **Calcified pleural thickening associated with tuberculosis.** The parietal and visceral pleura are densely calcified. Residual fluid is evident in the pleural space, and loculated collections anteriorly *(arrows)* reflect active infection.

can be localized to the parietal pleura, because only parietal pleura is present. Pleural plaques along the mediastinum have been considered unusual in patients with asbestos-related pleural disease, but they are visible on CT scans in about 40% of patients. Paravertebral pleural thickening is also common.

Although it is unusual, pleural thickening can involve a fissure and result in a localized intrapulmonary pleural plaque. These may simulate a lung nodule on CT unless the plane of the fissure is identified.

Pleural Effusion Associated with Malignancy

In patients with malignancy, pleural effusion can result from tumor involvement of the pleura or lymphatic obstruction in the hila or mediastinum. In both instances, an exudate is typically present. Effusions may be large.

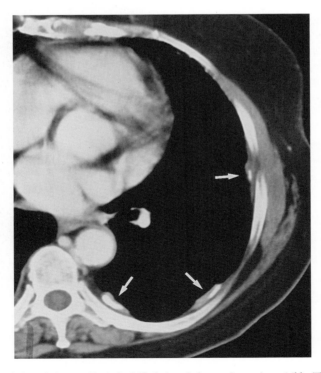

FIGURE 7-17 **Asbestos-related pleural plaques.** Typical calcified pleural plaques *(arrows)* are visible. They are often internal to ribs.

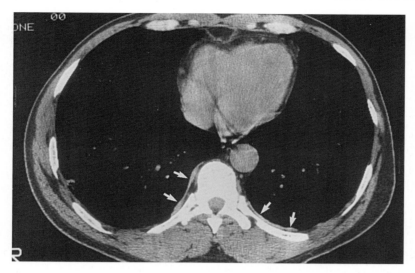

FIGURE 7-18 **No change. Asbestos-related pleural thickening.** Linear pleural thickening *(arrows)* can be seen with asbestos exposure or other causes of pleural disease, such as rheumatoid arthritis. The thickened pleura is visible internal to the ribs.

The term *malignant effusion* means that malignant cells are present in the fluid. It can be present with pleural metastases or mesothelioma. In patients with malignant effusion, pleural thickening may or may not be visible on contrast–enhanced CT (Fig. 7-19).

CT findings that strongly suggest the diagnosis of malignant involvement of the pleura (Fig. 7-20) include:

1. Nodular pleural thickening
2. A pleural thickness of more than 1 cm
3. Thickening that concentrically involves the pleura, encasing the lung
4. Thickening of the mediastinal pleura

Mesothelioma

Mesothelioma (also known as diffuse or malignant mesothelioma) is a highly aggressive neoplasm with an extremely poor prognosis. It is characterized morphologically by gross

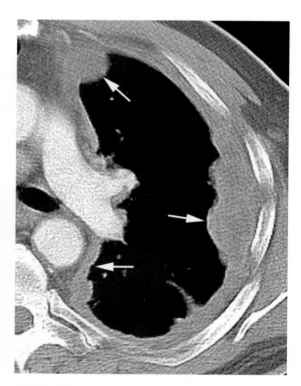

FIGURE 7-20 **Mesothelioma.** There is circumferential, nodular pleural thickening involving the left hemithorax *(arrows)*. The mediastinal pleura is involved, and the pleural thickening exceeds 1 cm. These findings suggest a malignant process.

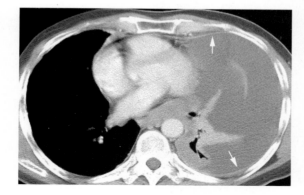

FIGURE 7-19 **Malignant effusion caused by metastatic carcinoma.** A large left pleural effusion is associated with left lung atelectasis, mediastinal displacement to the left, and pleural thickening *(arrows)*.

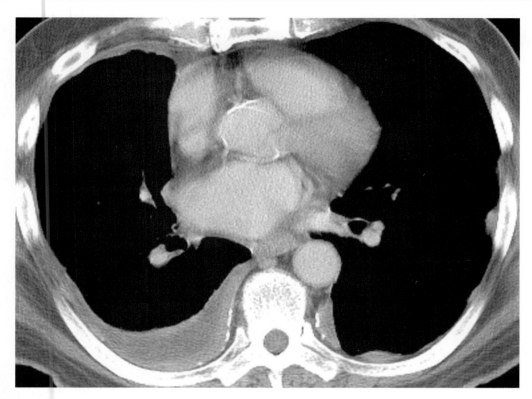

FIGURE 7-21 **Mesothelioma in a patient with asbestos exposure.** Pleural plaques on the left and bilateral calcification of the parietal pleura reflect asbestos exposure. A new right pleural effusion indicates the presence of mesothelioma but is nonspecific.

and nodular pleural thickening. However, hemorrhagic pleural effusion is often present and may obscure the underlying pleural thickening, which, in early cases, can be minimal. Mesothelioma spreads most commonly by local infiltration of the pleura. In most patients, mesothelioma is related to asbestos exposure; although it is rare in the general population, the incidence in workers heavily exposed to asbestos is about 5%.

In patients with mesothelioma, CT can expedite the initial diagnosis and define the extent of tumor. Usually, irregular or nodular pleural thickening is visible (see Fig. 7-20), although a new pleural effusion may be the only recognizable finding (Fig. 7-21). Often, pleural thickening is most pronounced in the inferior thorax. Contrast infusion can allow tumor to be distinguished from associated fluid collections. Scans with the patient in the prone or decubitus position can also help in distinguishing underlying mesothelioma from pleural fluid.

Although mesothelioma is visible most frequently along the lateral chest wall, mediastinal pleural thickening or concentric pleural thickening is seen with extensive disease (see Fig. 7-20). The abnormal hemithorax can appear contracted and fixed, with little change in size on inspiration. Thickening of the fissures, particularly the lower part of the major fissures, can reflect tumor infiltration. Malignant mesothelioma typically spreads by local invasion, involving the mediastinum and sometimes the chest wall, but hematogenous pulmonary metastases and distant metastases do occur.

Localized Fibrous Tumor of the Pleura

Localized fibrous tumor of the pleura, previously termed *benign mesothelioma,* is uncommon. It is usually detected incidentally on chest radiographs but can be associated with chest pain, hypoglycemia, and hypertrophic pulmonary osteoarthropathy. About 70% of tumors are benign and 30% are malignant.

Localized fibrous tumor usually arises from the visceral pleura and most commonly involves the costal pleural surface (Fig. 7-22); occasionally, it can be seen within a fissure (see Fig. 7-21). On CT, these tumors are solitary,

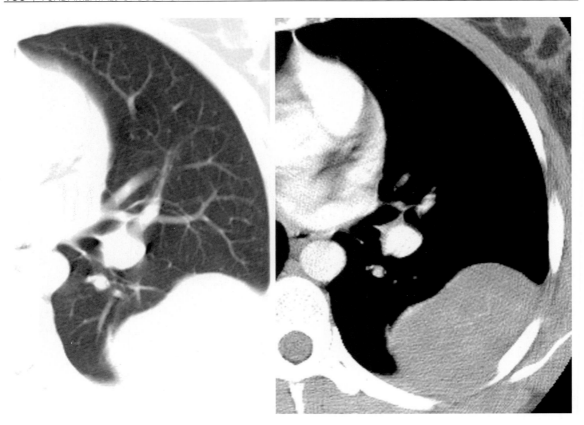

FIGURE 7-22 Localized fibrous tumor of the pleura. The large homogeneous mass is smooth and sharply defined. Slight beak-shaped pleural thickening is seen adjacent to the mass, probably related to a small amount of pleural fluid.

smooth, sharply defined, often large lesions, contacting a pleural surface (see Figs. 7-22 and 7-23).

Usually, a localized fibrous tumor will appear homogeneous on CT, but necrosis can result in a multicystic appearance with or without

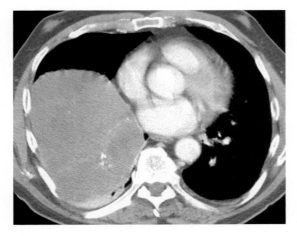

FIGURE 7-23 Localized fibrous tumor of the pleura. A large inhomogeneous and calcified mass appears smooth and sharply defined.

contrast infusion. Although it is generally believed that pleural abnormalities result in obtuse angles at the point of contact of the lesion and chest wall, localized fibrous tumors may show acute angles with slightly tapered pleural thickening adjacent to the mass (see Fig. 7-22). This thickening may reflect a small amount of fluid accumulating in the pleural space at the point where the visceral and parietal pleural surfaces are separated by the mass. A similar "beak" or "thorn" sign is often visible on plain radiographs in patients with a localized fibrous tumor in a fissure.

Metastases

Malignant pleural effusion may not be associated with visible pleural thickening. However, metastases to the pleura can also result in nodular pleural thickening visible on CT; pleural metastases are more easily seen on contrast–enhanced scans, being greater in attenuation than the fluid (Figs. 7-24 and 7-25). Usually, pleural effusion masks the underlying pleural mass or

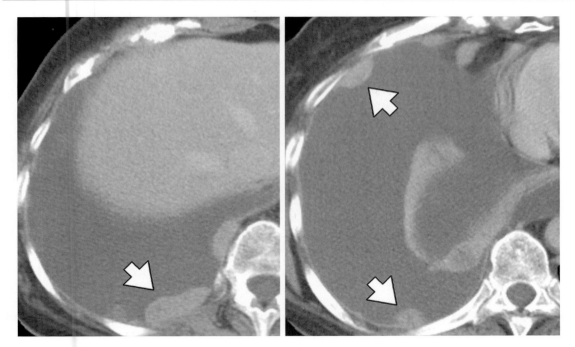

FIGURE 7-24 **Pleural metastases from colon carcinoma.** On a contrast-enhanced CT scan, focal nodular pleural masses *(arrows)* are visible arising from the parietal pleura. A large pleural effusion is also present.

masses on plain radiographs. Invasive thymoma and some other tumors can result in pleural nodules that are not associated with pleural effusion.

Pleural metastases can diffusely infiltrate the pleura, resulting in an appearance indistinguishable from that of mesothelioma (Fig. 7-26). Extension into the fissures can also be seen.

Lymphoma

Pleural effusions occur in 15% of patients with Hodgkin's disease and usually reflect lymphatic or venous obstruction by mediastinal or hilar tumor, rather than by pleural involvement; effusions in Hodgkin's disease tend to resolve after local mediastinal or hilar radiation. Pericardial effusions, however, present in 5% of patients,

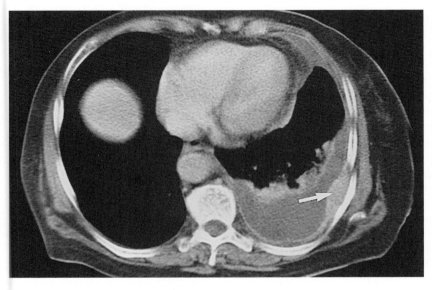

FIGURE 7-25 **Pleural metastasis.** Pleural thickening is evident after contrast medium infusion. An enhancing pleural mass *(arrow)* and pleural effusion are visible.

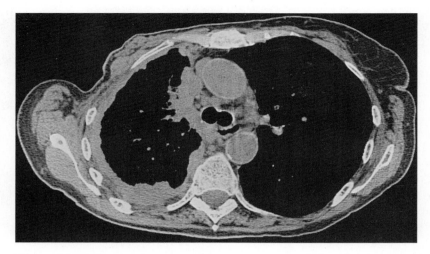

FIGURE 7-26 Pleural metastasis. Diffuse nodular pleural thickening in a patient with breast cancer simulates mesothelioma.

usually indicate direct involvement of the pericardium.

Pleural Calcification and Talc Pleurodesis

Pleural calcification may be seen with chronic empyema, particularly tuberculous in nature (see Fig. 7-16); resolved hemothorax; asbestos exposure (see Figs. 7-17 and 7-21); and some masses (see Fig. 7-23). Pleurodesis using talc can mimic pleural calcification. The talc is dense and typically accumulates in the posterior and inferior hemithorax (Fig. 7-27).

☐ CHEST WALL

Chest Wall Abnormalities

Lung Cancer with Chest Wall Invasion

Direct invasion of the chest wall by a peripheral bronchogenic carcinoma is common. Chest wall invasion by lung cancer does not rule out surgery unless there is invasion of great vessels (i.e., subclavian artery) or vertebral body. In the lung cancer staging system (see Table 4-3), resectable tumors invading chest wall are termed *T3*; unresectable invasive tumors are *T4*. Similarly, Hodgkin's disease can involve structures of the chest wall by direct invasion from the mediastinum or lung in a small percentage of cases. Malignant mesothelioma is a less common tumor that also can invade the chest wall.

The CT diagnosis of chest wall invasion can be difficult. A variety of CT findings can indicate

chest wall invasion. The most accurate CT findings of chest wall invasion (Fig. 7-28) are:

1. Extensive contact between the tumor and chest wall (>3 cm)
2. Obtuse angles at the point of contact between tumor and pleura
3. A ratio of the length of contact of tumor with chest wall to the tumor's maximum diameter that is greater than 0.7
4. Obliteration of extrapleural fat layers
5. A chest wall mass
6. Bone destruction

Diagnosing chest wall invasion when a tumor simply abuts the pleura should be avoided. Tumors adjacent to the pleura, even when associated with focal pleural thickening and pleural effusion, may not be invasive. In a patient with bronchogenic carcinoma, pleural

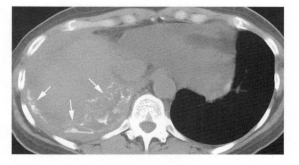

FIGURE 7-27 Talc pleurodesis. Streaky high-attenuation opacities in the posterior right hemithorax represent talc injected for pleurodesis *(arrows)*. This appearance mimics pleural thickening with calcification.

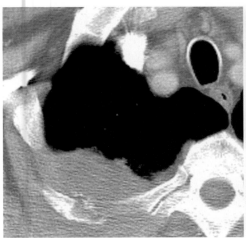 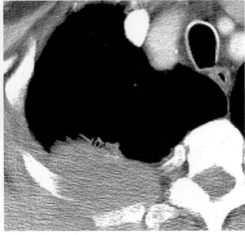

FIGURE 7-28 **Lung carcinoma with chest wall invasion.** Findings that suggest or are diagnostic of chest wall invasion in this patient include more than 3 cm of contact between the tumor and chest wall, obtuse angles of the lung mass with the pleura, a ratio of the length of contact of tumor with the chest wall to the tumor's maximum diameter greater than 0.7, obliteration of extrapleural fat layers posteriorly, a chest wall mass, and bone destruction.

effusion can occur for a variety of reasons, including obstructive pneumonia and lymphatic or pulmonary venous obstruction by tumor. Only those patients with demonstration of tumor cells in the pleural fluid are considered to have unresectable disease.

Superior Sulcus (Pancoast) Tumors

Invasive tumors arising in the superior pulmonary sulcus produce the characteristic clinical findings of Horner's syndrome and shoulder and arm pain; this presentation is termed *Pancoast's syndrome.* Previously, tumors of the superior sulcus had a poor prognosis, but combined therapy with radiation, followed by resection of the upper lobe, chest wall, and adjacent structures, has resulted in 5-year survival rates of up to 30%. In patients being considered for this combined therapy, CT scans can provide information on the anatomic extent of tumor spread that is useful in planning both the radiation therapy and the surgical approach to the tumor. However, magnetic resonance imaging has been shown to be more accurate than CT in showing the apical extent of tumor.

Extension of tumor posteriorly or laterally at the lung apex primarily involves the chest wall (Fig. 7-29). Although such chest wall invasion does not prevent resection, extensive chest wall and bone involvement makes surgical treatment difficult, and the prognosis for patients with extensive chest wall disease is poor. Inva-

sion of tumor posteromedially involves the ribs or vertebral bodies. This occurs in one third to one half of cases and usually can be seen on CT scans. Anterior and medial extension of tumor can involve the esophagus, trachea, and brachiocephalic vessels. Invasion of these structures or the vertebral body precludes resection.

☐ AXILLARY SPACE

Anatomy

As usually defined, the axilla is bordered by the fascial coverings of the following muscles: the pectoralis major and pectoralis minor anteriorly; the latissimus dorsi, teres major, and subscapularis posteriorly; the chest wall and serratus anterior medially; and the coracobrachialis and biceps laterally. However, when patients are scanned with their arms above their heads, the axilla is open laterally.

The axilla contains the axillary artery and vein, branches of the brachial plexus, some branches of the intercostal nerves, and a large number of lymph nodes, all surrounded by fat. The axillary vessels and the brachial plexus extend laterally, near the apex of the axilla, close to the pectoralis minor muscle. In general, the axillary vein lies below and anterior to the axillary artery, whereas the brachial plexus is largely above and posterior to the artery. Although these vessels usually can be seen on

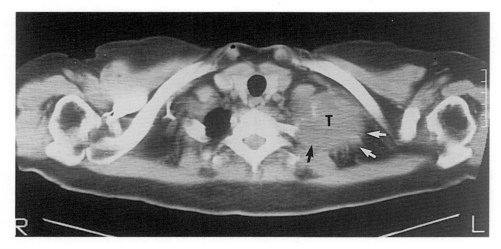

FIGURE 7-29 **Pancoast tumor.** A patient with a superior sulcus tumor (T) has rib destruction *(black arrow)* and invasion of fat by tumor *(white arrows).*

CT scans, in many healthy individuals, it is impossible to distinguish artery and vein within the axilla, unless the vein is opacified by contrast medium.

Lymphadenopathy or Mass

Axillary lymph nodes, usually up to 1 cm but occasionally 1.5 cm in diameter, can be seen in normal subjects. Lymph nodes larger than 1 cm (short axis or least diameter) should be considered suspicious when an abnormality can be suspected on clinical grounds; lymph nodes 2 cm in diameter are considered pathologic regardless of history. Axillary lymphadenopathy is seen most frequently in patients with lymphoma or metastatic carcinoma. Lymph node masses are detected most easily by observing both axillae for symmetry. Enlarged lymph nodes high within the axilla lie beneath the pectoral muscles and may not be palpable, but these nodes can be detected by CT. Axillary masses in relation to nerves of the brachial plexus can also be demonstrated using CT.

☐ BREAST

Soft tissues of the breasts are seen on CT scans of female patients in the supine position. Localized breast masses are occasionally visible, but their CT appearance is usually nonspecific. Breast masses detected incidentally on CT images generally should be evaluated by physical examination and mammography.

Breast Carcinoma

CT has not become an established technique for the routine evaluation of patients with breast cancer. However, CT can aid the planning of radiation therapy by providing an accurate measurement of chest wall thickness and by detecting internal mammary lymph node metastases.

Mastectomy

In women who have had a mastectomy, characteristic alterations in chest wall anatomy are seen, depending on the surgical procedure performed. CT is sometimes used to evaluate suspected local tumor recurrence and to guide needle biopsy.

A radical mastectomy consists of complete removal of the breast tissue and pectoralis major and pectoralis minor muscles and extensive axillary lymph node dissection. On CT, although most of the pectoralis muscles are absent, residual pectoralis major muscle is sometimes seen at its sternal or costal attachment. This should not be misinterpreted as recurrent tumor.

A typical modified radical mastectomy consists of removal of the breast and pectoralis minor muscle and an axillary lymph node dissection. The precise techniques for this procedure can vary among surgeons, and a discussion with the surgeon concerning the procedure performed is advisable before interpreting the CT scans. In patients who have undergone a modified radical mastectomy, the amount of pectoralis minor muscle remaining is variable. Without careful clinical correlation, it is sometimes difficult to distinguish postsurgical changes from tumor recurrence. This is a particular problem when the patient has difficulty elevating both arms symmetrically for the CT examination. With the arms raised, asymmetry of the pectoralis muscles is accentuated, and the scans often are difficult to interpret. It is therefore best to obtain scans with the patient's arms at her sides.

A simple mastectomy consists of removal of only breast tissue; the underlying musculature remains intact. Residual breast tissue will remain when segmental or partial mastectomy is performed. Lumpectomy results in focal abnormalities.

☐ DIAPHRAGM

Anatomy

Because of the transaxial plane of CT, the central portion of the diaphragm does not appear as a distinct structure, and its position can only be inferred by the position of the lung base above and the upper abdominal organs below. However, as the more peripheral portions of the diaphragm extend caudad toward their sternal and costal attachments, the anterior, posterior, and lateral portions of the diaphragm become visible adjacent to retroperitoneal fat (Fig. 7-30). Where the diaphragm is contiguous with the liver or spleen, it cannot usually be delineated by CT unless thin-collimation CT is used and a subdiaphragmatic fat layer is present.

Diaphragmatic Crura

The right and left diaphragmatic crura are tendinous structures arising inferiorly from the anterior surfaces of the upper lumbar vertebral bodies and intervening discs and continuous with the anterior longitudinal ligament of the spine. The crura ascend anterior to the spine, on each side of the aorta, and then pass medially and anteriorly, joining the muscular diaphragm anterior to the aorta, to form the aortic hiatus (see Fig. 7-30). The right crus, which is larger and longer than the left, arises from the first three lumbar vertebral levels; the left crus arises from the first two lumbar segments.

The diaphragmatic crura can be mistaken for enlarged lymph nodes or masses because of their rounded appearance; para-aortic lymph nodes can indeed be seen in a similar position. However, on contiguous CT scans, the crura merge gradually with the diaphragm at more cephalad levels. The diameter of the crura also will vary with lung volume, increasing in thickness at full inspiration compared with expiration.

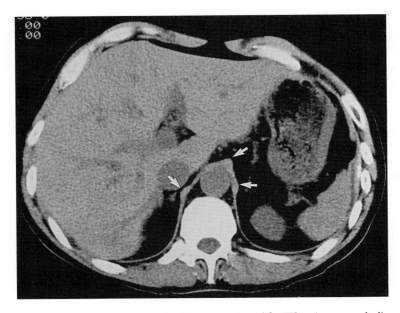

FIGURE 7-30 **Normal diaphragm.** The diaphragm is outlined by retroperitoneal fat. Where it contacts the liver and spleen it is not usually visible as a discrete structure. The diaphragmatic crura can appear quite lumpy *(arrows)*. Here they pass anterior to the aorta to form the aortic hiatus.

Openings in the Diaphragm

The diaphragm is perforated by several openings that allow structures to pass from the thorax to the abdomen. The aortic hiatus is posterior; it is bounded posteriorly by the vertebral body and anteriorly by the crura. Through it pass the aorta, the azygos and hemiazygos veins, the thoracic duct, the intercostal arteries, and the splanchnic nerves. The esophageal hiatus is situated more anteriorly, in the muscular portion of the diaphragm. Through it pass the esophagus, the vagus nerves, and small blood vessels. The foramen of the inferior vena cava pierces the fibrous central tendon of the diaphragm anterior and to the right of the esophageal hiatus.

Of these three structures, the aortic hiatus is defined most easily. On CT scans, the esophageal foramen is visible as an opening at the junction of the esophagus and stomach. The foramen of the inferior vena cava must be inferred from the position of the inferior vena cava. The foramina of Morgagni and of Bochdalek are not visible on CT scans in normal individuals.

Diaphragmatic Abnormalities

Hernias

Abdominal or retroperitoneal contents can herniate into the chest through congenital or acquired areas of weakness in the diaphragm or through traumatic diaphragmatic ruptures. Hernias of the stomach through the esophageal hiatus are the most common.

Hernias through the foramen of Bochdalek were thought to be uncommon in adults; however, CT has shown that small Bochdalek defects may occur in as many as 5% of healthy adult subjects. This is the most common type of diaphragmatic hernia in infants. Most are left sided; and although they are often located in the posterolateral diaphragm, they can occur anywhere along the posterior costodiaphragmatic margin (Fig. 7-31). Bochdalek hernias in adults usually contain retroperitoneal fat or, much less commonly, kidney.

Parasternal hernias through the foramen of Morgagni are relatively rare. Most Morgagni hernias occur on the right and, in contrast to Boch-

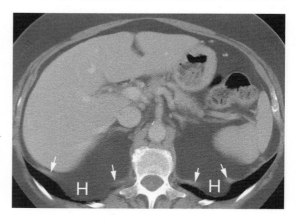

FIGURE 7-31 **Bochdalek hernias.** In this patient, bilateral Bochdalek hernias (H) consist of retroperitoneal fat. The edges of the diaphragm *(arrows)* outline the defects leading to herniation.

dalek hernias, usually contain an extension of the peritoneal sac. Their contents can include omentum, liver, or bowel.

An understanding of the anatomy of the anterior portion of the diaphragm is essential in correctly diagnosing a Morgagni hernia. The presence of bowel anterior to the heart can suggest the presence of a hernia, but this is not usually the case.

Diaphragmatic rupture can result from penetrating or nonpenetrating trauma to the abdomen or thorax. In nearly all cases, the left hemidiaphragm is affected, with ruptures of the central or posterior diaphragm being the most frequent. Omentum, stomach, small or large intestine, spleen, or kidney may all herniate through the diaphragmatic rent.

Diaphragmatic Eventration

Local eventration of the right hemidiaphragm and superior displacement of the liver can be confused radiographically with a peripheral pulmonary or pleural mass. CT scans after infusion of contrast medium can demonstrate opacification of normal intrahepatic vessels in the apparent mass, allowing its identification. In addition, scans reformatted in the coronal plane can show that the "mass" has the same attenuation as liver.

SUGGESTED READING

ABERLE DR, GAMSU G, RAY CS, FEUERSTEIN IM: Asbestos-related pleural and parenchymal fibrosis: Detection with high-resolution CT. Radiology 166:729–734, 1988.

ADLER BD, PADLEY SPG, MÜLLER NL: Tuberculosis of the chest wall: CT findings. J Comput Assist Tomogr 17:271–273, 1993.

AQUINO SL, WEBB WR, GUSHIKEN BJ: Pleural exudates and transudates: Diagnosis with contrast-enhanced CT. Radiology 192:803–808, 1994.

BERKMEN YM, DAVIS SD, KAZAM E, et al: Right phrenic nerve: Anatomy, CT appearance, and differentiation from the pulmonary ligament. Radiology 173:43–46, 1989.

CHOI JA, HONG KT, OH YW, et al: CT manifestations of late sequelae in patients with tuberculous pleuritis. AJR Am J Roentgenol 176:441–445, 2001.

DYNES MC, WHITE EM, FRY WA, GHAHREMANI GG: Imaging manifestations of pleural tumors. Radiographics 12:1191–1201, 1992.

FEDERLE MP, MARK AS, GUILLAUMIN ES: CT of subpulmonic pleural effusions and atelectasis: Criteria for differentiation from subphrenic fluid. AJR Am J Roentgenol 146:685–689, 1986.

FERRETTI GR, CHILES C, CHOPLIN RH, COULOMB M: Localized benign fibrous tumors of the pleura. AJR Am J Roentgenol 169:683–686, 1997.

HALVORSEN RA, FEDYSHIN PJ, KOROBKIN M, et al: Ascites or pleural effusion? CT differentiation: Four useful criteria. Radiographics 6:135–149, 1986.

IM J-G, WEBB WR, ROSEN A, GAMSU G: Costal pleura: Appearances at high-resolution CT. Radiology 171:125–131, 1989.

KAWASHIMA A, LIBSHITZ HI: Malignant pleural mesothelioma: CT manifestations in 50 cases. AJR Am J Roentgenol 155:965–969, 1990.

LEUNG AN, MÜLLER NL, MILLER RR: CT in differential diagnosis of diffuse pleural disease. AJR Am J Roentgenol 154:487–492, 1990.

MCLOUD TC, FLOWER CDR: Imaging the pleura: Sonography, CT, and MR imaging. AJR Am J Roentgenol 156:1145–1153, 1991.

MÜLLER NL: Imaging the pleura. Radiology 186:297–309, 1993.

NAIDICH DP, MEGIBOW AJ, HILTON S, et al: Computed tomography of the diaphragm: Peridiaphragmatic fluid localization. J Comput Assist Tomogr 7:641–649, 1983.

NAIDICH DP, MEGIBOW AJ, ROSS CR, et al: Computed tomography of the diaphragm: Normal anatomy and variants. J Comput Assist Tomogr 7:633–640, 1983.

STARK DD, FEDERLE MP, GOODMAN PC, et al: Differentiating lung abscess and empyema: Radiography and computed tomography. AJR Am J Roentgenol 141:163–167, 1983.

TAKASUGI JE, GODWIN JD, TEEFEY SA: The extrapleural fat in empyema: CT appearance. Br J Radiol 64:580–583, 1991.

WAITE RJ, CARBONNEAU RJ, BALIKIAN JP, et al: Parietal pleural changes in empyema: Appearances at CT. Radiology 175:145–150, 1990.

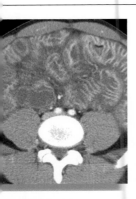

PART TWO

THE ABDOMEN AND PELVIS

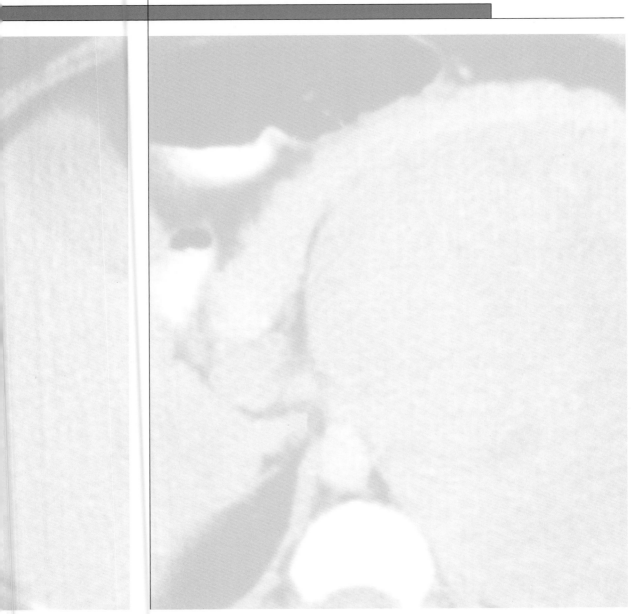

PART TWO

THE ABDOMEN
AND PELVIS

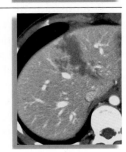

Introduction to CT of the Abdomen and Pelvis

William E. Brant, M.D.

In the early 1990s, helical (spiral) CT rejuvenated the role of CT in body imaging, further entrenching CT as the primary imaging modality for the abdomen and pelvis. In the mid–1990s, dual-detector row CT was introduced. Since that time multidetector row CT (MDCT) has progressed through 4-row (quad), 8-row, 16-row, 32-row, to 64-row scanners. MDCT has enabled remarkably fast CT scanning using thin sections that provide volumetric data acquisition and allow reconstruction of excellent quality images in any anatomic plane. MDCT allows long area coverage and multiphase imaging during contrast administration to provide assessment of organ and lesion vascularity and perfusion. MDCT is superior to single-slice helical CT for virtually all clinical applications. Temporal and spatial resolutions are improved, and intravenous contrast material can be delivered at a faster rate, improving conspicuity of arteries, veins, and pathologic conditions characterized by high blood flow. CT angiography and virtual endoscopy are now a reality.

Evaluation of the abdomen and pelvis by CT requires greater attention to patient preparation, technique, and individualization than CT evaluation of any other area of the body. The best quality studies are produced when the radiologist is present to evaluate the patient clinically, to assess the nature of the imaging problem, and to tailor the study to optimize the information that the examination provides.

☐ APPROACH

When a request is presented for an abdomen and pelvis CT scan, the radiologist should assess the clinical problem to be evaluated by reviewing available patient history and all pertinent previous imaging studies. Medical history of importance to CT examination includes the current indication for the study, contrast agent allergies, cardiac and renal impairments, past abdominal surgeries, history of prior malignancies and radiation therapy, and findings and availability of previous imaging studies. Previous imaging studies are reviewed to ensure that all previously identified abnormalities and questionable findings are appropriately re-evaluated.

Decisions to be made to individualize the examination include:

- Contrast medium to be administered: intravenous, oral, rectal, or intracavitary
- Intravenous contrast medium concentration, administration rates, method of administration, and scan timing

- Area scanned: anatomic landmarks and scan extent
- Multiphase scanning and timing: arterial, venous, and delayed
- Reconstruction intervals, reconstruction planes, and three-dimensional image reconstructions

□ GASTROINTESTINAL CONTRAST AGENTS

Nearly all CT scans of the abdomen require the administration of intraluminal contrast agents to demonstrate the lumen and to distend the gastrointestinal tract. Radiopaque agents may be dilute concentrations of barium or iodinated contrast agents. Iodine agent concentrations of 1% to 3% are optimal for CT compared with the 30% to 60% solutions used for fluoroscopy. Barium mixtures and water-soluble iodinated agents are equally effective as oral contrast agents. A number of commercial preparations are available specifically for CT. For routine bowel preparation for CT, 1500 to 1600 mL oral contrast is given over 3 to 4 hours.

Air and water are excellent as low-attenuation contrast agents. Air or carbon dioxide can be instilled into the rectum to insufflate the colon. Effervescent crystals with a small volume of water are given orally to distend the stomach with gas. Water serves as an excellent low-density contrast agent for the upper gastrointestinal tract. Urine in the distended bladder provides excellent contrast for bladder lesions.

□ INTRAVENOUS CONTRAST AGENTS

Intravenous contrast agents improve the quality of abdominal CT by opacifying blood vessels, increasing the CT density of vascular abdominal organs, and improving image contrast between lesions and normal structures. MDCT allows multiphase imaging to demonstrate the passage of contrast through the arterial system, organs and tumors, and venous system. Delayed images show contrast excretion by the kidneys, late enhancement, or prolonged retention of intravenous contrast agent. For most applications, intravenous contrast agents are administered by power injectors that provide accurate control of rate and volume of administration.

Low-osmolar, "nonionic," iodine-based agents are the intravenous contrast media of choice for most abdominal scanning because of their lower rate of adverse reactions. Compared with older "ionic" contrast agents, nonionic contrast provides a significantly decreased risk for adverse reactions and an improved margin of safety.

Sterile iodinated contrast agents approved for intravenous injection can be injected into indwelling catheters, drainage tubes, sinus tracts, and fistulas to evaluate extent of disease. Dilution of the contrast agent to a concentration of 1% to 3% is usually adequate for CT. High-osmolar, ionic, meglumine-based agents are satisfactory for this application.

□ HOW TO INTERPRET CT SCANS OF THE ABDOMEN AND PELVIS

When just beginning to learn interpretation of body CT it is useful to develop a checklist to ensure that all structures are inspected and that all key observations are noted to make accurate and comprehensive diagnoses. Because of the dramatic increase in the number of images obtained by MDCT, image viewing is now best performed on a computer workstation using the digital images directly from the CT scanner. Image display workstations allow rapid scrolling through serial images, the ability to conveniently change window level and window width settings, and the ability to perform rapid image reformatting in multiple planes and with three-dimensional techniques.

Each CT image of the abdomen contains much more information than can be displayed by any one window width and level setting. Routine "soft-tissue windows" (window width, ~400; window level, 30–50) define most abdominal anatomy. However, the liver may also be inspected using narrower "liver windows" (window width, ~100–150; window level, 70–80) to increase image contrast within the liver and to improve visibility of subtle lesions. The lung bases are included on scans through the upper abdomen and should be inspected using "lung windows" (window width, 1000–2000; window level, 600–700). Lastly, inspection of the bones using "bone windows" (window width, ~2000; window level, ~600) may yield important clues to pathologic findings within the abdomen and pelvis (Fig. 8-1).

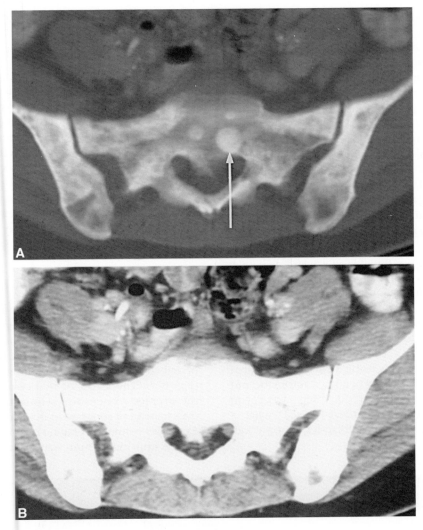

FIGURE 8-1 **Bone windows.** Metastatic lesions *(arrow)* from prostate carcinoma to the sacrum and iliac bones are obvious on "bone window" *(A)* but cannot be seen on routine "soft-tissue window" *(B).*

Each organ and structure should be systematically examined on serial images obtained through all phases of the CT examination. No interpretation will be accurate without considering the "phase" of contrast enhancement — (arterial, venous, cortical, nephrogram, and so forth). For example:

- Lung bases: nodules, infiltrates, scars, pleural effusions, atelectasis
- Liver: size, homogeneous parenchymal attenuation, uniform enhancement, portal veins, hepatic veins, hepatic arteries
- Biliary tree and gallbladder: visible bile ducts, wall thickness, presence and disten-

tion of the gallbladder, low-density stones, high-density stones
- Spleen: size (normal up to 14 cm), inhomogeneous enhancement early, homogeneous enhancement late, splenules, splenic vein, splenic artery
- Adrenals: Y or V shape, limb thickness less than 1 cm, no convex margins
- Pancreas: size and position, head, neck, body, tail, visible pancreatic duct, patent splenic vein, lucent peripancreatic fat
- Kidneys: size 9 to 13 cm in adults, symmetric enhancement, calyces and pelvis and ureter, position and orientation

- Lymph nodes: retroperitoneum, mesentery, omentum, porta hepatis, pelvis
- Blood vessels: aorta, inferior vena cava, celiac axis, superior and inferior mesenteric arteries, renal arteries, renal veins, splenic vein, superior mesenteric vein, portal vein
- Stomach: position, distention, wall thickness, fold thickness
- Duodenum and small bowel: position, distention, wall thickness, surrounding fat, mesentery
- Colon and rectum: position, distention, wall thickness, luminal contents, diverticula
- Uterus and ovaries: size, position, appropriate for age and phase of the menstrual cycle, masses
- Prostate and seminal vesicles: size, calcifications
- Bladder: distension, wall thickness, luminal contents
- Bones: degenerative changes, metastatic disease, mineralization

After consistently using a checklist, detailed inspection of the images becomes automatic and familiar. Remember that you "see" what you look for and that it is hardest to "see" what is not there (e.g., absent gallbladder, ectopic kidney, among others).

ARTIFACTS IN BODY CT

Patient Motion

Patient movement during CT scanning causes anatomic structures to be displaced, distorted, and blurred. Anomalous white bands and dark spots may be displayed on the image. The rapid scan times of modern CT scanners diminishes but does not totally eliminate the effect of cardiac motion, vessel pulsation, and bowel peristalsis. Most patients can hold their breath for the 20 seconds or less required to scan the abdomen. Uncooperative patients may breathe or move during scanning, causing severe artifacts and limiting diagnostic information (Fig. 8-2).

Volume Averaging

By design a CT scanner irradiates a three-dimensional slab of tissue to create a two-dimensional image. All CT images are "volume averaged" in that a finite thickness of patient tissue is summated to create the two-dimensional image (Fig. 8-3). The effect of this error is to display the average of densities within the slice thickness instead of separate individual densities. For example, volume averaging of opaque oral contrast within duodenum may create the appear-

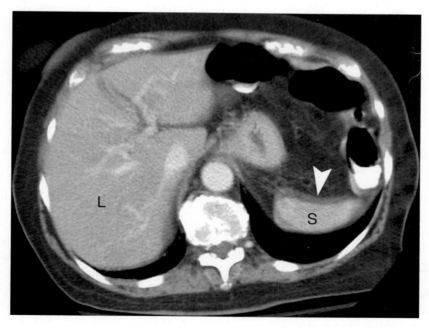

FIGURE 8-2 **Motion artifact.** Despite a scan acquisition time of less than 1 second, patient breathing motion has caused blurring *(arrowhead)* of the margin of the spleen (S), simulating a subcapsular collection. Careful inspection of the image of the liver (L) indicates indistinctness of the hepatic vessels and the outline of the liver.

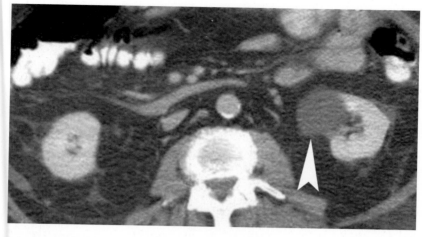

FIGURE 8-3 **Volume-averaging artifact.** The margin *(arrowhead)* of the cyst extending from the left kidney is blurred because its contour is rounded and attenuation of the cyst is averaged with attenuation of the adjacent fat within this 5-mm CT slice.

ance of a high-density stone in the gallbladder when no stone is present. Volume averaging is diminished and spatial resolution is increased by using thin slices. MDCT has the capability to obtain a large number of thin slices over a short period to minimize volume-averaging artifacts.

Beam Hardening

Beam hardening refers to an increase in the mean energy of the x-ray beam when it passes through an object. Low-energy x-ray photons are preferentially absorbed, and high-energy x-ray photons are more likely to pass through the structure. Radiographically dense structures that strongly absorb x-ray photons "harden the beam" and may produce streak artifacts on the CT image. This artifact is most commonly seen in body CT between the bones of the hips (Fig. 8-4) and those of the shoulders. Dense metallic objects such as surgical clips, bullets, and orthopedic hardware produce dramatic beam hardening and prominent streak artifact (Fig. 8-5).

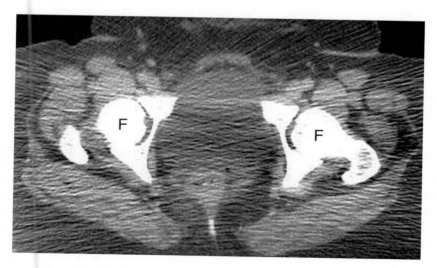

FIGURE 8-4 **Beam hardening artifact.** The alternating light and dark streaks of beam hardening artifact are prominent on this CT image of the pelvis in an obese patient. The dense bone of the femoral heads (F) and acetabuli selectively absorb lower energy x-ray photons resulting in greater average energy of the transmitted x-ray beam. The artifact is accentuated by the increased absorption of radiation in the "thicker" patient.

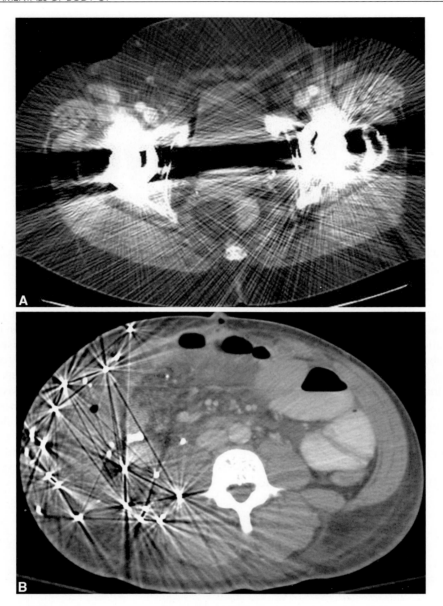

FIGURE 8-5 **Metal artifact.** *A,* Bilateral metallic hip prostheses ruin the CT image of the pelvis with dense dark and light bands and streaks. *B,* Similar effect is produced by lead buckshot in this patient who was shot by a shotgun.

Noise: Quantum Mottle

Image reconstruction in CT requires a large amount of data to produce an adequate image. The data are generated by x-ray photons striking CT detectors. The more x-ray photons that strike the detectors, the better are the data; the smaller the number of x-ray photons, the more limited are the data. Reducing slice thickness to improve resolution and decrease volume-averaging effect will reduce the number of photons used to create the image and will cause quantum mottle artifact. When the CT x-ray technique is reduced to decrease radiation exposure to the patient, data collection may be limited to the extent that the resulting image decreases in quality. Quantum mottle noise resulting from photon-poor imaging technique results in a low-resolution, salt-and-pepper appearance of the CT image (Fig. 8-6). With MDCT, choices must be made to find the balance between radiation dose to the patient and acceptable noise in the image.

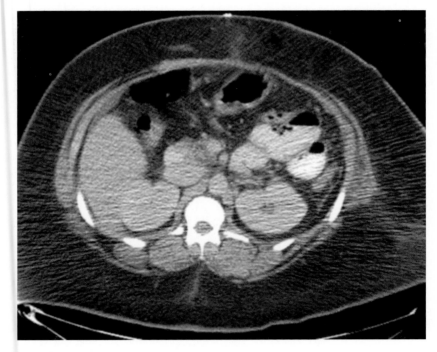

FIGURE 8-6 **Quantum mottle artifact.** CT image of the abdomen in an obese patient shows a generalized prominent "salt-and-pepper" *(light and dark dots)* appearance to the image. This is called quantum mottle or noise artifact and is created by a deficiency in the number of photons used to create the image. Low-dose CT technique (mA), reduced slice thickness, and large size of the patient are factors that increase image noise.

RADIATION DOSE IN CT

The continuing expansion of the use of CT for diagnostic imaging combined with the popularity and widespread use of MDCT has caused a dramatic increase in radiation exposure to patients. CT now accounts for more than 40% of all radiation exposure to patients from diagnostic imaging. There may be as many as 65 million CT examinations performed each year in the United States. Approximately 11% of these examinations are performed on infants and children who are more susceptible to the adverse effects of radiation. The radiation dose profile for MDCT is 27% greater than for single-detector helical CT. The individual doses to the kidneys, uterus, ovaries, and pelvic bone marrow may be 92% to 180% greater with MDCT than with single-detector helical CT. The dose "penalty" with MDCT increases with decreasing slice thickness. These considerations mandate a responsibility for the radiologist and the ordering physician to limit CT to definitive indications, provide dose-efficient CT imaging protocols, offer alternative imaging techniques for young children who are at the greatest risk from radiation, work with manufacturers to limit radiation dose, and educate patients and health care providers on the potential risks of low-dose radiation.

SUGGESTED READING

FRUSH DP, APPLEGATE K: Computed tomography and radiation: Understanding the issues. J Am Coll Radiol 1:113–119, 2004.

KALRA MK, MAHER MM, TOTH TL, et al: Strategies for CT radiation dose optimization. Radiology 230:619–628, 2004.

MCNITT-GRAY MF: Radiation dose in CT. Radio-Graphics 22:1541–1553, 2002.

RYDBERG J, BUCKWALTER KA, CALDEMEYER KS, et al: Multisection CT: Scanning techniques and clinical applications. Radiographics 20:1787–1806, 2000.

THORTON FJ, PAULSON EK, YOSHIZUMI TT, et al: Single versus multi-detector row CT: Comparison of radiation doses and dose profiles. Acad Radiol 10:379–385, 2003.

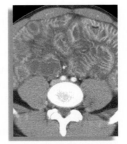

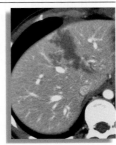

9

Peritoneal Cavity, Vessels, Nodes, and Abdominal Wall

William E. Brant, M.D.

☐ PERITONEAL CAVITY

Anatomy

The various recesses and spaces of the peritoneal cavity are easiest to recognize on CT when ascites is present. Identifying the precise compartment that an abnormality is in goes a long way toward identifying the nature of the abnormality and deciding on a plan for intervention. Whereas all the spaces of the peritoneal cavity potentially communicate with one another, diseases, such as abscesses, tend to loculate within one or more specific locations. The right subphrenic space communicates around the liver with the anterior subhepatic and posterior subhepatic (Morison's) space. The left subphrenic space communicates freely with the left subhepatic space. The right and left subphrenic spaces are separated by the falciform ligament and do not communicate directly. The lesser sac is the isolated peritoneal compartment between the stomach and the pancreas. It communicates with the rest of the peritoneal cavity (greater sac) through the small opening of the foramen of Winslow.

The right subphrenic and subhepatic spaces communicate freely with the pelvic peritoneal cavity by means of the right paracolic gutter. The phrenicocolic ligament prevents free communication between the left subphrenic/subhepatic spaces and the left paracolic gutter. Free fluid, blood, infection, and peritoneal metastases commonly settle in the pelvis because the pelvis is the most dependent portion of the peritoneal cavity and communicates with both sides of the abdomen.

The small-bowel mesentery suspends the jejunum and ileum and contains branches of the superior mesenteric artery and vein, as well as mesenteric lymph nodes. The mesentery extends like a fan obliquely across the abdomen from the ligament of Treitz in the left upper quadrant to the region of the right sacroiliac joint. Disease originating from above the ligament is directed toward the right lower quadrant. Disease originating from below the ligament has open access to the pelvis.

The greater omentum is a double layer of peritoneum that hangs from the greater curvature of the stomach and descends in front of the abdominal viscera. The greater omentum encloses fat and a few blood vessels. It serves as fertile ground for implantation of peritoneal metastases.

Fluid in the Peritoneal Cavity

Fluid in the peritoneal cavity originates from many different sources and varies greatly in composition. *Ascites* refers to accumulation of serous fluid within the peritoneal cavity and results from cirrhosis, hypoproteinemia, congestive heart failure, or venous obstruction. Exudative ascites is associated with inflammatory processes such as pancreatitis, peritonitis, and bowel perforation. Neoplastic ascites is caused by intraperitoneal tumor. Chylous ascites is caused by obstruction or traumatic injury to the thoracic duct or cisterna chyli. Urine and bile may spread through the peritoneal cavity because of obstruction or injury to the urinary or biliary tracts. *Hemoperitoneum* is an important sign of abdominal injury in blunt trauma. When the anatomy of the peritoneal cavity is known, recognition of fluid density within its recesses on CT is easy. Paracentesis is required for precise differentiation of the exact type of fluid present in the peritoneal cavity. However, CT can offer some clues, such as:

- Free intraperitoneal fluid occupies and distends the recesses of the peritoneal cavity. Bowel loops tend to float to the central abdomen. The diaphragm may be elevated or even inverted by a large volume of ascites.
- Serous ascites has an attenuation value near water (−10 to +15 H) and tends to accumulate in the greater peritoneal space, sparing the lesser sac.

- Hemoperitoneum has a larger attenuation value, averaging 45 H, and is usually greater than 30 H. Blood tends to accumulate, with the greatest amount of accumulation at about the site of hemorrhage.
- Exudative ascites caused by pancreatitis tends to accumulate preferentially within the lesser sac. Exudative and neoplastic ascites have intermediate attenuation values that overlap those of both serous ascites and blood. With peritonitis (Fig. 9-1), the peritoneum appears thickened and enhances after intravenous contrast administration.
- Loculations of peritoneal fluid caused by benign or malignant adhesions may simulate cystic abdominal masses. Tense loculated ascites may accumulate in confined spaces such as the lesser sac and compress and displace bowel loops. Loculated ascites, however, tends to conform to the general shape of the space it occupies. Cystic masses make their own space, cause greater displacement of adjacent structures, and have more varied internal consistency.
- Pseudomyxoma peritonei is an unusual complication of mucocele of the appendix or of mucinous cystadenocarcinoma manifested by filling of the peritoneal cavity with gelatinous mucin. The mucinous fluid is typically loculated and causes scalloping and

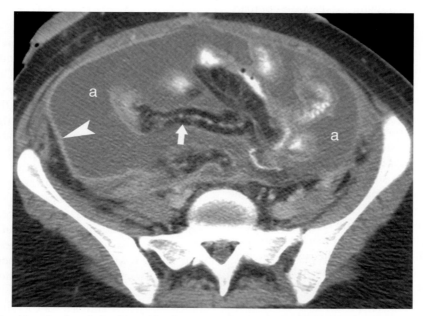

FIGURE 9-1 **Peritonitis and ascites.** Ascites (a) resulting from pancreatitis occupies and distends peritoneal recesses. Small-bowel loops float within the fluid suspended on fat-filled mesentery *(arrow)*. The parietal peritoneum *(arrowhead)* is thickened and enhances after intravenous contrast administration.

mass effect on the liver and adjacent bowel. Septations, mottled densities, and calcification within the fluid may be seen on CT (Fig. 9-2).

Free Air in the Peritoneal Cavity

Free air within the peritoneal cavity is an important sign of perforated viscus but may be surprisingly difficult to recognize on CT. The diagnosis is based on recognizing that the air is outside of the bowel lumen (Fig. 9-3). Images should be routinely examined at "lung windows" (window level, −400 to −600 H; window width, 1000–2000 H) for free intraperitoneal air. Free intraperitoneal air is easiest to recognize anterior to the liver and in nondependent recesses that do not contain bowel. The thin wall of distended bowel may be difficult to recognize. A clue is that the air within bowel appears confined, whereas free intraperitoneal air is not confined. Rolling the patient into a decubitus position and rescanning will assist in interpretation of difficult cases. Before ascribing pneumoperitoneum to bowel perforation, a thoracic source, such as pneumothorax or mechanical ventilation, or an iatrogenic source, such as recent paracentesis or recent surgical procedure, should also be considered.

Peritoneal Carcinomatosis

Diffuse metastatic seeding of the peritoneal cavity occurs commonly with abdominopelvic tumors. The most common tumors to spread by this method are ovarian carcinoma in female patients and stomach, pancreas, and colon carcinoma in both sexes. The preferential sites for tumor implantation are the pouch of Douglas, the right paracolic gutter, and the greater omentum. CT findings with peritoneal tumor seeding include:

- Ascites is usually presented and is commonly loculated.
- Tumor nodules appear as soft-tissue masses or thickening of the parietal peritoneum (Fig. 9-4).
- "Omental cake" describes the thickened nodular appearance of tumor involving the greater omentum. The tumor cake displaces bowel away from the anterior abdominal wall (Fig. 9-5).
- Tumor nodules and enlarged lymph nodes may be seen in the mesentery (Fig. 9-6).
- Thickening and nodularity of the bowel wall is caused by serosal tumor implantations.
- Minute implants, which may be painfully obvious and diffuse at surgery, are commonly missed by CT because of their small size. The presence of ascites in patients with

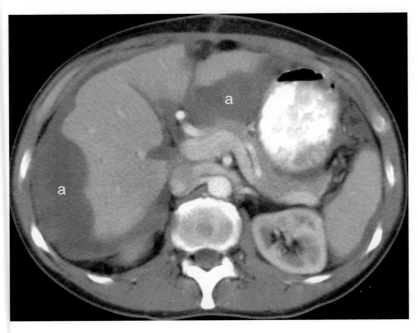

FIGURE 9-2 Pseudomyxoma peritonei. High-attenuation gelatinous ascites (a) is loculated in peritoneal recesses and causes mass effect on adjacent organs. The cause was mucinous adenocarcinoma of the stomach metastatic to the peritoneum.

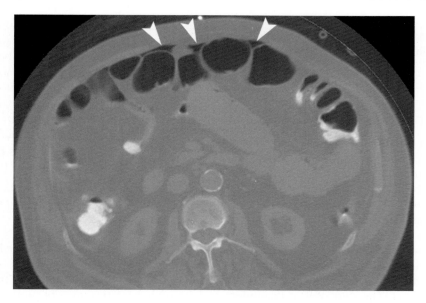

FIGURE 9-3 **Pneumoperitoneum.** Free intraperitoneal air is recognized by its characteristic triangular and linear appearance *(arrowheads)* between bowel loops in the nondependent areas of the abdomen. Note the more rounded appearance of air within bowel confined by the thin bowel wall.

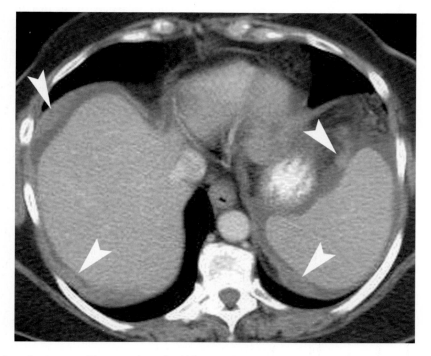

FIGURE 9-4 **Peritoneal metastases.** Metastases *(arrowheads)* from ovarian carcinoma to the peritoneum appear as focal areas of peritoneal thickening and nodules.

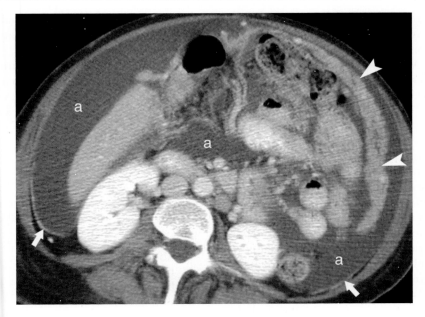

FIGURE 9-5 Omental cake. Ascites (a) is present throughout the peritoneal cavity. The parietal peritoneum *(arrows)* is thickened and enhances after intravenous contrast administration, indicating that the ascites is neoplastic or inflammatory. Omental cake *(arrowheads)* manifests as a layer of irregular soft tissue that displaces bowel away from the anterior abdominal wall.

known abdominopelvic tumor, especially ovarian carcinoma, should be regarded as suspicious for peritoneal seeding. Calcification of tumor implants may aid in their CT identification.

Peritoneal Mesothelioma

About 20% to 40% of mesotheliomas arise within the abdomen, but it remains a rare type of tumor with a rapidly fatal course. CT shows an enhancing solid tumor in the mesentery, omen-

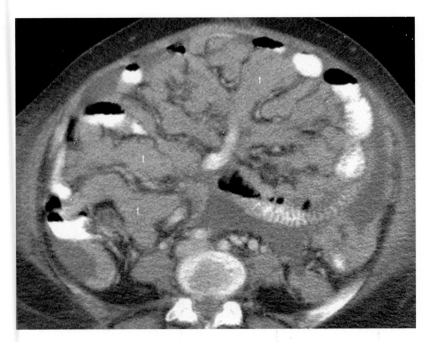

FIGURE 9-6 Mesenteric carcinomatosis. Tumor nodules (t) from intraperitoneal spread of ovarian cancer cause diffuse thickening of the folds of the small-bowel mesentery.

tum, or on peritoneal surfaces (Fig. 9-7). It may cause diffuse, irregular thickening of the peritoneal surfaces, multiple small nodules, or an infiltrating mass. Multilocular cystic forms of the tumor also occur. Ascites is present in most cases.

Abscess

CT is commonly performed to search for and plan for percutaneous drainage of abdominal and pelvic abscesses. Once found, percutaneous aspiration confirms the diagnosis and provides material for culture. Image-directed catheter placement is commonly used for drainage ("pus busting"). Most abscesses occur as complications of abdominal trauma, surgery, pancreatitis, or bowel perforation (ruptured appendicitis, diverticulitis). Intraperitoneal abscesses are commonly located in the pelvic cavity and the subphrenic and subhepatic spaces. CT features of abscess include:

- Most abscesses appear as loculated fluid collections, often with internal debris, fluid–fluid levels, septations, and sometimes air–fluid levels or bubbles of air (Fig. 9-8).
- Definable wall with irregular thickening is usually identifiable.
- Nearby fascia is thickened and fat planes are obliterated because of inflammation.

- Ascites, pleural effusions, and lower lobe pulmonary infiltrates commonly accompany abdominal abscesses.
- Any fluid collection within the abdomen is suspect in patients in whom abscess is suggested clinically. Fine-needle aspiration is a safe and definitive way to exclude or confirm the diagnosis.

Cystic Abdominal Masses

Cystic masses in the abdomen commonly present challenges in diagnosis. Differential considerations include:

- Abscess
- Loculated ascites
- Pancreatic pseudocyst
- Ovarian cyst/cystic tumor
- Lymphocele: a cystic mass containing lymphatic fluid that occurs as a complication of surgery or trauma that disrupts lymphatic channels; it may be of any size and appear days to years after surgery
- Cystic lymphangioma: a congenital counterpart of lymphocele believed to arise because of congenital obstruction of lymphatic channels (Fig. 9-9); most are thin walled and multiloculated; attenuation ranges from water to fat density; *mesenteric cysts* are

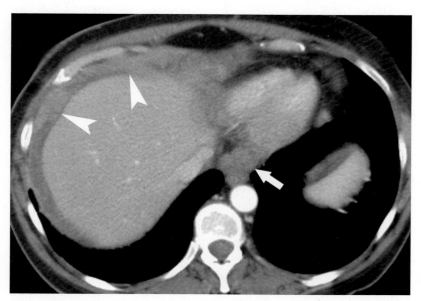

FIGURE 9-7 **Peritoneal mesothelioma.** Tumor nodules *(arrowheads)* on peritoneal surfaces are apparent. The appearance is indistinguishable from peritoneal carcinomatosis, but biopsy confirmed peritoneal mesothelioma. Adenopathy *(arrow)* is seen adjacent to the esophagus.

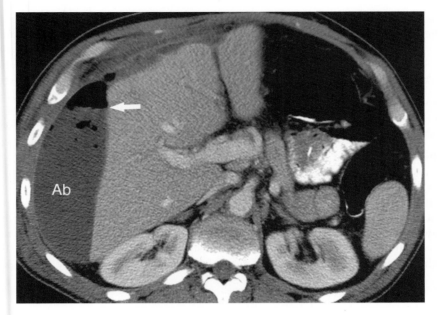

FIGURE 9-8 **Subphrenic abscess.** A postoperative abscess (Ab) is seen as a fluid collection between the diaphragm and the liver. Mass impression on the liver is evidence of fluid loculation. An air–fluid level *(arrow)* caused by gas-producing *Escherichia coli* is evident. This abscess was successfully treated using CT-guided percutaneous catheter drainage.

cystic lymphangiomas of the mesentery; *omental cysts* are less common cystic lymphangiomas of the greater omentum

- Enteric duplication cysts: cysts lined with gastrointestinal mucosa and usually attached to normal bowel
- Cystic teratoma: may arise in the retroperitoneum, mesentery, or omentum; CT shows a complex cystic and solid mass with areas of water and fat attenuation and calcifications

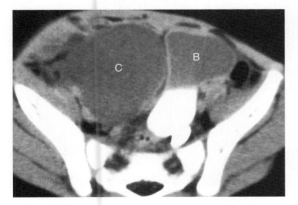

FIGURE 9-9 **Cystic lymphangioma.** A fluid-filled mass (C) displaces the bladder (B) in a 2-year-old boy. Pathology after surgical removal revealed a cystic lymphangioma.

☐ VESSELS

Anatomy

The abdominal aorta descends anterior to the left side of the spine to its bifurcation at the level of the iliac crest. The normal aorta does not exceed 3 cm in diameter and tapers progressively as it proceeds distally. The inferior vena cava lies to the right of the aorta. Its shape varies from round to oval to slitlike depending on breath holding technique and intravascular fluid balance. The common iliac arteries and veins appear oval in cross section as they diverge from the midline. The common iliac vessels bifurcate at the pelvic brim, which is identified by noting the shape of the sacrum change from convex anteriorly (the sacral promontory) to concave. The external iliac vessels course anteriorly to the inguinal triangle, whereas the internal iliac (hypogastric) vessels have many small branches in the posterior pelvis. The iliac arteries normally do not exceed 1.5 cm in diameter.

The celiac axis originates from the anterior aspect of the aorta at the level of the aortic hiatus in the diaphragm. The superior mesenteric artery originates anteriorly from the aorta 1 cm below the celiac axis. The renal arteries arise from the lateral aspect of the aorta within 1 cm of the superior mesenteric artery. The inferior mesenteric artery is a tiny anterior branch off the aorta just above the bifurcation.

Anatomic Variations

A number of vascular anomalies must be recognized to avoid misinterpretation as abnormalities. Variations include:

- Above the popliteal fossa the veins of the lower limbs and abdomen are usually solitary and slightly larger than the accompanying artery.
- Duplication of the inferior vena cava (Fig. 9-10) may be identified extending between the left common iliac vein and the left renal vein on the left side of the aorta.

- Left renal veins may course posterior instead of anterior to the aorta (retroaortic left renal vein) (Fig. 9-11), or duplicated left renal veins may course both anterior and posterior to the aorta (circumaortic left renal vein).
- The intrahepatic segment of the inferior vena cava may be absent, with drainage continuing to the superior vena cava by means of the azygos system.

Technical Considerations

MDCT combined with three-dimensional reconstruction techniques have made CT angiography a reality. CT angiography offers several advan-

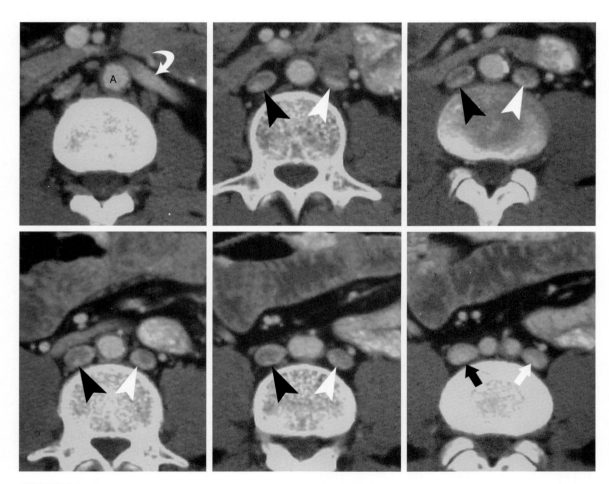

FIGURE 9-10 Duplication of the inferior vena cava (IVC). The persistent left IVC *(white arrowheads)* extends as the continuation of the left common iliac vein *(white arrow)* along the left side of the aorta (A) to end in the left renal vein *(curved arrow).* The normal right IVC *(black arrowheads)* extends from the right common iliac vein *(black arrow)* to follow its normal course through the liver. Blood flow from the left IVC flows into the right IVC through the left renal vein.

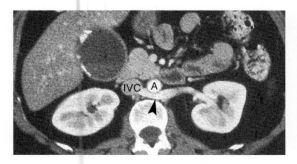

FIGURE 9-11 **Retroaortic left renal vein.** The left renal vein *(arrowhead)* courses posterior instead of anterior to the aorta (A) to join the inferior vena cava (IVC).

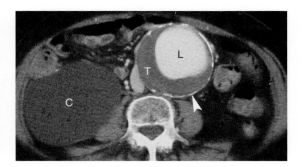

FIGURE 9-12 **Aneurysm abdominal aorta.** A large aortic aneurysm is evident. The aorta exceeds 5 cm in diameter. A large amount of thrombus (T) partially surrounds the patent, contrast-enhancing, lumen (L). Note the atherosclerotic calcification *(arrowhead)* in the wall of the aneurysm. A large cyst (C) extends from the right kidney.

tages over conventional catheter angiography. CT angiography is less invasive, is less expensive, can be performed more quickly, and is capable of demonstrating important nonvascular abnormalities that would be missed by conventional angiography.

CT venography of the lower limbs may be combined with CT angiography of the pulmonary arteries to allow complete evaluation for venopulmonary thromboembolism. CT venography has reported sensitivity of 89% to 100% with specificity of 94% to 100% for venous thrombosis. Optimal venous enhancement of the lower limbs is obtained at 3 minutes 30 seconds after onset of intravenous contrast injection into the upper extremity. Images are viewed at 3- to 5-mm slice thickness. Three-dimensional reconstructions may be created.

Abdominal Aortic Aneurysm

Aneurysms are defined as circumscribed dilatations of an artery. A true aneurysm involves all three layers of the arterial wall (intima, media, and adventitia). Most are caused by atherosclerotic disease that weakens the vessel wall and allows it to dilate as a result of high intra-aortic blood pressure. Up to 9% of the population older than 65 years has an abdominal aortic aneurysm. CT findings, of abdominal aortic aneurysm include:

- Fusiform, saccular, or spherical dilatation of the aorta is the key finding (Fig. 9-12). Care must be taken to avoid overestimation of aortic size because the vessel is tortuous and imaged obliquely.
- Outer-to-outer diameter of the abdominal aorta greater than 3 cm is evidence of aneurysm. Risk for rupture depends on the size

of the aneurysm. The risk is about 5% for abdominal aortic aneurysms less than 5 cm, 16% for those greater than 6 cm, and 76% for those greater than 7 cm.
- Failure of the aorta to taper distally is another sign of aneurysm. Distal dilatation is evidence of aneurysm even if the diameter is less than 3 cm.
- The iliac arteries are aneurysmal when their diameter exceeds 1.5 cm (Fig. 9-13).
- The patent lumen enhances with intravenous contrast. Thrombus within the abdominal aortic aneurysm remains low in density.
- Calcification in the wall of the aorta and in the wall of the aneurysm is common.

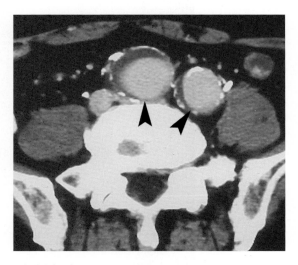

FIGURE 9-13 **Aneurysms of both common iliac arteries.** In this patient, an aneurysm of the abdominal aorta extends into both common iliac arteries *(arrowheads)*. Each vessel exceeds 15 mm in outer-to-outer diameter.

Occasionally, long-standing intraluminal thrombus may also calcify.

- The proximal extent of the aneurysm must be defined. Most (90%) begin below the origin of the renal arteries (infrarenal abdominal aortic aneurysm). Origin above the renal arteries must be identified because more complicated surgical repair is required.

- Inflammatory and fibrotic changes may be seen in the perianeurysmal soft tissues. These likely result from an immune response to atherosclerotic plaque and do not represent a chronic leak of the aneurysm. The inflammatory tissue may enhance after intravenous contrast administration. These changes may, however, envelop and obstruct the ureters.

Rupture of an Abdominal Aortic Aneurysm

Acute rupture of an abdominal aortic aneurysm is highly lethal (77% to 94% mortality rate). The classic presentation is abdominal pain, hypotension, and pulsatile abdominal mass. Because ruptured abdominal aortic aneurysms are commonly confused clinically with other diseases, CT is used to confirm the diagnosis. Unenhanced CT is adequate to confirm the diagnosis. Rapid intervention is needed. CT findings indicating rupture include:

- An abdominal aortic aneurysm, usually large, is evident.

- Adjacent periaortic hemorrhage dissects tissue planes of the pararenal and perirenal retroperitoneum (Fig. 9-14).

- Active arterial bleeding may be demonstrated with intravenous contrast administration. Streaks and puddles of contrast are seen outside of the aorta within the retroperitoneal hematoma.

- Iliac artery aneurysms, especially those larger than 3.5 cm, may also be the site of rupture producing similar findings.

- The *hyperattenuating crescent sign* refers to a crescent-shaped area of high attenuation within the wall or within the intraluminal thrombus of abdominal aortic aneurysm (Fig. 9-15). The sign is indicative of impending rupture of an abdominal aortic aneurysm. It is caused by acute blood dissecting into the intraluminal thrombus and dissecting to the outer weak wall of the aneurysm. Progressive damage of the wall leads to rupture.

Infected Aortic Aneurysms

Infected aneurysms are rare, difficult to suspect clinically, and highly prone to rupture (53% to 75%). Infected aneurysms are also called *mycotic*

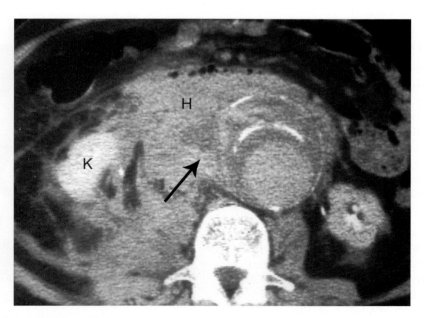

FIGURE 9-14 **Rupture of aortic aneurysm.** Postcontrast CT demonstrates prominent hemorrhage (H) extending into retroperitoneal tissues to the right kidney (K). Note the disruption *(arrow)* of the calcified wall of the aortic aneurysm.

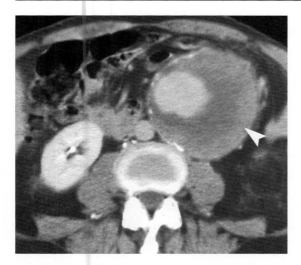

FIGURE 9-15 **Hyperattenuating crescent sign.** Routine follow-up CT documented a rapid increase in size of this aortic aneurysm. The crescent of increased density *(arrowhead)* in the periphery of the aneurysm is highly indicative of impending rupture.

aneurysms; however, this term does not imply fungal infection. Most infected aneurysms occur as a result of bacterial infection of the intima in a normal aortic wall or in a preexisting aneurysm, commonly in association with bacterial endocarditis. Urgent surgical repair is needed. Indications of infection include:

- The aneurysm is saccular in shape with lobulated contour in nearly all cases (Fig. 9-16). It may be found anywhere in the aorta. Gas is occasionally present in the soft tissues.

- Periaortic soft-tissue stranding and fluid is commonly present.
- Findings of osteomyelitis may be seen in the adjacent vertebral body.

Aortic Dissection

Dissection of blood into the media through a tear in the intima results in a dilated segment of artery with two lumina. Branch vessels may be occluded by the process or may be fed by the new (false) or the original (true) lumen. Most dissections begin in the thoracic aorta but commonly extend into the abdominal aorta. Indications of aortic dissection include:

- The key finding is an intimal flap separating the true and false lumens (Fig. 9-17).
- Thrombosis of the false lumen may preclude visualization of the intimal flap.
- Differentiation of the true and false lumens is important in treatment planning. The false lumen is usually larger and commonly contains a thrombus. Thrombus is generally not seen in the true lumen. The junction of the flap with the outer wall of the false lumen produces an acute angle, called the "beak sign." Intimal calcifications may be seen on the intimal flap and in the wall of the true lumen.
- Internal displacement of intimal plaque calcification may be present.

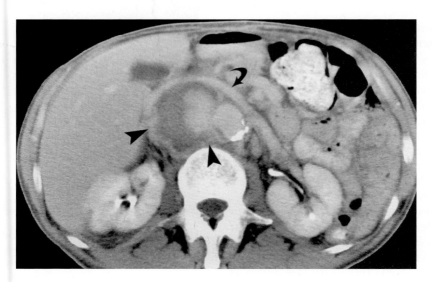

FIGURE 9-16 **Mycotic aneurysm.** CT in this drug abuser with abdominal pain showed a saccular aneurysm *(arrowheads)* of the abdominal aorta. The left renal vein *(curved arrow)* is stretched and draped over the aneurysm.

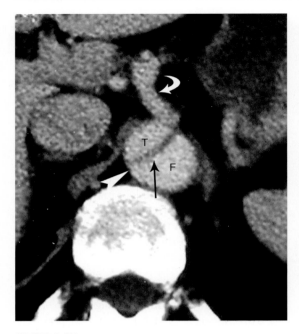

FIGURE 9-17 Aortic dissection. A dissection of the thoracic aorta extends into the abdominal aorta. The intimal flap *(straight arrow)* is readily apparent within the enhancing aorta. The true lumen (T) supplies the celiac axis *(curved arrow)*. The false lumen (F) is identified by the "beak sign" *(arrowhead)*.

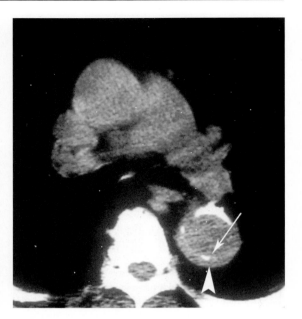

FIGURE 9-18 Intramural hematoma. Noncontrast CT demonstrates high-attenuation hemorrhage *(arrowhead)* in the wall of the descending thoracic aorta. Atherosclerotic calcification *(arrow)* that serves as a marked of the location of the intima is displaced toward the lumen.

- Compression of the true lumen by expanding hematoma in the false lumen may be present.
- Branch vessels may be compressed or occluded resulting in ischemia or infarction of supplied organs.
- Ischemia or infarction of organs supplied by branch arteries.
- *Intramural hematoma* refers to aortic dissection without rupture of the intima. It is caused by hemorrhage of the vasa vasorum that weakens the media but does not tear the intima. Noncontrast CT shows high-attenuation blood within the wall of the aorta (Fig. 9-18). Intimal calcifications are displaced toward the aortic lumen. The luminal surface is smooth compared with the irregular surface of the more common intraluminal thrombus. Intramural hematomas may resolve or progress.
- *Penetrating atherosclerotic ulcer* is an atherosclerotic lesion with ulceration that is a precursor to intramural hemorrhage. CT shows a focal ulcer extending into a subintimal hematoma (Fig. 9-19). Treatment is controversial but may involve graft replacement of the affected section of the aorta.

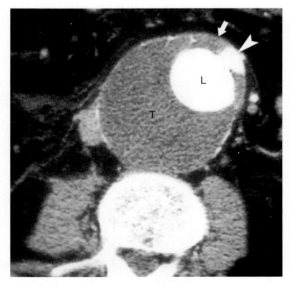

FIGURE 9-19 Penetrating atherosclerotic ulcer. Contrast CT shows a focal, contrast-defined ulceration *(arrowhead)* within a high-attenuation intramural thrombus *(arrow)*. The ulcer communicates with the contrast-enhancing lumen (L) of the aortic aneurysm. A large volume of intraluminal thrombus (T) is also present.

Deep Venous Thrombosis

Venous thrombi may be bland, septic, or associated with tumor invasion. For example,

- Thrombus appears as a filling defect within the vein, causing complete or partial obstruction (Fig. 9-20). Dilatation of the vein at the site of thrombosis is evidence that the process is acute.
- Upstream veins may be dilated compared with the contralateral side, and soft tissues may show streaks and strands of edema.
- The wall of the affected vein may show contrast enhancement provided by the vasa vasorum.
- Chronic thrombosis appears as an irregular intraluminal clot that may calcify. The wall of the affected vein is commonly thickened.
- Flow artifacts and layering of contrast medium may mimic thrombosis. Confirmation with venous compression and Doppler ultrasound may be needed in questionable cases.
- Extrinsic displacement and compression may also be difficult to differentiate from thrombosis. Tumors most likely to extend into the inferior vena cava are renal, hepatic, and adrenal carcinomas.

☐ **NODES**

Anatomy

Normal lymph nodes are oblong and homogeneous in CT attenuation. Most are oriented parallel to their accompanying vessels. Abdominoaortic nodal groups surround the aorta and inferior vena cava and are commonly involved in abdominal and pelvic malignancy. Visceral nodes drain adjacent organs and include mesenteric, hepatic, splenic, and pancreaticoduodenal nodal groups.

Nodal Metastases

Size is the major criterion for diagnosis of abnormal lymph nodes. Nodes are considered to be pathologically enlarged when they exceed 10 mm in short axis in the abdomen or pelvis or 6 mm in the retrocrural and porta hepatis region. Multiple 8- to 10-mm nodes in the abdomen or pelvis are considered suspicious. Interpretation must always be made in clinical context. Even minimally enlarged nodes should be viewed with suspicion when present in an area where a known malignancy is highly likely to metastasize.

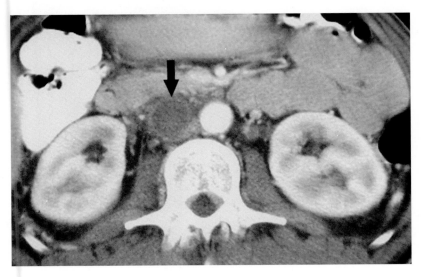

FIGURE 9-20 **Thrombosis of the inferior vena cava (IVC).** Thrombus fills and distends the inferior vena cava *(arrow).* Note the enhancement of the wall of the IVC that serves as additional evidence that this represents true thrombosis and not a flow defect.

Unfortunately, involvement of nodes with metastatic tumor does not usually change the CT attenuation of the node and, in some cases, will not enlarge the node sufficiently to be interpreted as pathologic by size criteria. Nodes may be enlarged because of benign disease (false-positive interpretation) or may be of normal size and yet be involved (false-negative interpretation). Low attenuation within enlarged nodes is seen uncommonly and usually represents necrosis. Calcification of nodes may occur with some calcifying tumors or with tumor necrosis after treatment.

Lymphoma

Lymphomas are divided into Hodgkin's and non–Hodgkin's types. Hodgkin's lymphoma accounts for about 40% of lymphomas and tends to spread in an orderly, contiguous manner. Non–Hodgkin's lymphoma is a mixed group of diseases with a confusing array of changing names and classifications. Noncontiguous spread and involvement of the gastrointestinal tract is characteristic of non–Hodgkin's lymphoma. CT features of lymphoma in the abdomen and pelvis include:

- Multiple enlarged individual nodes (Fig. 9-21)

- Coalescence of enlarged nodes to form rounded multilobular masses that may encase vessels, displace organs, and obstruct ureters (Fig. 9-22)
- Conglomerate nodal masses: these masses are typical of lymphoma and are rarely seen with other conditions

Acquired Immunodeficiency Syndrome

Acquired immunodeficiency syndrome (AIDS) is characterized on abdominal CT by signs of intra-abdominal opportunistic infections, AIDS-related lymphoma, and Kaposi's sarcoma. Most CT findings are a manifestation of a complicating disease rather than human immunodeficiency virus infection alone. The most common findings on CT include:

- Lymphadenopathy involving the retroperitoneal, pelvic, and mesenteric nodes is caused by disseminated *Mycobacterium avium-intracellulare* infection (30%), AIDS-related lymphoma (30%), Kaposi's sarcoma, or other infection. Lymph node enlargement is unlikely to be caused by human immunodeficiency virus infection alone. Unexplained adenopathy warrants biopsy.

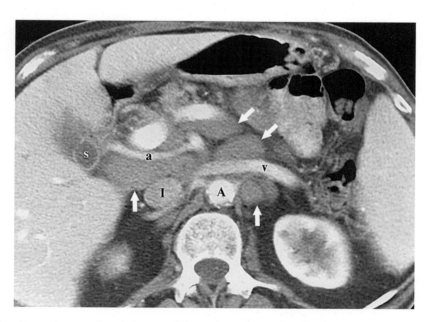

FIGURE 9-21 **Lymphoma.** CT image through the upper abdomen demonstrates enlarged nodes *(arrows)* surrounding the hepatic artery (a), left renal vein (v), aorta (A), and inferior vena cava (I). The patient also has a gallstone(s).

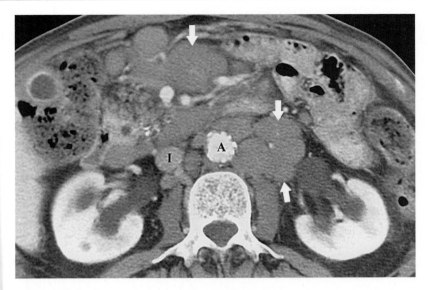

FIGURE 9-22 **Lymphoma.** Enlarged lymph nodes *(arrows)* surround the aorta (A) and inferior vena cava (I) and are seen in the small-bowel mesentery.

- Hepatosplenomegaly without focal lesions may result from *M. avium-intracellulare* infection, histoplasmosis, and hepatocellular disease.
- Focal, small (<1 cm), low-attenuation lesions in the liver are usually caused by *Mycobacterium tuberculosis,* AIDS-related lymphoma, Kaposi's sarcoma, or histoplasmosis.
- Focal, small (< 1 cm), low-attenuation lesions in the spleen are caused by *M. tuberculosis, M. avium-intracellulare,* coccidiomycosis, candidiasis, bacillary peliosis, Kaposi's sarcoma, AIDS-related lymphoma, and *Pneumocystis carinii* infection.
- Focal bowel wall thickening or focal bowel mass is nearly always caused by AIDS-related lymphoma.
- Calcifications in spleen, lymph nodes, and liver usually result from *P. carinii* infection.
- Nephromegaly with striated nephrogram after contrast agent administration is a sign of human immunodeficiency virus nephropathy.
- *Mycobacterial infections* cause lymph node enlargement; small, low-density lesions in solid organs; hepatosplenomegaly; and bowel wall thickening.
- *P. carinii* infections cause punctate or nodular calcifications in solid organs and lymph nodes and low-attenuation lesions in the spleen.

- *Kaposi's sarcoma* causes adenopathy and hepatosplenomegaly. Less common findings include focal bowel wall thickening, low-density nodules in the liver, and intrahepatic low-density bands in the periportal region.
- *AIDS-related lymphoma* must be suspected for any solid mass anywhere in the abdomen. Additional findings include multiple sites of adenopathy, bowel involvement with wall thickening and focal masses, and focal masses in the spleen, liver, and kidney.

☐ ABDOMINAL WALL

Anatomy

CT is an excellent imaging technique for evaluation of abnormalities of the abdominal wall. The muscles of the abdominal wall are outlined by subcutaneous and extraperitoneal fat. The rectus abdominis muscles are anterior within the rectus sheath. The flanks are defined by three muscle layers formed by the external and internal oblique and transversus abdominis muscles. The posterior muscles are the latissimus dorsi, the quadratus lumborum, and the paraspinal muscles.

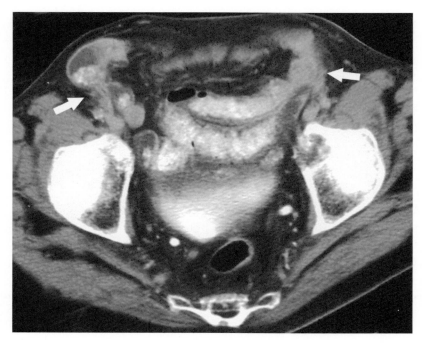

FIGURE 9-23 **Bilateral indirect inguinal hernias.** Bowel protrudes through the internal inguinal rings *(arrows)* and into the inguinal canal bilaterally.

Abdominal Wall Hernia

Obesity makes hernias of the abdominal wall difficult to detect clinically. Hernias may cause intermittent pain or bowel obstruction. Hernia sacs contain fat, which is usually omentum, bowel, and occasionally ascites.

- *Incisional hernias* are common ventral hernias with protrusion of abdominal contents through the abdominal wall weakened by a surgical incision.
- *Inguinal hernias* are classified as indirect or direct. Indirect hernias are congenital lesions seen to protrude anterior to the spermatic cord (in male patients) or round ligament (in female patients) and lateral to the inferior epigastric vessels (Fig. 9-23). Direct inguinal hernias are always acquired and are seen to occur medial to the inferior epigastric vessels.
- *Paraumbilical hernias* protrude through the linea alba in the region of the umbilicus (Fig. 9-24).
- *Spigelian hernias* are uncommon but carry a high risk for bowel incarceration and strangulation. They protrude through the linea semilunaris at the lateral edge of the rectus abdominis (Fig. 9-25).

Abdominal Wall Hematoma

Bleeding into the abdominal musculature may complicate bleeding disorders or anticoagulant therapy or result from trauma. Hematomas enlarge the involved muscle, are hyperdense acutely, and progressively decrease in attenuation

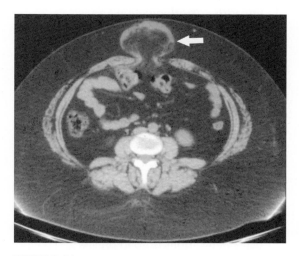

FIGURE 9-24 **Paraumbilical hernia.** CT of an obese woman shows a paraumbilical hernia *(arrow)* containing fat-density greater omentum.

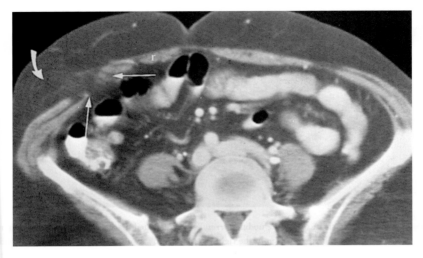

FIGURE 9-25 **Spigelian hernia.** Fat-density omentum and blood vessels *(curved arrow)* protrude through a defect *(straight arrows)* in the anterior abdominal wall at the lateral edge of the rectus abdominis (r).

with time (Fig. 9-26). Hematomas or seromas are commonly visualized in surgical wounds during the postoperative period. Infection results in abscess formation with increased stranding densities in subcutaneous fat, gas formation, and fluid levels. Confirmation of infection requires percutaneous aspiration.

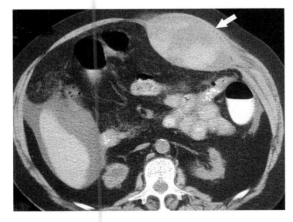

FIGURE 9-26 **Rectus hematoma.** The left rectus muscle *(arrow)* is markedly enlarged and shows irregular high attenuation indicative of intramuscular hematoma. Bleeding occurred as a complication of dialysis. This patient also has ascites.

Subcutaneous Nodules

Fatty tissue provides an optimal background for CT demonstration of nodules and masses in the subcutaneous tissues. Diagnostic considerations include:

- Hematogenous metastases to the skin are characteristic of malignant melanoma (Fig. 9-27). Other primary diagnoses to consider include breast, stomach, ovary, renal, and lung carcinomas. Nodules are usually well defined and enlarge over time.
- Injection hematomas and granulomas are usually seen in the lower anterior abdominal wall.
- Sebaceous cysts vary in size and are attached to the skin surface.
- Enlarged subcutaneous vessels are round, oval, or tubular in shape. They may be related to portal hypertension or venous thrombosis. Contrast administration shows enhancement.
- Endometriomas result from implants of endometrium in surgical scars. They characteristically bleed and become painful with menstruation.

the presence of blood flow and provides the best detection of lacerations and hematomas, which may be isodense in unenhanced organs. All trauma CT scans must include both the abdomen and pelvis. Extensive hemorrhage may settle dependently in the pelvis and be barely detectable on scans confined to the abdomen. All CT images should be viewed with lung windows to detect pneumothorax and pneumoperitoneum, with bone windows to detect bone injuries, and with routine soft-tissue windows to demonstrate organ injury.

The use of oral contrast before trauma CT scans remains controversial; an increasing number of institutions are switching to CT scanning without oral contrast in the setting of trauma. Extended patient preparation with oral contrast may inappropriately delay CT scanning. Patients may vomit or aspirate oral contrast. Oral contrast may interfere with performance of angiography, if needed in the treatment of active hemorrhage. Contrast is often poorly distributed through the bowel because of ileus induced by trauma. At my institution, scanning without oral contrast is routinely performed in acute trauma patients. A number of studies, including my own, have documented no significant change in the accuracy of trauma CT without the use of oral contrast. When possible and without causing delay in obtaining the CT scan, 400 to 700 cc iodinated contrast agent is given orally or through nasogastric tube.

Single-slice or multislice helical CT allows rapid scanning of the chest, abdomen, and pelvis during the same rapid intravenous contrast bolus. Scans are obtained at 5- to 7-mm collimation using single-slice spiral technique and at 2.5–3.0 mm collimation using multislice spiral technique. The 2.5-mm multislice images are routinely viewed as 5-mm slices. The 150 cc of intravenous contrast is given at 2.5 to 3.0 cc per second with scanning initiated at 70 seconds after onset of injection. Delayed images should be obtained at 3 to 5 minutes after contrast injection to evaluate the excretory phase of the kidneys for injuries to the collecting system.

CT cystography is performed by instilling 250 to 350 cc of 3% to 5% iodinated contrast agent into the bladder through a Foley catheter. Scans are obtained through the pelvis before and after contrast instillation using 5-mm collimation. Scans obtained after bladder drainage are not necessary.

☐ CT FINDINGS OF TRAUMATIC INJURY

CT findings of traumatic injury within the abdomen or pelvis include:

- *Hemoperitoneum.* Blood within the peritoneal cavity is a highly reliable sign of intra-abdominal injury (Fig. 10-1). Fresh, unclotted blood measures 30 to 45 H compared with 0 to 15 H ascites or serum. Separation of clotted blood and serum may result in visible fluid layers (hematocrit effect). Fresh blood flows from the area of injury to dependent recesses in the abdomen and pelvis.
- *Sentinel clot.* A focal collection of clotted blood (>60 H) is an accurate marker of injury to the adjacent organ (see Figs. 10-1*A* and 10-2). Occasionally, the sentinel clot is the only positive finding of organ injury. The higher density clot stands out in relief compared with lower density unclotted blood or serum.
- *Active bleeding.* Active hemorrhage may be detected by scanning during the arterial phase of dynamic intravenous contrast administration, which is routinely obtained by using power injectors and helical CT scanners. Active bleeding is identified as hyperdense foci within areas of lower density liquid blood (Fig. 10-3). The attenuation of active hemorrhage ranges from 85 to 370 H and is usually within 20 H of the attenuation of nearby arteries such as the aorta. This finding is a sign of life-threatening hemorrhage and often necessitates immediate angiographic or surgical therapy.
- *Free air.* Free air in the peritoneal cavity is a sign of transmural bowel laceration (Fig. 10-4). Unfortunately, this sign is neither sensitive nor specific. Extraluminal air is found in only 32% to 55% of cases of bowel laceration. Free air may also result from DPL, barotrauma, or mechanical ventilation. Additional findings of bowel injury must be present before definitively ascribing this finding to bowel perforation. Free air is usually best detected on lung windows.
- *Free contrast.* Free contrast in the peritoneal cavity may occur with extravasation of oral contrast through a bowel perforation or from leakage of contrast-opacified urine from the urinary tract (Fig. 10-5). Extra-

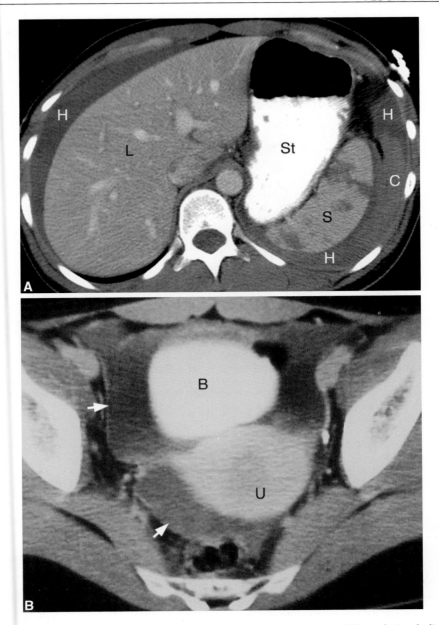

FIGURE 10-1 Hemoperitoneum. *A,* Scan through the upper abdomen shows hemoperitoneum (H) enveloping the liver (L) and spleen (S). Multiple lacerations of the spleen are evident. Higher density blood clot (C) is seen adjacent to the spleen. This patient received oral contrast, which distends the stomach (St). *B,* CT image of the pelvis shows blood *(arrows)* settling in the peritoneal recesses of the pelvis surrounding the bladder (B) and uterus (U).

luminal oral contrast is found in only 14% of bowel transections. Additional findings such as bowel wall thickening and blood in the mesentery confirm bowel injury as the source of extraluminal contrast. Extravasated contrast-containing urine should be seen on delayed images after the ureter and bladder fill with contrast agent.

- *Subcapsular hematomas.* These hematomas appear as crescent-shaped collections that flatten and indent the organ parenchyma (Fig. 10-6). Density is less than that of contrast-enhanced parenchyma. The outer border of the collection is sharply defined by the organ capsule. The inner margin compresses adjacent parenchyma.

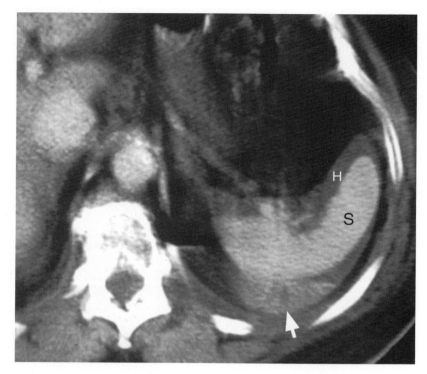

FIGURE 10-2 **Sentinel clot.** A high-attenuation blood clot *(arrow)* serves as a marker of a poorly visible laceration of the spleen (S). Lower attenuation blood (H) is seen in the recesses of the peritoneal cavity around the spleen.

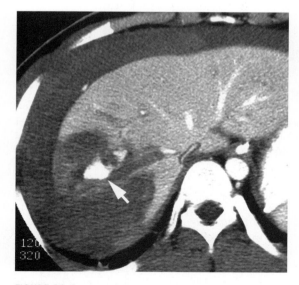

FIGURE 10-3 **Active hemorrhage.** Trauma CT of the liver shows a focus of active hemorrhage *(arrow)* seen as an amorphous extravascular collection of contrast within a low-attenuation hepatic hematoma. Extensive hemoperitoneum is evident.

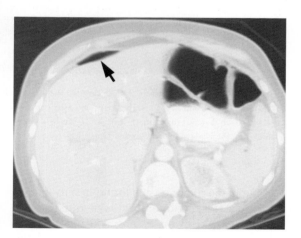

FIGURE 10-4 **Pneumoperitoneum.** CT of the abdomen shown with lung windows demonstrates an extraluminal collection of air *(arrow)* anterior to the liver. This patient had a traumatic laceration of the jejunum. Serial images are inspected to assure that no bowel is in this area.

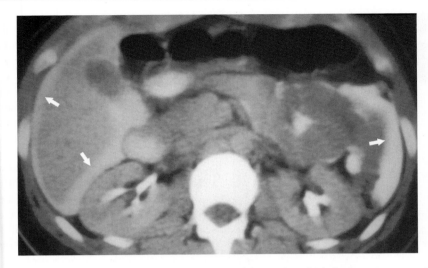

FIGURE 10-5 **Free intraperitoneal contrast.** Image through the upper abdomen shows high-density contrast agent in the peritoneal recesses *(arrows)*. This patient had an intraperitoneal rupture of the bladder. Contrast excreted in the urine extravasated through the hole in the bladder into the peritoneal cavity.

- *Intraparenchymal hematomas.* These hematomas are seen as irregularly shaped, rounded, low-density collections within contrast-enhanced parenchyma (Fig. 10-7). Small intraparenchymal hematomas are commonly called *contusions.*
- *Lacerations.* Lacerations are jagged linear defects in organ tissue that are defined by lower density blood within the laceration (Fig. 10-8). Most lacerations extend through the organ capsule and are associated with hemoperitoneum.

- *Shattered organs.* Shattered organs are disrupted by multiple lacerations (Fig. 10-9). They are frequently associated with multiple infracted segments of parenchyma. Portions of enhancing and nonenhancing organ parenchyma may be widely dispersed by hematoma.
- *Absence of parenchymal enhancement.* This is an indication of loss of vascular supply (Fig. 10-10). The supplying artery may be lacerated or thrombosed. The entire

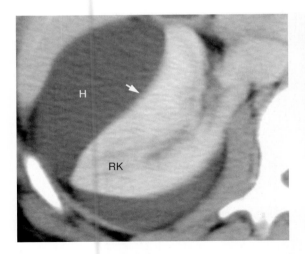

FIGURE 10-6 **Subcapsular hematoma.** The contour *(arrow)* of the right kidney (RK) is compressed and distorted by a hematoma (H) confined within the restricted space bounded by the renal capsule. This finding is indicative of subcapsular location of the hematoma.

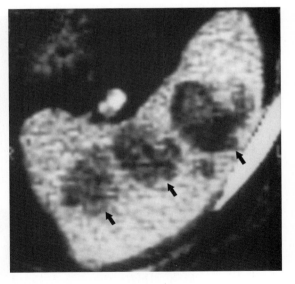

FIGURE 10-7 **Intraparenchymal hematomas.** Multiple intraparenchymal hematomas *(arrows)* are seen as low-attenuation defects within the splenic parenchyma.

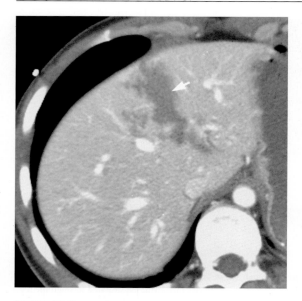

FIGURE 10-8 **Liver laceration.** Traumatic laceration *(arrow)* of the liver is seen as a jagged low-density defect with the enhanced liver parenchyma. Blood and fluid within the laceration are responsible for the low attenuation of the laceration.

organ, or only a portion of the organ, may be affected.

- *Infarctions.* Infarctions are seen as sharply demarcated, often wedge-shaped areas of decreased contrast enhancement that extend to the organ capsule (Fig. 10-11). Infarctions are caused by thrombosis or lacerations of segmental arteries.

Spleen Trauma

The spleen is the most frequently injured abdominal organ. Current management strives to avoid splenectomy. Patients who undergo splenectomy have a significantly increased risk for infection and overwhelming sepsis. Patients who are hemodynamically stable may be treated conservatively with close observation. *Delayed rupture of the spleen* may occur up to 10 days after trauma. Delayed rupture is associated with low-grade splenic injuries including intraparenchymal and subcapsular hematomas. Surgery is reserved for patients who have active bleeding, large nonperfused portions of the spleen, or who have formed pseudoaneurysms. Up to 40% of patients with splenic injury have associated left lower rib fractures. Extraperitoneal hemorrhage may be present in association with splenic injury and intraperitoneal hemorrhage. Blood tracks into the anterior pararenal space along the splenic vessels and pancreas. With rapid bolus administration of intravenous contrast and the rapid scanning of multislice CT, early irregular enhancement of the spleen (Fig. 10-12) is a common normal finding. Contrast diffuses relatively slowly through the pulp of the spleen. These defects in enhancement must not be mistaken for splenic abnormalities. Delayed images will demonstrate uniform splenic enhancement.

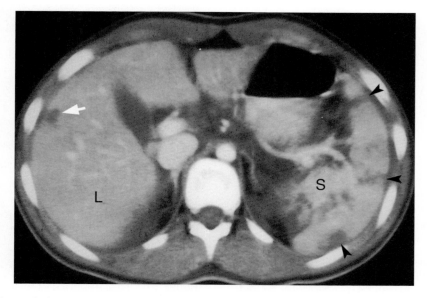

FIGURE 10-9 **Shattered spleen.** Multiple lacerations *(black arrows)* are seen as jagged defects in the parenchyma of the spleen (S). A focal laceration *(white arrow)* of the liver (L) is also evident.

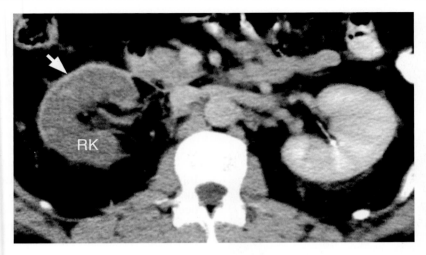

FIGURE 10-10 **Renal pedicle injury.** The right kidney (RK) shows a diffuse lack of enhancement compared with the left kidney. Failure of an organ to enhance with intravenous contrast is evidence of injury to the vascular supply. In this case, the right left renal artery thrombosed because of a traumatic tear of the intima. Faint enhancement of the periphery of the kidney is seen demonstrating the cortical rim sign *(arrow)*. Arteries supplying the renal capsule do not arise from the main renal artery, and thus remain patent when the main renal artery is occluded. These capsular branches provide blood supply to a thin rim of peripheral cortex.

Liver Trauma

The liver is the second most commonly injured abdominal organ. However, liver laceration is associated with twice the morbidity of spleen laceration. Up to 45% of patients with liver injury also have spleen injury. When the liver capsule is intact, the liver will usually heal within 1 to 6 months. Liver lacerations tend to parallel the course of the hepatic arteries. For example,

- *Periportal low attenuation* (Fig. 10-13) may be found with blood tracking adjacent to portal vessels or with dilated periportal lymphatics associated with increased central venous pressure caused by vigorous fluid resuscitation. Injuries to the biliary tree or intrahepatic lymphatic system are additional causes of periportal low attenuation. This nonspecific finding does not preclude nonsurgical management of liver trauma.

- Diffuse, fatty infiltration makes identification of lacerations and hematoma more difficult. Hematomas may appear high in density rather than low in density relative to enhanced liver parenchyma.

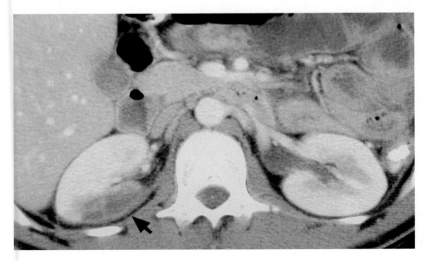

FIGURE 10-11 **Renal infarction.** A wedge-shaped portion *(arrow)* of the right kidney fails to enhance. This is evidence of renal infarction resulting from occlusion or tear of a renal artery branch. The left kidney enhances normally.

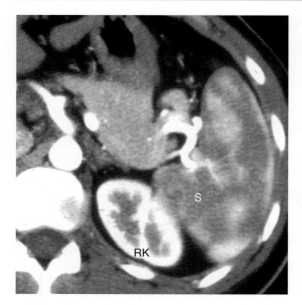

FIGURE 10-12 **Early mottled enhancement of the spleen.** Multislice CT image obtained during arterial enhancement shows irregular enhancement of the splenic parenchyma (S) caused by normal diffusion of contrast through the splenic pulp. Compare with the image of the shattered spleen in Figure 10-9. RK, right kidney.

• Delayed complications affect up to 20% of liver injuries. Bile in liver hematomas delay healing and may result in bilomas. Vascular injury may result in pseudoaneurysms or arterioportal fistulas. Mass effect of bilomas or hematomas may cause obstructive jaundice.

Pancreas Trauma

Injury to the pancreas is uncommon but carries a high morbidity rate and is frequently clinically occult. Penetrating trauma (e.g., knife and gunshot wounds) causes most (75%) pancreatic injuries. Blunt abdominal trauma, often associated with child abuse, is the most common cause of pancreatitis in children. The body of the pancreas is compressed against the spine and is prone to contusion, laceration (Fig. 10-14), transection, pancreatitis, and focal hemorrhagic necrosis. CT findings in pancreas trauma include:

• Tissue displacement may be minimal, making pancreatic lacerations difficult to identify. Fluid tracking adjacent to the splenic vein,

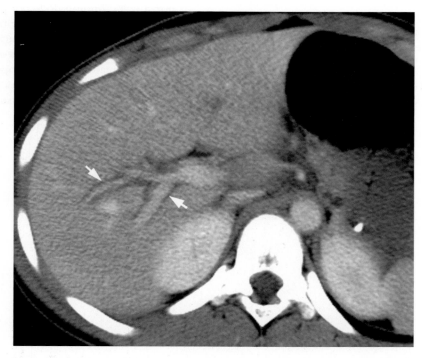

FIGURE 10-13 **Periportal low attenuation.** Trauma CT image of a 10-year-old child shows linear low attenuation *(arrows)* adjacent to the enhancing portal veins. A careful search must be made for additional evidence of liver laceration. In this case, the periportal low attenuation was caused by aggressive intravenous hydration.

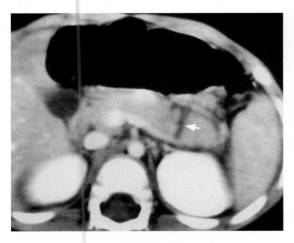

FIGURE 10-14 **Pancreas laceration.** Trauma CT of a 2-year-old girl shows a laceration *(arrow)* extending between the body and the tail of the pancreas.

unexplained thickening of the anterior renal fascia, and fluid in the lesser sac or anterior pararenal space are CT clues to possible pancreatic injury. The sensitivity of CT for pancreatic injury is reported to be 67% to 90%.

- Complications of traumatic injury to the pancreas are common with mortality rates as high as 20%. Complications include pseudocyst formation, hemorrhagic pancreatitis, abscess, and fistula.

Bowel and Mesentery Trauma

Injuries to the bowel and mesentery occur in about 5% of patients after blunt abdominal trauma. CT findings associated with these injuries are often subtle and are easily overlooked. Accuracy of CT in diagnosis of bowel and mesentery injuries is reported to be 77% to 93%. CT findings of bowel and mesentery trauma include:

- As mentioned earlier, free intraperitoneal air and oral contrast are highly suggestive but not specific signs of bowel injury. Many cases of bowel injury lack these findings.
- Hemoperitoneum in the absence of detected solid organ injury should promote a diligent search for subtle abnormalities of the bowel and mesentery. Fluid between bowel loops is highly suggestive of bowel injury.
- Focal mesenteric hematoma (Fig. 10-15) in association with focal thickening of the bowel wall indicates a high likelihood of significant bowel injury requiring surgery.
- Focal mesenteric hematoma without focal thickening of the bowel wall is a nonspecific finding associated with lesions that require surgery, as well as those that do not. Isolated mesenteric hematoma does not require surgery.
- Thickening of the bowel wall may be circumferential or eccentric (Fig. 10-16). High-density hematoma within the bowel

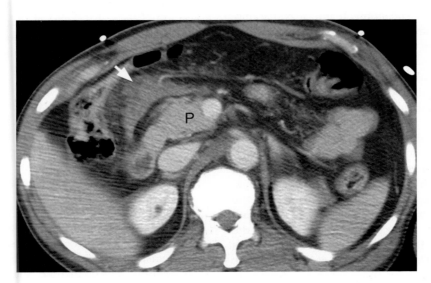

FIGURE 10-15 **Mesenteric hematoma.** A focal hematoma *(arrow)* in the mesentery is seen as an amorphous density enveloping mesenteric blood vessels. The head of the pancreas (P) is seen adjacent to the hematoma. In this case, the mesenteric hematoma was an isolated injury.

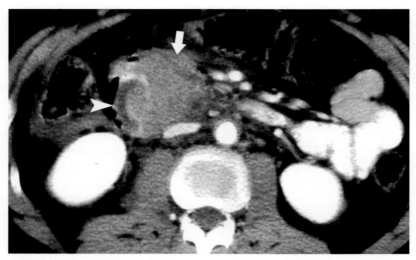

FIGURE 10-16 **Torn duodenum.** The descending duodenum is filleted open by an extended longitudinal tear. A large hematoma *(arrow)* occupies its lumen and extends around retroperitoneal vessels. The duodenal wall *(arrowhead)* is thickened. This is a retroperitoneal injury without hemoperitoneum.

wall is highly indicative of bowel injury. Wall thickening of more than 3 mm with the lumen well distended is considered to be abnormal.

- Intense enhancement of the bowel wall associated with bowel wall thickening and free intraperitoneal fluid is strongly indicative of bowel perforation and peritonitis.

- Retroperitoneal air or oral contrast is highly indicative of laceration of the duodenum.

- Wall thickening of the transverse duodenum is highly indicative of intramural duodenal hematoma. The stomach and proximal duodenum may be obstructed.

- Laceration or transection of the jejunum or ileum results in peritonitis and dilated small bowel within about 12 hours. Free air is seen in only about 50% of cases. Subtle findings include focal wall thickening and sentinel clot.

- Colonic injury may result in intraperitoneal or extraperitoneal findings.

- *Shock bowel* results from severe hypotension and hypoperfusion in trauma patients. CT findings include diffuse dilatation of the small bowel with wall thickening and increased contrast enhancement of the bowel wall (Fig. 10-17). The colon remains normal. The inferior vena cava is flattened, and the kidneys show intense contrast enhancement of the parenchyma.

- Fluid overload resulting from aggressive fluid resuscitation may cause diffuse edema of the small bowel wall associated with dilatation of the inferior vena cava, periportal edema, and normal enhancement of the bowel wall and renal parenchyma.

Renal Trauma

The kidneys are injured in 8% to 10% of patients with blunt trauma abdominal injuries. Minor injuries are most common (75% to 85%) and are managed without surgery. Minor injuries include contusions, subcapsular hematomas, and minor lacerations with limited perinephric hematomas, and small cortical infarcts. Hematuria is frequently present with minor renal injuries.

- Injury to the renal collecting system is diagnosed on delayed images by extravasation of contrast-opacified urine into the renal sinus and medial perirenal space (Fig. 10-18). Deep renal lacerations may be associated with urine leakage into the lateral perirenal space. Urinary extravasation will heal spontaneously as long as there is no obstruction to antegrade urine flow. Obstruction requires stent placement or surgical repair.

- Catastrophic injuries require surgical intervention. These include shattered kidneys and injuries to the renal vascular pedicle.

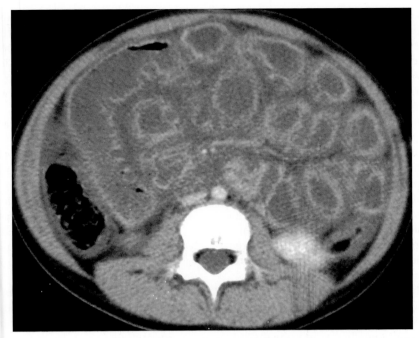

FIGURE 10-17 **Shock bowel.** CT image of the mid abdomen of a 7-year-old girl injured in a motor vehicle collision shows diffuse distension of small bowel with striking enhancement of the bowel wall. The small-bowel lumen is filled with fluid, and ascites is present.

Shattered kidneys (Fig. 10-19) have multiple lacerations, severe impairment of contrast excretion, extensive hemorrhage, lacerations of the renal collecting system with urine leakage, and often active arterial bleeding. Devitalized segments of kidney may be present.

- Thrombosis of the main renal artery is caused by stretching of the renal pedicle

with tearing of the intima, which is less elastic than the media and adventitia. The intimal flap initiates thrombosis, which propagates distally. The entire kidney, or a segmental portion of the kidney, fails to enhance (see Fig. 10-10). Abrupt termination of the renal artery may be visualized

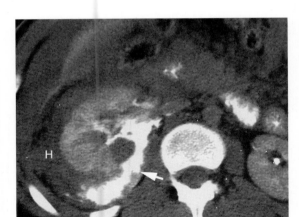

FIGURE 10-18 **Tear of the renal collecting system.** Delayed image through the right kidney shows extravasation of contrast *(arrow)* from the renal pelvis into the perirenal space already distended with blood (H) and urine. Early postcontrast images showed no early contrast extravasation, excluding active bleeding.

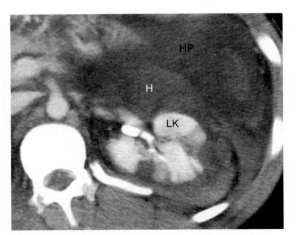

FIGURE 10-19 **Shattered kidney.** The left kidney (LK) demonstrates multiple lacerations and foci of parenchyma that does not enhance indicating devascularization. A large perirenal hematoma (H) is present. Hemoperitoneum (HP) caused by a spleen laceration is also evident. This severely damaged kidney was removed.

with high-quality helical CT. Most occlusions occur in the proximal 2 cm of the renal artery. This injury usually occurs in the absence of perirenal hematoma. The *cortical rim sign* is a delayed finding of renal arterial occlusion, appearing several days after the acute renal artery thrombosis (see Fig. 10-10). Only the periphery of the kidney, supplied by collaterals to the renal capsule, enhances. The bulk of the kidney supplied by the renal artery, which lacks collateral pathways, does not enhance.

- Avulsion of the renal artery is rare and usually results in the patient's death. Patients with avulsion who survive to be examined have absent renal enhancement and large perinephric hematomas and may show arterial extravasation.

- Ureteropelvic junction injuries are caused by sudden deceleration, which tears the ureteropelvic junction. Urinomas are seen medially or occasionally surrounding the kidney, but no perinephric hematoma is usually present. Complete transections show contrast in the renal pelvis but not in the distal ureter. Ureteropelvic junction lacerations are characterized by visualization of contrast in both the renal pelvis and the distal ureter. Absence of CT visualization of contrast in the ureter is an indication for retrograde pyelography.

Bladder Trauma

Rupture of the bladder occurs in up to 10% of patients with pelvic fractures. In most patients (80%), the bladder is lacerated by a spicule of fractured bone, and urine (and contrast) leaks into extraperitoneal spaces. Rupture of the bladder into the peritoneal cavity (20%) occurs as a result of a blow to the lower abdomen when the bladder is distended. The sudden increase in intracystic pressure ruptures the bladder at its dome, resulting in leakage of urine into the peritoneal cavity. Both types of bladder rupture are effectively demonstrated by CT after contrast administration either intravenously or by bladder catheter. However, the bladder must be distended to at least a volume of 250 cc to reliably demonstrate small ruptures. CT indications of bladder trauma include:

- The presence of free fluid or hematoma in the pelvis, or fractures of the pubic rami,

sacrum, or ileum suggests possible bladder injury. CT cystography should be considered.

- *Extraperitoneal bladder rupture* is characterized by contrast leakage into the retropubic space with extension along fascial planes into the abdominal wall, scrotum, thigh, and retroperitoneum. The contrast collections tend to be linear and poorly defined.

- *Intraperitoneal bladder rupture* is characterized by contrast leakage into the peritoneal cavity surrounding loops of bowel and extending along the paracolic gutters. The contrast collections are sharply defined by visceral and parietal peritoneum.

- Combined extraperitoneal and intraperitoneal ruptures occur in about 5% of patients (Fig. 10-20).

- *Bladder contusions* appear as focal areas of thickening of the bladder wall. Hemorrhage in the bladder wall may produce focal high attenuation.

- *Urethral injuries* should be suspected in patients with pelvic fractures, bladder injuries, and pelvic hematomas. Clinical findings include blood at the urethral meatus and inability to void. Urethral injuries are diagnosed by retrograde urethrogram.

Adrenal Trauma

Hemorrhage into the adrenal gland is seen in about 2% of adults with severe trauma. Post-traumatic hemorrhage has a striking propensity to involve the right adrenal gland (90% of patients). The predilection for the right adrenal gland has been attributed to compression of the gland between the liver and spine. Hemorrhage is bilateral in 25% of cases. Bilateral hemorrhage places the patient at risk for development of adrenal insufficiency. CT indications of adrenal trauma include:

- Acute hemorrhage produces a hyperdense (50–75 H) round-to-oval mass replacing the affected adrenal gland (Fig. 10-21).

- Fat adjacent to the adrenal gland is infiltrated with streaks of soft-tissue density representing bleeding into the periadrenal fat.

- The hemorrhage decreases in density and shrinks over time. Calcifications may develop in the gland within a few months.

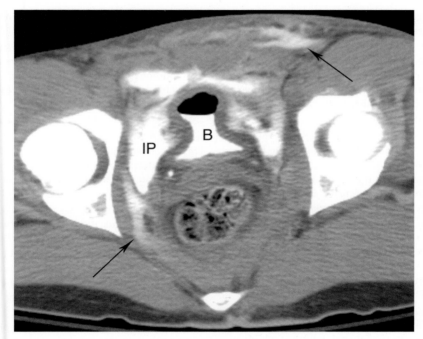

FIGURE 10-20 **Intraperitoneal and extraperitoneal bladder rupture.** CT cystogram demonstrates free spill of contrast from the bladder (B) into the peritoneal cavity (IP) and extraperitoneal spaces *(arrows)*.

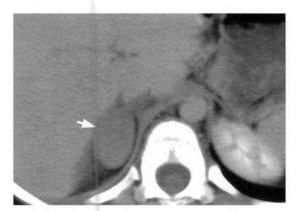

FIGURE 10-21 **Adrenal hemorrhage.** A solid mass *(arrow)* replaces the right adrenal gland in a patient with multiple injuries from a motor vehicle accident. Follow-up CT confirmed the return of the right adrenal gland to a normal appearance.

▢ SUGGESTED READING

BODE PJ, EDWARDS MJR, KRUIT MC, VAN VUGT AB: Sonography in a clinical algorithm for early evaluation of 1671 patients with blunt abdominal trauma. AJR Am J Roentgenol 172:905–911, 1999.

BRODY JM, LEIGHTON DB, MURPHY BL, et al: CT of blunt trauma bowel and mesenteric injury: Typical findings and pitfalls in diagnosis. Radiographics 20:1525–1536, 2000.

BUTELA ST, FEDERLE MP, CHANG PJ, et al: Performance of CT in detection of bowel injury. AJR Am J Roentgenol 176:129–135, 2001.

CERNIGLIARO J, SIRAGUSA D, PRESLEY J, et al: A review of gastrointestinal and pancreatic injuries. Radiologist 6:163–171, 1999.

CLANCY TV, RAGOZZINO MW, RAMSHAW D, et al: Oral contrast is not necessary in the evaluation of blunt abdominal trauma by computed tomography. Am J Surg 166:680–685, 1993.

DONNELLY LF, FRUSH DP, O'HARA SM, et al: CT appearance of clinically occult abdominal hemorrhage in children. AJR Am J Roentgenol 170: 1073–1076, 1998.

DOWE MF, SHANMUGANATHAN K, MIRVIS SE, et al: CT findings of mesenteric injury after blunt trauma: Implications for surgical intervention. AJR Am J Roentgenol 168:425–428, 1997.

HARRIS A, ZWIREWICH C, LYBURN I, et al: CT findings in blunt renal trauma. Radiographics 21: S201–S214, 2001.

KAWASHIMA A, SANDLER CM, CORL FM, et al: Imaging of renal trauma: A comprehensive review. Radio-Graphics 21:557–574, 2001.

KULZER LM, DECARVALHO VL, EPSTEIN RE: Helical CT evaluation of traumatic bowel and mesenteric injuries. Radiologist 9:55–61, 2002.

LANE MJ, KATZ DS, SHAH RA, et al: Active arterial contrast extravasation on helical CT of the abdomen, pelvis, and chest. AJR Am J Roentgenol 171:679–685, 1998.

LEVINE CD, PATEL UJ, SILVERMAN PM, WACHSBERG RH: Low attenuation of acute traumatic hemoperitoneum on CT scans. AJR Am J Roentgenol 166:1089–1093, 1996.

MCGAHAN J, RICHARDS J, GILLEN M: The focused abdominal sonography for trauma scan. J Ultrasound Med 2002:789–800, 2002.

MIRVIS S, SHANMUGANATHAN K, ERB R: Diffuse small-bowel ischemia in hypotensive adults after blunt trauma (shock bowel): CT findings and clinical significance. AJR Am J Roentgenol 163: 1375–1379, 1994.

MORGAN DE, NALLAMALA LK, KENNEY PJ, et al: CT cystography: Radiographic and clinical predictors of bladder rupture. AJR Am J Roentgenol 174: 89–95, 2000.

NEISH AS, TAYLOR GA, LUND DP, ATKINSON CC: Effect of CT information on the diagnosis and management of acute abdominal injury in children. Radiology 206:327–331, 1998.

ORWIG D, FEDERLE MP: Localized clotted blood as evidence of visceral trauma on CT: The sentinel clot sign. AJR Am J Roentgenol 153:747–749, 1989.

PAO DM, ELLIS JH, COHAN RH, KOROBKIN M: Utility of routine trauma CT in the detection of bladder rupture. Acad Radiol 7:317–324, 2000.

PATRICK EL, TURNER BI, ATKINSON GO, WINN KJ: Pediatric blunt abdominal trauma: Periportal tracking at CT. Radiology 183:689–691, 1992.

PENG MY, PARISKY YR, CORNWELL EE III, et al: CT cystography versus conventional cystography in evaluation of bladder injury. AJR Am J Roentgenol 173:1269–1272, 1999.

SHANMUGANATHAN K, MIRVIS SE, AMEROSA M: Periportal low density on CT in patients with blunt abdominal trauma: Association with elevated venous pressure. AJR Am J Roentgenol 160: 279–283, 1992.

SHUMAN WP: CT of blunt abdominal trauma in adults. Radiology 205:297–306, 1997.

SIVIT CJ, FRAZIER AA, EICHELBERGER MR: Prevalence and distribution of extraperitoneal hemorrhage associated with splenic injury in children. AJR Am J Roentgenol 172:1015–1017, 1999.

STROUSE PJ, CLOSE BJ, MARSHALL KW, CYWES R: CT of bowel and mesenteric injuries in children. Radiographics 19:1237–1250, 1999.

TSANG BD, PANACEK EA, BRANT WE, WISNER DH: Effect of oral contrast administration for abdominal computed tomography in the evaluation of acute blunt trauma. Ann Emerg Med 30:7–13, 1997.

VACCARO JP, BRODY JM: CT cystography in the evaluation of major bladder trauma. Radiographics 20:1373–1381, 2000.

WILLMANN J, ROOS J, PLATZ A, et al: Multidetector CT: Detection of active hemorrhage in patients with blunt abdominal trauma. AJR Am J Roentgenol 179:437–444, 2002.

YAO D, JEFFREY R Jr, MIRVIS S, et al: Using contrast-enhanced helical CT to visualize arterial extravasation after blunt abdominal trauma: Incidence and organ distribution. AJR Am J Roentgenol 178: 17–20, 2002.

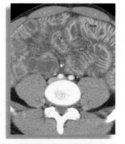

Liver

William E. Brant, M.D.

□ ANATOMY

The Couinaud (pronounced "kwee-NO") International Classification System divides the liver into eight independent segments (Fig. 11-1; Table 11-1). Each segment is a self-contained unit that can be surgically resected without damaging the remainder of the liver. Each segment has its own dual vascular inflow (hepatic artery and portal vein), its own biliary drainage, and a shared vascular outflow (hepatic veins). The portal triads (bile ducts, hepatic arteries, and portal veins) course through the center of each segment, whereas the hepatic veins define the periphery of the segment and the plane of surgical dissection. This segmental anatomy provides a useful and widely accepted method for identification of the location of lesions seen on CT and other imaging studies.

The right, middle, and left hepatic veins enter the intrahepatic inferior vena cava (IVC) just before it pierces the diaphragm about 2 cm below the right atrium. Whereas the right hepatic vein usually enters the IVC separately, the middle and left hepatic veins often (65% to 85%) form a common trunk before joining the IVC. In most patients, these three major hepatic veins drain the entirety of the liver except for the caudate lobe. Short hepatic veins drain the cau-

date lobe separately directly into the IVC. As an anatomic variant, accessory hepatic veins drain segments V or VI independently into the IVC.

The portal vein is formed by the junction of the splenic vein with the superior mesenteric vein just anterior to the IVC and just posterior to the neck of the pancreas. It ascends behind the duodenum in company with the hepatic artery and common bile duct to the porta hepatis where it divides into a short, fat, right portal vein and a longer, thinner, left portal vein.

The hepatic artery has variable anatomy. In its "classic" form (55%), the right and left hepatic arteries branch from a proper hepatic artery that is a continuation of the common hepatic artery arising from the celiac axis. In 10% of individuals, the left hepatic artery arises as a branch of the left gastric artery. In 11% of individuals, the right hepatic artery arises from the superior mesenteric artery. In this case, the "replaced" right hepatic artery passes through the portocaval space from the superior mesenteric artery to the right hepatic lobe.

Division of the liver into eight segments is based on a concept of three vertical planes and one transverse plane. A vertical plane through the middle hepatic vein, IVC, and gallbladder fossa divides the liver into right and left lobes. A vertical plane through the right hepatic vein divides the right lobe into anterior (VII and V) and posterior (VII and VI) segments. A vertical plane through the left hepatic vein divides the left lobe into medial (IVa and IVb) and lateral (II and III) segments. A transverse plane through the left portal vein divides the left lobe into superior (IVa and II) and inferior (IVb and III) segments. An oblique transverse plane through

the right portal vein divides the right lobe into superior (VIII and VII) and inferior (V and VI) segments (see Table 11-1).

Segment I is the caudate lobe, which is separated from the rest of the liver by the fissure of the ligamentum venosum anteriorly and the IVC posterolaterally. It is supplied by branches of both right and left hepatic arteries and portal

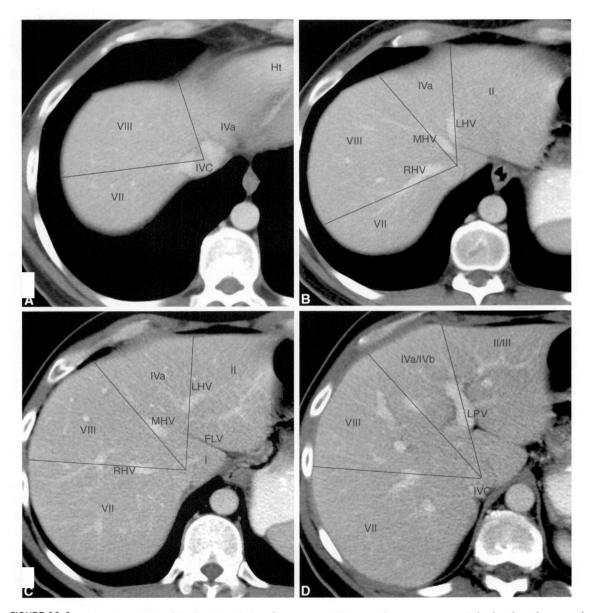

FIGURE 11-1 **Anatomic segments of the liver.** *A–I,* Series of postcontrast CT images demonstrate anatomic landmarks and segmental anatomy of the liver. Segments are labeled I through VIII. The vertical planes defined by the right (RHV), middle (MHV), and left (LHV) hepatic veins are shown as straight lines. Other key landmarks are identified. *Black arrowhead* indicates posterior branch of the right portal vein (RPV); *white arrowhead* indicates anterior branch of the RPV. This patient has had a cholecystectomy. Note the difficulty of applying straight geometric planes to curving vessels. FLT, fissure of the ligamentum teres; FLV, fissure of the ligamentum venosum; GBF, gallbladder fossa; Ht, heart; IVC, inferior vena cava; LPV, left portal vein; MPV, main portal vein.

Continued

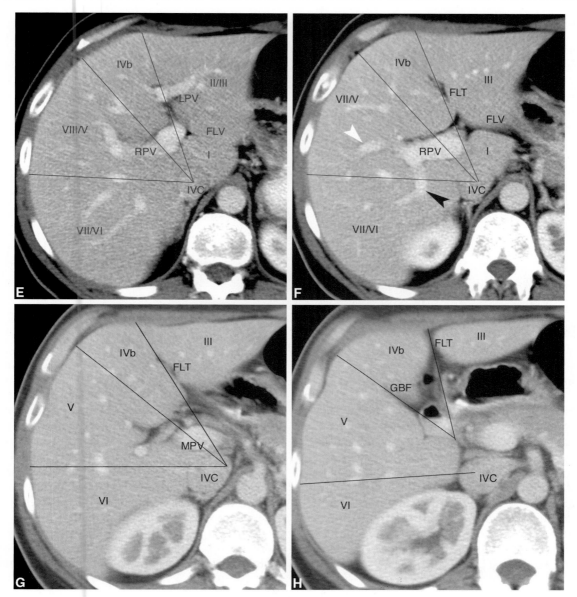

FIGURE 11-1 Cont'd   *Continued*

veins and drains venous blood directly into the IVC by numerous small hepatic veins. The papillary process of the caudate lobe extends toward the lesser sac and may appear separate from the rest of the caudate lobe, simulating a mass or enlarged lymph node.

Segments II and *III* make up the lateral division of the left lobe. The plane of the left portal vein divides segments II and III. Segment II makes up the left superior and lateral contour of the liver. Segment III makes up the left inferior and lateral contour of the liver. *Segment IV* makes up the medial division of the left lobe.

The plane of the left portal vein divides the medial segment of the left lobe into segments IVa (superior) and IVb (inferior). Segment IV was previously called the quadrate lobe.

The anterior segments (V and VIII) of the right lobe are separated from the posterior segments (VI and VII) by the plane of the right hepatic vein. The lateral contour of the anterior right lobe is formed by *segment VIII* superiorly and *segment V* inferiorly. *Segment VII* lies posterior to segment VIII, and *segment VI* lies posterior to segment V. The plane of the right portal vein separates anterior segment VIII from

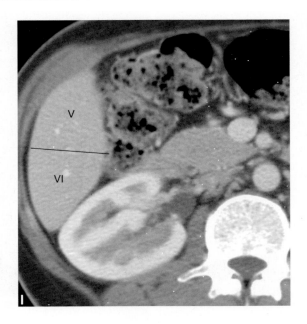

FIGURE 11-1 Cont'd

segment V and separates posterior segment VII from segment VI.

Unfortunately, natural anatomic variation in blood supply does not adhere perfectly to the concept of flat geometric planes dividing the segments (Fasel and colleagues, 1998). In reality, the vascular territorial boundaries between segments have more variable and curving undulations to their borders than the concept of flat planes indicate. In addition, many three-dimensional drawings in the literature are misleading as to the location of the lobes. Segment VII is posterior to and hidden by segment VIII in a frontal projection, rather than lateral to

segment VIII as shown in some drawings. Likewise, segment VI is posterior, not lateral, to segment V. The axial images in Figure 11-1 are an attempt to localize the segments as demonstrated by CT. Correlate the anatomic description of the lobes in Table 11-1 with their location as shown in Figure 11-1 to learn the segments. Recognize that anatomic variation in blood supply makes localization of lesions to specific segments rather inaccurate. Also, many liver lesions will involve two or more segments.

Several fissures and ligaments deserve special mention either because they are particularly prominent or because they define important

TABLE 11-1

Nomenclature for Anatomic Segments of the Liver

Couinaud Segment	Anatomic Description	Traditional Nomenclature
I	Caudate lobe	Caudate lobe
		Left lobe
II	Left lateral superior subsegment	Lateral segment
III	Left lateral inferior subsegment	Lateral segment
IVa	Left medial superior subsegment	Medial segment
IVb	Left medial inferior subsegment	Medial segment
		Right lobe
V	Right anterior inferior subsegment	Anterior segment
VIII	Right anterior superior subsegment	Anterior segment
VI	Right posterior inferior subsegment	Posterior segment
VII	Right posterior superior subsegment	Posterior segment

perihepatic spaces. The falciform ligament consists of two closely applied layers of peritoneum extending from the umbilicus to the diaphragm in a parasagittal plane. The caudal free end of the falciform ligament contains the ligamentum teres, which is the remnant of the obliterated umbilical vein. The reflections of the falciform ligament separate over the posterior dome of the liver to form the coronary ligaments that define the "bare area" of the liver not covered by peritoneum. The coronary ligaments reflect between liver and diaphragm and prevent access of intraperitoneal fluid from covering the bare area of the liver. The absence of fluid over the bare area is an important sign in the differentiation of ascites from pleural effusion on CT. The remainder of the falciform ligament and ligamentum teres continues into the liver to form a prominent fat-filled fissure that defines the left intersegmental fissure dividing the medial and lateral segments of the left lobe.

The fissure of the ligamentum venosum contains the remnant of the ductus venosus, which in fetal life carried oxygenated blood from the umbilical vein to the IVC. This fissure is commonly fat filled and prominent on CT, separating the caudate lobe and the left lobe.

The lesser omentum suspends the lesser curve of the stomach and the duodenal bulb from the inferior surface of the liver, attaching within the fissure of the ligamentum venosum. The lesser omentum is subdivided into the gastrohepatic and the hepatoduodenal ligaments. The gastrohepatic ligament contains coronary veins that serve as an important sign of portal hypertension when they become dilated. The right free edge of the hepatoduodenal ligament carries the portal vein, hepatic artery, and common bile duct between the porta hepatis and the duodenum. The hepatoduodenal ligament provides the anterior border of the foramen of Winslow, which opens into the lesser sac.

The normal liver is homogeneous in attenuation, measuring 40 to 70 H on unenhanced CT. The unenhanced liver parenchymal density is normally greater than that of blood vessels and 7 to 8 H greater than splenic parenchyma. Anemia reduces the CT density of blood vessels and may make the liver parenchyma appear falsely increased in density. The contour of the liver is smooth and convex adjacent to the diaphragm with a sharp inferior border and a concave undersurface. Fissures may be fat filled and prominent. The right lobe is usually larger than the left lobe

and may extend far caudad as a Riedel's lobe. The left lobe is more variable in size, and its lateral segment may extend far to the left and wrap partially around the spleen. Congenital absence of the left lobe is a rare anomaly. Diaphragmatic slips are infoldings of the diaphragm that indent the normal smooth contour of the liver (Fig. 11-2). These invaginations of diaphragmatic muscle occur with increasing frequency with age older than 60 years and should not be mistaken for masses in the liver or on the diaphragm.

☐ TECHNICAL CONSIDERATIONS

Multidetector CT allows scanning of the entire liver with thin collimation during a single 10- to 25-second breath hold. Acquisition is routinely repeated several times during various phases of contrast medium enhancement.

Dynamic contrast-enhanced liver CT offers the opportunity to accurately characterize lesion enhancement patterns and significantly improve the specificity of diagnosis. Various lesions are detected best, or sometimes only, in specific phases of postcontrast scanning. Intravenous contrast is administered by power injector using a contrast concentration of 300 mg I/mL at a rate of 2.5 to 4 mL/second for a volume of 100 to 150 mL. Routine scan delays for multidetector CT are 25 seconds after initiation of contrast injection for arterial phase and 65 seconds after initiation of contrast injection for portal venous phase. With multidetector CT, images are routinely acquired at 1.25- to 2.50-mm collimation but are viewed at 5-mm slice thickness. Enhancement of the normal liver is homogeneous throughout the parenchyma on all enhancement phases. For example,

- *Noncontrast scans* are commonly obtained to provide a baseline for degree of lesion enhancement. Many liver lesions are detected, but small lesions are often mistaken for unopacified vessels. Noncontrast scans are superior to postcontrast scans for diagnosis of fatty infiltration and other alterations of parenchymal attenuation.
- *Arterial phase* acquisition is optimal for visualization of hypervascular lesions supplied by the hepatic artery such as hepatoma, carcinoid metastases, and focal nodular hyperplasia. Lesions are conspicuous because

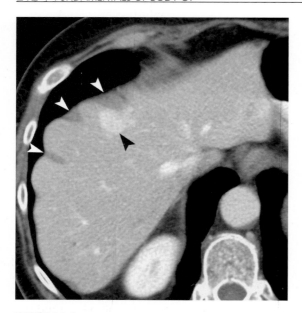

FIGURE 11-2 **Diaphragmatic slips.** Folds in the diaphragm *(white arrowheads)* in this 78-year-old woman create defects in the liver. These diaphragmatic slips are more common in older patients. They are recognized by their peripheral location and characteristic linear appearance. An enhancing hemangioma *(black arrowhead)* is partially visualized.

they enhance more than the surrounding parenchyma. A variety of perfusion abnormalities are seen only on arterial phase images.

- *Portal venous phase* imaging shows the overall best lesion detection because parenchymal enhancement is maximum during this phase. Lesions are conspicuous because they are low in attenuation within a background of maximally enhanced liver parenchyma.
- *Equilibrium phase* occurs at 2 to 3 minutes after initiation of contrast injection. During equilibrium phase, the concentration of contrast agent is approximately equal between the intravascular and extravascular spaces, rendering most liver lesions invisible.
- *Delayed phase* images, acquired 10 to 20 minutes after contrast injection, are to demonstrate delayed contrast fill-in of hemangiomas and to detect fibrotic tumors such as cholangiocarcinoma.

☐ LIVER HEMODYNAMICS AND PERFUSION ABNORMALITIES

The liver has a distinctive dual blood supply with ~25% of its blood volume normally coming from the hepatic artery and ~75% arriving from

the portal vein. Although this distribution holds for the liver as a whole, this distribution pattern is not uniform throughout the liver. Alterations in arterial and venous supply to portions of the liver result in transient perfusion abnormalities that are demonstrated on postcontrast CT. Some perfusion abnormalities result from transient conditions, whereas others are congenital or chronic conditions that cause metabolic alterations in the liver resulting in abnormalities such as focal steatosis or focal sparing in diffuse fatty liver. Temporary conditions that may cause transient perfusion abnormalities include compression of the liver capsule by ribs or by infoldings of the diaphragm (slips) during breath hold for CT. Variations in vascular supply, termed *third inflow,* are chronic conditions that may result in focal metabolic changes in the liver parenchyma. Third inflow refers to small areas of the liver that are supplied by aberrant systemic veins, in addition to the usual hepatic artery and portal venous supply.

Perfusion defects usually represent an increase of arterial blood flow to a portion of the liver in response to a decrease in portal venous flow. In most cases, the perfusion abnormality manifests as increased enhancement of a segment or subsegment of the liver during arterial phase with normal parenchymal enhancement during portal venous phase. When the blood flow anomaly is persistent, the metabolic abnormality manifests as focal steatosis or focal fatty sparing. Most perfusion disorders are asymptomatic but must be recognized to avoid mistaking them for significant lesions.

Third inflow by systemic veins causes perfusion abnormalities in predictable areas of the liver, which thus are relatively easy to recognize. Systemic veins communicate with portal venous branches to focally decrease portal venous flow and cause an increase in hepatic arterial flow in the same area. These are prime areas for focal steatosis or focal sparing. For example,

- The liver parenchyma adjacent to the gallbladder in segments IV and V is sometimes supplied by the cholecystic vein draining the gallbladder.
- The dorsal aspect of segment IV adjacent to the porta hepatis may be supplied by the parabiliary veins draining the distal stomach and head of the pancreas.

- The anterior aspect of segments IV and III adjacent to the fissure of the ligamentum teres is often supplied by the epigastric-paraumbilical veins draining blood from the anterior abdominal wall directly into the liver (Fig. 11-3). This venous plexus may be enlarged and prominently visualized on CT when obstruction to either the superior vena cava or IVC is present. In portal hypertension, these collaterals are enlarged and blood flow may reverse to drain out of, rather than into, the liver.

Extrinsic compression of the liver capsule causes low-attenuation defects with the following features:

- A poorly marginated low-attenuation defect is seen during portal venous phase beneath a concave indentation of the liver capsule.
- No abnormalities are seen in the same area on unenhanced, arterial phase, equilibrium phase, or delayed images.
- The offending ribs or diaphragmatic slips are evident. Metastatic disease on the peritoneal surface of the liver and subcapsular fluid collections may cause similar perfusion findings.

Tumors may affect perfusion in adjacent liver parenchyma in several ways, including:

- Hypervascular tumors may have intratumoral arterioportal shunts. These produce transient, peripheral, wedge-shaped enhancement zones during arterial phase in the parenchyma peripheral to the tumor and early enhancement of peripheral portal vein branches before the main portal vein is enhanced. The peripheral enhancement may be mistaken for additional tumor, resulting in overestimation of tumor size.
- Tumor invasion, compression, or induced thrombosis may obstruct the portal vein. This results in decreased attenuation of affected parenchyma on noncontrast scans because of edema and in transient increased enhancement during arterial phase because of increased arterial flow (Fig. 11-4). Thrombi may be seen in portal veins.
- Hypervascular tumors, such as large hepatocellular carcinomas (HCCs), may parasitize and enlarge regional hepatic arteries. The tumor may either "steal" blood from adjacent parenchyma or cause increased arterial blood flow to adjacent parenchyma. Thus, on arterial phase, parenchyma adjacent to large hypervascular tumors may show either increased or decreased enhancement.

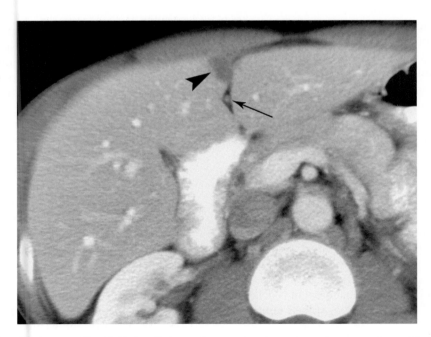

FIGURE 11-3 **Pseudolesion caused by third inflow.** Early portal venous phase image shows a low-attenuation nodular focus *(arrowhead)* adjacent to the fissure of the ligamentum teres *(arrow)*. This should be recognized as a common pseudolesion related to third inflow. The remnant of the falciform ligament is seen as a soft-tissue density within the fissure.

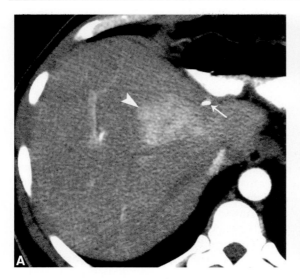 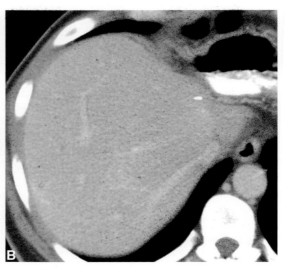

FIGURE 11-4 **Transient arterial perfusion abnormality.** *A,* Arterial phase image of the liver in a patient who has had a left hepatic lobectomy shows a poorly marginated area of bright arterial enhancement *(arrowhead).* Serial images showed no evidence of a mass in this region. A metallic staple *(arrow)* placed during surgery is noted. *B,* Portal venous phase image through same region shows normal parenchymal enhancement. This perfusion defect was believed to be caused by occlusion of portal venous branches to this area, resulting in a compensatory increase in hepatic arterial flow.

☐ DIFFUSE LIVER DISEASE

Fatty Liver

Fatty infiltration of the liver (steatosis) is one of the most common abnormalities diagnosed by liver CT. Fatty infiltration is a nonspecific response of hepatocytes to a variety of insults, including alcoholism, obesity, diabetes, chemotherapy, corticosteroid therapy, hyperalimentation, and malnutrition.

- *Fatty infiltration.* Fatty infiltration reduces the CT attenuation of the involved liver parenchyma. The findings are most accurately assessed on noncontrast CT. The normal liver attenuation is at least 10 H greater than that of the spleen. With fatty infiltration, involved liver is at least 10 H lower than that of the spleen. Hepatic vessels course through areas of fatty infiltration unchanged. Fatty change is more difficult to judge on postcontrast CT because of the variability of timing of the scan and the fact that maximum liver enhancement is delayed compared with maximum spleen enhancement.
- *Diffuse fatty infiltration.* In most cases, the entire liver is uniformly reduced in density (Fig. 11-5). Vessels stand out in prominent

relief but run their normal course through the liver without displacement by mass effect. The liver is usually enlarged, and the parenchyma enhances minimally. This pattern is the most common and is the easiest to recognize. In some cases, the fatty infiltration is diffuse throughout the liver but is nonuniform and patchy in severity.

- *Focal fatty infiltration.* A geographic or fan-shaped portion of the liver shows fat infiltration, whereas the remainder of the liver is of normal density (Fig. 11-6). The low density may extend to the liver surface, but no bulge in contour is seen. Vessels run their normal course through the area of involvement. Margins between fat-infiltrated and normal liver are frequently straight and well defined. Fat infiltration is confined to segments and subsegments. Areas of the liver supplied by third inflow systemic veins are commonly affected—adjacent to the gallbladder, the fissure of the ligamentum teres, and the porta hepatis.
- *Multifocal fatty infiltration.* Patchy areas of decreased attenuation are scattered through the liver (Fig. 11-7). Tumors may be simulated by the islands of fatty infiltration surrounded by normal parenchyma or by islands of normal parenchyma surrounded by fatty infiltration. The pattern

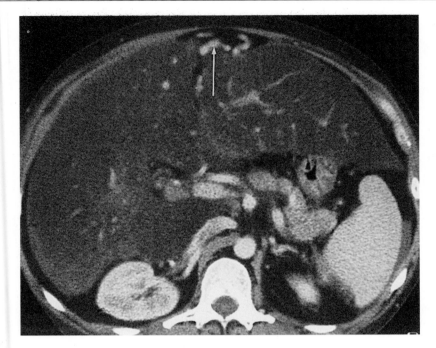

FIGURE 11-5 **Diffuse fatty infiltration.** The liver parenchyma is diffusely and markedly lower in density than the spleen parenchyma, indicating diffuse hepatocellular fatty infiltration. Enlarged paraumbilical veins *(arrow)* are evidence of portal hypertension.

tends to be geographic with straight margins, rather than rounded masses. Areas of involvement may interdigitate with normal parenchyma.

- *Focal sparing*. Islands of normal parenchyma are surrounded by large areas of diffuse fatty infiltration and may simulate neoplasms (Fig. 11-8). As mentioned earlier, the pattern of focal steatosis and focal sparing is related to chronic perfusion abnormalities such as systemic venous drainage into the liver. Focal sparing is most common in the same areas of the liver most often affected by focal steatosis.

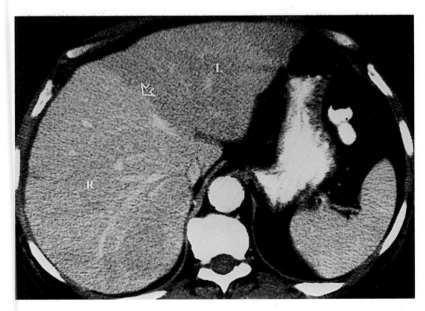

FIGURE 11-6 **Focal fatty infiltration.** The left lobe of the liver (L) is lower in density than the right lobe of the liver (R) and the spleen. A strikingly sharp boundary *(arrow)* separates the left and right lobes. This appearance is characteristic of focal fatty infiltration.

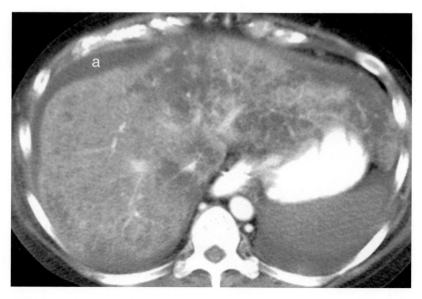

FIGURE 11-7 **Multifocal fatty infiltration.** Patchy areas of low-attenuation fatty infiltration permeate the liver parenchyma. The intrahepatic blood vessels follow a normal course without mass effect. Ascites (a) is present.

The following findings are most useful in making a confident diagnosis of fatty infiltration:

- Angulated geometric margins (nonspherical shape)
- Interdigitating margins with slender fingers of normal or fatty tissue
- Absence of mass effect or vessel displacement

- Rapid change over time; fatty changes can be seen within 3 weeks after the insult and can resolve within 6 days after removing the insult
- Further confirmation of fatty replacement can be provided by other imaging tests; ultrasonography will show the areas of fatty infiltration as corresponding areas of increased parenchymal echogenicity, which

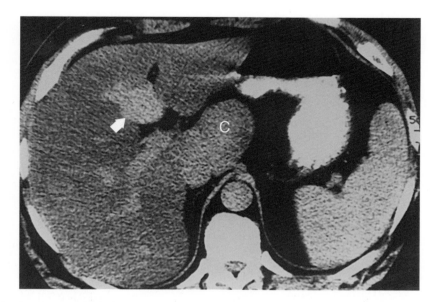

FIGURE 11-8 **Focal sparing.** An island of normal parenchyma *(arrow)*, in segment IVb, simulates a mass lesion in a liver with extensive fatty infiltration. The caudate lobe (C) is hypertrophied. The image is photographed with narrow "liver" windows to accentuate the findings.

gives rise to the "flip-flop" sign: fat is dark on CT and is bright on ultrasonography; chemical shift magnetic resonance with in-phase and out-of-phase images may demonstrate the presence of fat; percutaneous biopsy is an option in difficult cases.

Increased Liver Attenuation

Normal liver attenuation on unenhanced CT is 40 to 70 H and is at least 10 H greater than the attenuation of the spleen. Increased liver attenuation is usually in the range of 75 to 140 H. Portal and hepatic veins stand out as dark tubular structures in a background of bright liver parenchyma. Causes of increased liver attenuation include:

- Amiodarone is toxic to the liver and increases its attenuation by deposition of iodine-containing metabolites (Fig. 11-9).
- Hemochromatosis increases liver attenuation by deposition of iron. Primary hemochromatosis is characterized by increased intestinal absorption of iron with deposition of hemosiderin in hepatocytes and the parenchyma of the pancreas and other organs, eventually causing cellular injury and loss of function. In secondary hemochromatosis (also called hemosiderosis), iron overload from multiple blood transfusions is taken up by reticuloendothelial cells in the liver, spleen, and bone marrow. Hemochromatosis commonly progresses to cirrhosis. Magnetic resonance is excellent

for confirming the presence of iron excess in the liver.

Cirrhosis

Cirrhosis is a chronic diffuse liver disease characterized by progressive destruction of hepatocytes with distortion of hepatic architecture by extensive collagen deposition and nodular regeneration of liver tissue. The common forms of cirrhosis are Laënnec's caused by alcoholism, postnecrotic caused by various types of hepatitis and toxic injury to the liver, and biliary caused by chronic intrahepatic cholestasis. In Western countries, alcohol abuse causes 60% to 70% of cirrhosis cases. Patients with cirrhosis show the following CT findings:

- The liver may appear healthy on CT in the earliest stages of cirrhosis.
- Fatty infiltration with hepatomegaly is evidence of active hepatocyte injury.
- Heterogeneous parenchymal attenuation is caused by patchy fatty infiltration and irregular fibrosis (Fig. 11-10). Contrast enhancement is heterogeneous as well and accentuates the heterogeneous appearance of the liver tissue.
- The surface contour of the liver is irregular lobulated or finely nodular because of areas of atrophy and regenerative nodules.
- Atrophy of the right lobe with hypertrophy of the left and caudate lobes is common in alcoholic (Laënnec's) micronodular cirrhosis.
- With progressive cirrhosis, liver volume decreases and the liver becomes shrunken and deformed.
- The size and prominence of the porta hepatis and intrahepatic fissures increases because of atrophy of adjacent liver tissue.
- Ascites, splenomegaly, and other signs of portal hypertension are commonly present.
- Serous cysts may develop adjacent to intrahepatic and extrahepatic bile ducts. These peribiliary cysts may mimic biliary dilatation when present in a linear configuration. More typically they appear as a row of cysts with thin but visible cyst walls.
- Enlarged lymph nodes (>1 cm) are commonly seen in the porta hepatis and portocaval space in patients with end-stage cirrhosis. These are usually benign, are associated with cirrhosis, and are not indicative of a malignant process.

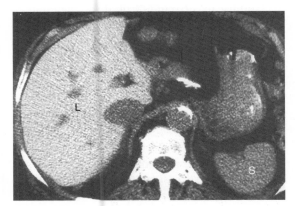

FIGURE 11-9 **High-attenuation liver.** Noncontrast CT demonstrates markedly high attenuation of the liver (L) compared with the spleen (S) in this patient receiving chronic amiodarone therapy for cardiac arrhythmias.

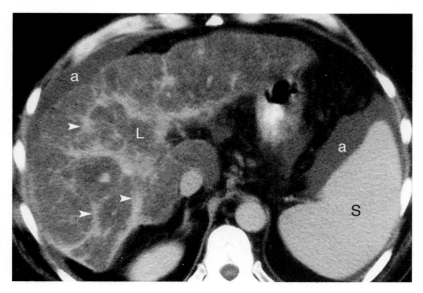

FIGURE 11-10 **Advanced cirrhosis with fatty infiltration.** Delayed portal venous phase CT demonstrates the liver (L) as misshapen and nodular in contour. Parenchymal density significantly less than that of the spleen (S) is indicative of fatty infiltration and continuing liver injury. Prominent scars and bands of fibrosis *(arrowheads)* are seen throughout the liver. Ascites (a) is present.

Nodules in Cirrhosis

Nodular lesions in cirrhosis are classified as regenerative nodules, dysplastic nodules, and nodules of HCC. Regenerative nodules are present in all cirrhotic livers but are visualized on CT in only 25% of cases. They represent a local reparative response to injury with focal proliferation of hepatocytes and supporting stroma. Dysplastic nodules are premalignant. A nodular collection of hepatocytes have cellular atypia and dysplastic features but no frank malignancy. HCC may develop spontaneously or as a result of progression of focal dysplasia. Confluent fibrosis may resemble HCC. CT findings of nodular lesions in cirrhosis include:

- Regenerative nodules usually are not demonstrated on noncontrast CT because they are isodense with surrounding tissue. However, they may accumulate iron and appear high attenuating on noncontrast CT (Fig. 11-11). These are termed *siderotic nodules.* Regenerative nodules typically do not enhance on arterial phase after contrast CT. On portal venous phase, regenerative nodules are either not seen because they enhance homogeneously with surrounding tissue or appear hypodense because they enhance less than surrounding tissue (Fig. 11-12). Visualized regenerative nodules are typically smaller than 10 mm.

- Dysplastic nodules are usually not demonstrated on CT. When seen, dysplastic nodules are slightly hypoattenuating or hyperattenuating on noncontrast CT. Siderotic nodules larger than 10 mm are considered dysplastic. On postcontrast CT, most dysplastic nodules enhance homogeneously with surrounding liver tissue on both arterial and portal venous phase and are not detectable. A small number of dysplastic nodules demonstrate homogeneous enhancement on arterial phase and are distinguishable from HCC only by biopsy.

- Small HCC nodules are hypointense or isointense to surrounding tissue on noncontrast CT. Hyperintense homogeneous enhancement on arterial phase is the key finding that suggests HCC. This hallmark finding should mandate consideration of biopsy. Enhancement decreases and visibility is variable on portal venous phase images. Up to 50% of small HCC nodules are not detectable because they are isodense to parenchyma on all phases.

- Diffuse metastatic disease, especially associated with breast cancer, may mimic cirrhosis with nodules. Medical history usually provides the differentiation. Innumerable small metastases may also be seen with small-cell lung carcinoma, melanoma, carcinoid, and occasionally pancreatic carcinoma.

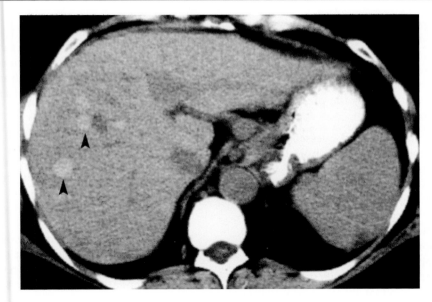

FIGURE 11-11 **Siderotic regenerative nodules.** Noncontrast CT demonstrates several high-attenuation nodules *(arrowheads)* within a cirrhotic liver. These represent siderotic regenerative nodules with high iron content.

- Hemangiomas are rarely seen in cirrhotic livers. The process of injury and scarring results in complete fibrosis of most hemangiomas, thus they are not detected. Hepatic cysts are present at the same frequency as noncirrhotic livers but are usually diagnosed easily.
- The hallmark finding of homogeneous enhancement during arterial phase may also be seen with benign conditions including

dysplastic nodules, focal fibrosis, arteriovenous shunts and pseudoaneurysms related to previous liver biopsy, and transient perfusion abnormalities discussed earlier.

Portal Hypertension

Portal hypertension results from progressive fibrosis of the hepatic vascular bed with development of portosystemic collateral vessels and

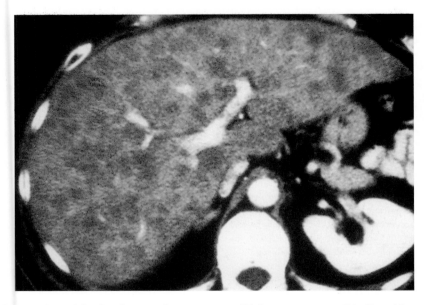

FIGURE 11-12 **Regenerative nodules.** Portal venous phase postcontrast CT shows numerous small (<10 mm) low-attenuation nodules in a cirrhotic liver. This represents unusually prominent visualization of regenerative nodules.

eventually hepatofugal flow (i.e., flow away from, instead of into, the liver). Portal hypertension causes major morbidity in patients with cirrhosis because of hepatic encephalopathy and variceal hemorrhage. Portal hypertension can be diagnosed on CT by the presence of the following anatomic signs:

- Portosystemic collateral vessels enlarge shunting blood between the portal and systemic veins (Fig. 11-13). Findings include esophageal, paraesophageal, and gastric varices; enlarged paraumbilical veins that connect with enlarged subcutaneous veins around the umbilicus (caput medusae); and splenorenal and perisplenic collaterals. Varices appear as well-defined, round, serpentine structures that enhance homogenously with contrast during portal venous and delayed phases (Fig. 11-14).
- The portal vein is enlarged (>13 mm).
- The splenic and superior mesenteric veins are enlarged (>10 mm).
- Splenomegaly is usually evident because of splenic congestion.
- Ascites is often present.
- The enlarged collateral vessels characteristic of portal hypertension may be subtle and easily missed, or they may be mistaken for other structures. You see what you are looking for!

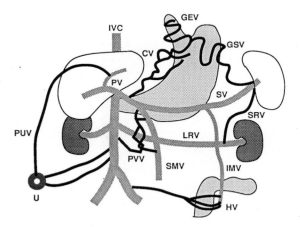

FIGURE 11-13 **Portosystemic collateral vessels.** Schematic representation of portosystemic collateral veins that may be seen in portal hypertension. CV, cardinal veins (in gastrohepatic ligament); GEV, gastroesophageal varices; GSV, gastrosplenic veins; HV, hemorrhoidal veins; IMV, inferior mesenteric vein; IVC, inferior vena cava; LRV, left renal vein; PUV, paraumbilical vein; PV, portal veins; PVV, paravertebral veins; SMV, superior mesenteric vein; SRV, splenorenal veins; SV, splenic vein; U, umbilicus.

Portal Vein Thrombosis

Thrombosis of the portal vein is usually found in association with cirrhosis, hepatoma, or mesenteric inflammation. Portal vein thrombosis can cause or exacerbate portal hypertension. Signs of acute thrombosis include:

- Low-density, nonenhancing, intraluminal thrombus fills the portal vein.
- The size of the portal vein is often increased.
- The portal vein does not enhance on postcontrast scans.
- Failure to visualize the portal vein suggests the diagnosis.
- Tumor thrombus within the portal vein may enhance during arterial phase (Fig 11-15).
- Cavernous transformation refers to the development of numerous periportal collateral veins in response to portal vein thrombosis, usually in patients with cirrhosis. CT demonstrates a nest of collateral vessels in the porta hepatis.
- Calcification may be seen within the portal vein when thrombus is chronic.

Passive Congestion

In the presence of right heart failure or constrictive pericarditis, the volume of returning venous blood exceeds the capacity of the right heart, causing an increase in central venous pressure and dilatation of the IVC and hepatic veins. Chronic congestion and stasis in the hepatic sinusoids causes ischemic injury to hepatocytes, resulting in fatty infiltration and eventually cirrhosis.

- The hepatic veins and IVC are distended because the failing heart cannot accommodate venous return (Fig. 11-16).
- Hepatic parenchyma may enhance in a mottled mosaic pattern similar to that seen with Budd–Chiari syndrome.
- Reflux of contrast into the hepatic veins during contrast injection into upper extremity veins is evidence of tricuspid regurgitation.
- Cardiomegaly, pleural and pericardial effusions, ascites, and hepatomegaly frequently are present.

Budd–Chiari Syndrome

Budd–Chiari syndrome refers to the manifestations of hepatic venous outflow obstruction,

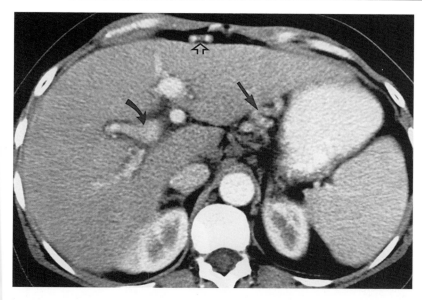

FIGURE 11-14 **Portal hypertension.** CT signs of portal hypertension are demonstrated in this slice through the porta hepatis. The portal vein *(curved arrow)* is enlarged, measuring 15 mm. Dilated and tortuous cardinal veins *(straight arrow)* are seen in the gastrohepatic ligament. The paraumbilical vein *(open arrow)* is enlarged. Visualization of a patent paraumbilical vein is the most specific CT sign of portal hypertension.

which include severe centrilobular congestion, hepatocellular necrosis, and atrophy. Acute thrombosis of the main hepatic veins or IVC is associated with pregnancy, oral contraceptive use, and polycythemia vera. Neoplastic obstruc-

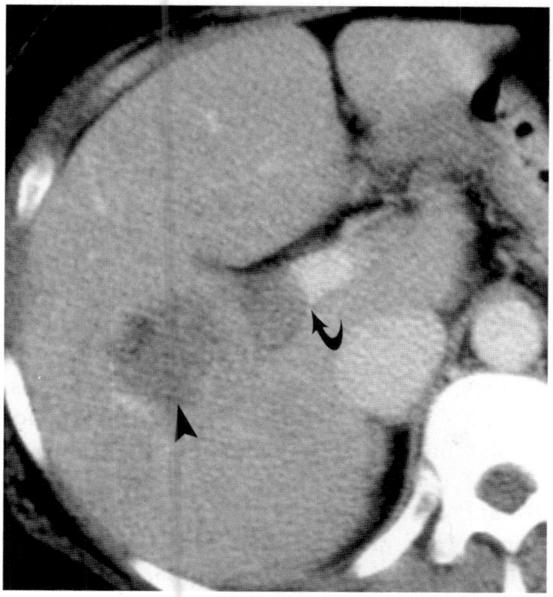

FIGURE 11-15 **Tumor thrombus portal vein.** Portal venous phase CT image shows a low-attenuation hepatocellular carcinoma *(arrowhead)* that invades the portal vein *(curved arrow)*.

tion of the hepatic veins or IVC occurs with hepatoma and renal cell and adrenal carcinoma. Chronic fibrosis is idiopathic and affects small sublobular and central hepatic veins. Congenital causes include webs or diaphragms that obstruct the IVC. CT findings include:

- The caudate lobe is enlarged. The caudate lobe is spared from injury because of its separate hepatic vein drainage.
- Hepatic veins and the IVC are narrowed or are not visualized.
- Parenchymal enhancement is inhomogeneous appearing as a mosaic pattern (Fig. 11-17). The central liver enhances early, and the peripheral liver enhances late.
- Intrahepatic collateral vessels are seen as comma-shaped enhancing vessels.

☐ FOCAL LIVER MASSES

Solid Liver Masses

A primary goal of liver imaging is to differentiate significant from insignificant liver masses. Clinically significant liver masses include metastases, hepatoma, and hepatic adenoma. Cavernous hemangioma, hepatic cyst, and focal nodular hyperplasia are nonsurgical liver masses that must be discriminated.

tumor (30%), and multinodular tumor (20%). Particularly characteristic is dominant mass surrounded by satellite lesions.

- Arterial hypervascularity is a hallmark CT finding of HCC (Fig. 11-19).
- Small tumors (<3 cm) typically demonstrate bright homogeneous enhancement on arterial phase postcontrast images. This finding is the hallmark for detection of HCC.
- Large HCCs are typically hypodense on noncontrast scans and enhance quite heterogeneously on both arterial phase and portal venous phase postcontrast scans.
- Areas of tumor necrosis are common, and calcification is present in 25%. A prominent fibrous capsule that is low in attenuation on noncontrast CT and enhances on portal venous phase and delayed images is uncommon but characteristic.
- Fatty metamorphosis within hepatomas is common histologically and has been reported on CT.
- Confluent fibrosis, appearing as an irregular mass replacing hepatic parenchyma, occurs

in up to a third of patients with cirrhosis. Typically, the mass of fibrosis is low in attenuation on noncontrast scans. On portal venous phase postcontrast CT, approximately 40% of lesions remain low in attenuation, whereas 50% of lesions become isoattenuating with surrounding tissue. In 10% of cases, the fibrosis distinctly enhances and biopsy is necessary to differentiate this lesion from HCC.

- Tumor invasion of hepatic and portal veins is frequent (see Fig. 11-15). A liver tumor seen in association with portal vein thrombosis is likely HCC.

Fibrolamellar Carcinoma

Fibrolamellar carcinoma is an entity distinct from HCC. This is a slow-growing tumor that usually arises in healthy liver. Patients are younger (usually <40 years) than most patients with hepatoma, and α-fetoprotein is not present in serum. Prognosis is good if the tumor is completely resected. CT findings of fibrolamellar carcinoma include:

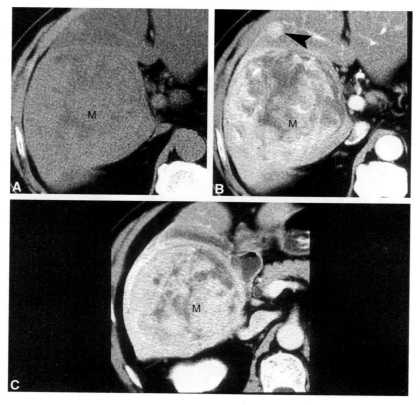

FIGURE 11-19 Hepatocellular carcinoma. Noncontrast (A), arterial phase (B), and portal venous phase (C) images demonstrate early heterogenous enhancement of this hepatocellular carcinoma. The tumor contained areas of hemorrhage and necrosis. A satellite tumor nodule *(arrowhead)* is seen on the arterial phase image.

- A large hepatic mass within a healthy liver in a young adult or adolescent is characteristic.
- Noncontrast CT demonstrates a large, low-attenuation, lobulated mass with well-defined margins.
- On postcontrast scans, the lesion enhances prominently and heterogeneously during both arterial and portal venous phases. Enhancement becomes more homogeneous and remains evident on delayed scans.
- Fibrous tissue extends through the mass separating the tumor into islands and commonly coalescing into a central scar (Fig. 11-20). The scar is visible on CT in up to 60% of cases. The scar may calcify (33–55%) and is best seen on delayed scans. Typically, the enhancement of the scar is not present on arterial and portal venous images but may be evident on delayed scans.
- Cirrhosis, vascular invasion, and multifocal disease common with HCC are rare with fibrolamellar carcinoma.
- Fibrolamellar carcinoma may be difficult to differentiate from focal nodular hyperplasia.

Lymphoma

The liver is involved in disease in more than half of all patients with both Hodgkin's and non–

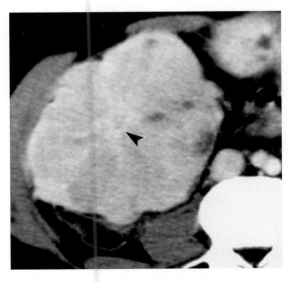

FIGURE 11-20 Fibrolamellar carcinoma. Portal venous phase image shows a fibrolamellar carcinoma in a 37-year-old man replacing most of the right lobe of the liver. An enhancing central scar *(arrowhead)* with enhancing radiating fibrous bands is faintly visualized.

Hodgkin's lymphoma; however, detection of involvement by CT is uncommon.

- Diffuse infiltration may cause only hepatomegaly without altering parenchymal density.
- Multiple well-defined, large, homogeneous, low-density nodules are the most characteristic finding (Fig. 11-21).
- Numerous small nodules resembling microabscesses occur with Hodgkin's lymphoma.
- The spleen is usually also involved, and abdominal adenopathy is usually present.

Hepatic Adenoma

Hepatocellular adenoma is a rare benign tumor seen most often in young women who use oral contraceptives, in men who take anabolic steroids, and in patients with glycogen storage disease. It is a significant lesion because of the risk for major hemorrhage associated with its presence. Hepatic adenomas are composed of neoplastic hepatocytes. Kupffer cells are occasionally present but are nonfunctional. Most patients are asymptomatic and have normal liver function study results. Surgical removal is often recommended because of the risk for rupture and malignant transformation. The imaging findings are:

- On unenhanced CT, many adenomas, consisting of well-differentiated hepatocytes, are isodense to normal liver parenchyma.
- However, in some tumors, the hepatocytes become filled with fat and the lesion approaches fat density. Lipid content may be focal or diffuse within the tumor.
- Hemorrhage may also be most apparent on noncontrast scans. Fresh hemorrhage is high in attenuation, whereas old hemorrhage appears as heterogeneous low attenuation. Intratumoral hemorrhage is common; it is seen in 25% to 40% of adenomas.
- Calcifications are seen in 10% of tumors.
- Arterial phase postcontrast scans show early homogeneous enhancement (Fig. 11-22).
- Contrast washes out relatively rapidly, and the tumors become near-isodense with liver parenchyma on portal venous phase and delayed postcontrast scans.
- Because Kupffer cells are few in number and dysfunctional, uptake of technetium–99m

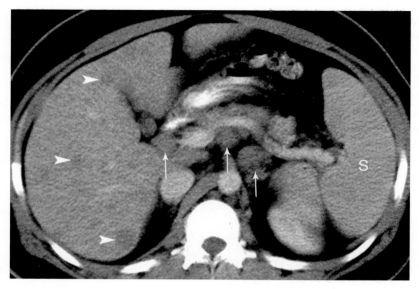

FIGURE 11-21 **Hepatic lymphoma.** Late portal venous phase CT image shows multiple subtle low-density nodules in the liver in this patient with non–Hodgkin's lymphoma. Numerous enlarged lymph nodes *(arrows)* are visualized, and the spleen (S) is enlarged.

sulfur colloid is absent within the tumor on radionuclide scans.

- Tumors are solitary in 70% to 80% of patients. Multiple tumors are seen in patients with glycogen storage disease type 1 and liver adenomatosis (see Fig. 11-22).
- Lesions vary in size from 1 to 15 cm.

Focal Nodular Hyperplasia

In contrast to hepatic adenoma, focal nodular hyperplasia contains all the histologic elements of normal liver, including Kupffer cells. It is the second most common benign liver tumor after cavernous hemangioma. Fibrous bands and central stellate fibrous scars are characteris-

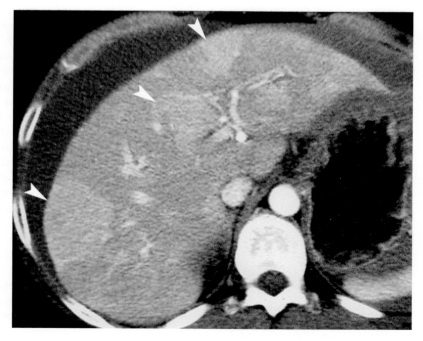

FIGURE 11-22 **Multiple hepatic adenomas.** Arterial phase image shows homogeneous enhancement of multiple hepatic adenomas *(arrowheads)* in this woman with liver adenomatosis. Ascites is present because of associated impaired liver function.

tic. Hemorrhage and necrosis are rare. Most patients are asymptomatic, and the tumor is discovered incidentally. Because the tumor is benign, no treatment is indicated. CT findings include:

- On unenhanced CT, lesions are isodense or slightly hypodense to normal liver parenchyma. The central scar may be hypodense (20%) or invisible (80%).
- The hallmark finding of immediate intense homogeneous enhancement is seen on arterial phase postcontrast CT. The central scar may remain hypodense (Fig. 11-23).
- On portal venous phase, the lesion becomes nearly isodense with enhanced parenchyma. Large draining veins result in rapid washout of contrast agent.
- On delayed phase, postcontrast images the lesion is usually isodense to parenchyma, but the central scar may show enhancement.
- Normal (40%) or increased (10%) radionuclide uptake within the tumor on technetium–99m sulfur colloid-labeled liver scan is the most specific finding. However, 50% of the lesions show a nonspecific cold defect.

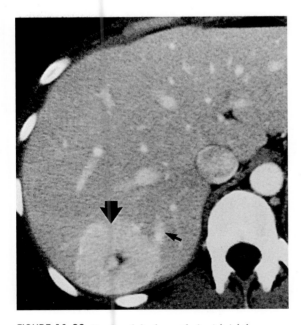

FIGURE 11-23 **Focal nodular hyperplasia.** A brightly enhanced mass *(large arrow)* in the posterior segment of the right hepatic lobe has a characteristic central low-density scar. A large draining vein *(small arrow)* indicates the hypervascular nature of the mass.

- Lesions are solitary (80% to 95%) and usually smaller than 5 cm.

Cavernous Hemangioma

Cavernous hemangiomas are the second most common focal mass lesion in the liver, exceeded in frequency only by metastases. They are the most common benign liver neoplasm, found in up to 7% of individuals. They are often discovered incidentally during hepatic imaging by ultrasonography or CT. They may be found at any age and are more common in women. Although most are solitary, 10% of the affected patients have multiple lesions easily mistaken for metastases. The tumors consist of large, thin-walled, blood-filled vascular spaces lined by epithelium and separated by fibrous septa. Blood flow through the complex of vascular spaces is slow, resulting in characteristic prolonged retention of contrast agents on CT. The majority of lesions are less than 5 cm, are asymptomatic, and pose no threat to the patient. Larger giant cavernous hemangiomas may cause symptoms by pressure effect, hemorrhage, or arteriovenous shunting. CT findings include:

- On unenhanced CT, hemangiomas appear as a well-defined hypodense mass of the same density as other blood-filled spaces, such as the IVC or portal vein.
- Postcontrast arterial phase images show early, peripheral nodules of contrast enhancement equal in density to the enhancement of the aorta (Fig. 11-24).
- Venous phase images show progressive fill-in enhancement from the periphery with the lesion becoming uniformly enhanced.
- Delayed images show prolonged enhancement because of the characteristic slow washout of contrast agent.
- Contrast enhancement usually persists within the lesion for 20 to 30 minutes after contrast injection.
- Because blood flow is slow through the lesion, thrombosis may occur, leading to irregular areas of fibrosis, which remain unenhanced through the postcontrast phases of CT. Occasionally, these fibrotic portions of the lesion may show particulate or dense calcification.
- Small hemangiomas, especially those less than 1 cm, may show immediate homogeneous enhancement during arterial phase,

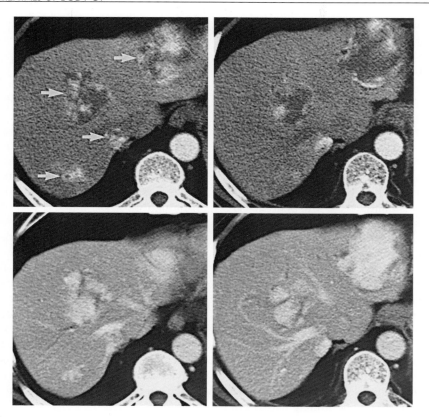

FIGURE 11-24 **Cavernous hemangioma.** Arterial phase *(top row)* and portal venous phase *(bottom row)* images demonstrate the characteristic enhancement pattern of multiple cavernous hemangiomas *(arrows)*. Early contrast medium enhancement appears nodular and at the periphery. Enhancement proceeds centrally to complete opacification, except for areas of fibrous scarring in large lesions.

mimicking HCCs and hypervascular metastases. Differentiation is made by observing the slow washout and persistent enhancement during portal venous phase and on delayed images characteristic of hemangiomas but not the other hypervascular tumors.

- Most hemangiomas remain stable in size over time.
- When classic findings are observed, the CT examination can be considered diagnostic of cavernous hemangioma with a high degree of confidence. In questionable cases, tagged red blood cell scintigraphy is usually diagnostic.

CYSTIC LIVER MASSES

Hepatic Cysts

Benign hepatic cysts are found in 5% to 10% of the population. They cause no symptoms and are usually discovered incidentally. They have no malignant potential but must be differentiated from significant lesions. Multiple tiny cysts may mimic early metastases.

- On unenhanced CT, cysts are well defined and low in density with internal attenuation of water (0–10 H). The cyst wall is not perceptible (Fig. 11-25). Size is a few millimeters to several centimeters. They may be solitary but are frequently multiple.
- Hepatic cysts tend to occur in clusters, which are lobulated in contour. The walls between cysts have the appearance of septa.
- No enhancement is seen on any phase of postcontrast scans.

Pyogenic Abscess

Bacterial hepatic abscess is a localized collection of pus and debris within an area of destroyed parenchyma. Bacterial seeding occurs by way of the portal vein, hepatic artery, biliary tree, by direct extension from adjacent infection, or as a

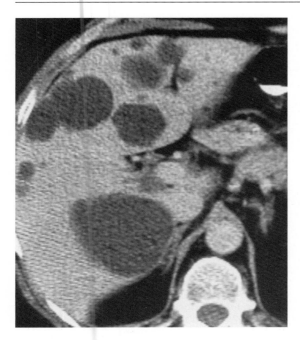

FIGURE 11-25 **Multiple simple hepatic cysts.** Simple hepatic cysts have uniform low internal density and sharp margins with the surrounding hepatic parenchyma. No cyst walls are evident. The lesions do not enhance with intravenous contrast medium.

result of trauma. Approximately 85% of liver abscesses in patients in the United States are pyogenic. Patients are usually clinically septic and are often jaundiced. CT findings include:

- Bacterial abscess is usually solitary but often multiloculated with thickened enhancing walls (Fig. 11-26). When multiple abscesses are present, lesions are often grouped and consist of many microabscesses. Masses are hypodense with a peripheral rim that usually enhances with contrast medium.
- Gas is present within the lesion in 20% of cases.
- Fine-needle aspiration is indicated for bacterial culture. Catheter or surgical drainage is needed.
- Biliary obstruction is the most common associated finding.

Amebic Abscess

Amebic abscess occurs in 3% to 7% of patients with amebiasis. Amebic abscesses account for 6% of liver abscesses in patients in the United States. Amebic serology is positive in 95% of cases. CT findings include:

- The abscess (Fig. 11-27) is usually solitary (85%) and in the right lobe (72%).
- The wall is well defined, sometimes nodular, and enhances with contrast administration. The liver parenchyma adjacent to the wall of the abscess also commonly enhances, producing a double-rim target appearance.
- Right pleural effusion and right lower lobe infiltration are often present.

Hydatid Cyst

Hydatid disease is produced by the larval stage of the tapeworm *Echinococcus*. The liver is the most common site of disease. The disease is not endemic in the United States, thus cases are seen in immigrants and travelers to endemic areas, primarily grazing areas in South America, New Zealand, Africa, the Middle East, Australia, and the Mediterranean. CT findings include:

- The appearance of the hydatid cyst (Fig. 11-28) depends on its stage of growth. The cyst may be unilocular, contain daughter cysts, or may be completely calcified (dead).
- The cyst wall is usually high in attenuation and is commonly calcified (50%). The

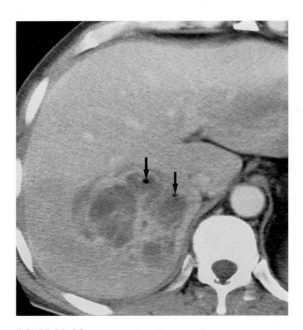

FIGURE 11-26 **Pyogenic liver abscess.** A liver abscess containing *Escherichia coli* has irregular septations and contains a few bubbles of air *(arrows)*. Because of the multiple loculations, this abscess did not respond to percutaneously placed catheter drainage but required surgical debridement.

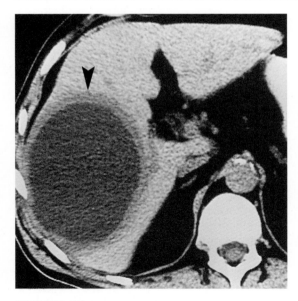

FIGURE 11-27 **Amebic abscess.** A 50-year-old American man living in Thailand returned to the United States with this mass in his liver. Although the internal density is homogeneously low, a distinct thick wall *(arrowhead)* is present and was observed to enhance with intravenous contrast medium administration. Serologic titers were positive for amebiasis.

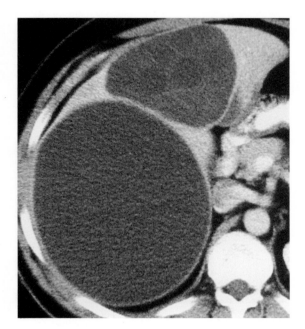

FIGURE 11-28 **Hydatid cysts.** Two hydatid cysts are seen in the right lobe of the liver. Although they appear unilocular on CT, ultrasound (not shown) showed thin internal membranes, a few daughter cysts, and hydatid sand.

internal fluid is usually near water attenuation. Layering debris (hydatid sand) is commonly present within the cysts. Detached floating membranes are sometimes evident.
- Daughter cysts present a cyst within a cyst appearance. The daughter cysts may be separated by a hydatid matrix that produces a spoke wheel appearance.

SUGGESTED READING

AUH YH, LIM JH, KIM KW, et al: Loculated fluid collections in hepatic fissures and recesses: CT appearance and potential pitfalls. Radiographics 14: 529–540, 1994.

BARON RL, PETERSON MS: Screening the cirrhotic liver for hepatocellular carcinoma with CT and MR imaging: Opportunities and pitfalls. Radio-Graphics 21:S117–S132, 2001.

BROWN JJ, NAYLOR MJ, YAGAN N: Imaging of hepatic cirrhosis. Radiology 202:1–16, 1997.

CARLSON SK, JOHNSON CD, BENDER CE, WELCH TJ: CT of focal nodular hyperplasia of the liver. AJR Am J Roentgenol 174:705–712, 2000.

CHEN W-P, CHEN J-H, HWANG J-I, et al: Spectrum of transient hepatic attenuation differences in biphasic helical CT. AJR Am J Roentgenol 172:419–424, 1999.

CHO KC, PATEL YD, WACHSBERG RH, SEEFF J: Varicies in portal hypertension: Evaluation with CT. Radiographics 15:609–622, 1995.

COLAGRANDE S, CENTI N, LA VILLA G, VILLARI N: Transient hepatic attenuation differences. AJR Am J Roentgenol 183:459–464, 2004.

DESSER TS, SZE DY, JEFFREY RB: Imaging and intervention in the hepatic veins. AJR Am J Roentgenol 180:1583–1591, 2003.

DODD GD: An American's guide to Couinaud's numbering system. AJR Am J Roentgenol 161:574–575, 1993.

DODD GDI, BARON RL, OLIVER JHI, FEDERLE MP: Spectrum of imaging findings of the liver in end-stage cirrhosis: Part I, gross morphology and diffuse abnormalities. AJR Am J Roentgenol 173:1031–1036, 1999.

DODD GDI, BARON RL, OLIVER JHI, FEDERLE MP: Spectrum of imaging findings of the liver in end-stage cirrhosis: Part II, focal abnormalities. AJR Am J Roentgenol 173:1185–1192, 1999.

DODD GDI, BARON RL, OLIVER JHI, et al: Enlarged abdominal lymph nodes in end-stage cirrhosis: CT-histopathologic correlation in 507 patients. Radiology 203:127–130, 1997.

FASEL JHD, SELLE D, EVERTSZ CJG, et al: Segmental anatomy of the liver: Poor correlation with CT. Radiology 206:151–156, 1998.

GALLEGO C, VELASCO M, MARCUELLO P, et al: Congenital and acquired anomalies of the portal venous system. Radiographics 22:141–159, 2003.

GAZELLE GS, HAAGA JR: Hepatic neoplasms: Surgically relevant segmental anatomy and imaging techniques. AJR Am J Roentgenol 158:1015–1018, 1992.

GORE RM, MATHIEU DG, WHITE EM, et al: Passive hepatic congestion: Cross-sectional imaging features. AJR Am J Roentgenol 162:71–75, 1994.

GRAZIOLA L, FEDERLE MP, BRANCATELLI G, et al: Hepatic adenomas: Imaging and pathologic findings. Radiographics 21:877–894, 2001.

GUERMAZI A, BRICE P, DE KERVILER E, et al: Extranodal Hodgkin disease: Spectrum of disease. Radiographics 21:161–179, 2001.

HORTON KM, BLUEMKE DA, HRUBAN RH, et al: CT and MR imaging of benign hepatic and biliary tumors. Radiograpics 19:431–451, 1999.

HUSSAIN SM, TERKIVATAN T, ZONDERVAN PE, et al: Focal nodular hyperplasia: Findings at state-of-the-art MR imaging, US, CT, and pathologic analysis. Radiographics 24:3–19, 2004.

ITO K, HIGUCHI M, KADA T, et al: CT of acquired abnormalities of the portal venous system. Radiographics 17:897–917, 1997.

JI H, MCTAVISH JD, MORTELE KJ, et al: Hepatic imaging with multidetector CT. Radiographics 21:S71–S80, 2001.

KAWAMOTO S, SOYER PA, FISHMAN EK, BLUEMKE DA: Nonneoplastic liver disease: Evaluation with CT and MR imaging. Radiographics 18:827–848, 1998.

LEE KHY, O'MALLEY MEO, KACHURA JR, et al: Hepatocellular carcinoma: Imaging and imaging-guided intervention. AJR Am J Roentgenol 180:1015–1022, 2003.

MCLARNEY JK, RUCKER PT, BENDER GN, et al: Fibrolamellar carcinoma of the liver: Radiologic-pathologic correlation. Radiographics 19:453–471, 1999.

MERGO PJ, ROS PR, BUETOW PC, BUCK JL: Diffuse disease of the liver: Radiologic-pathologic correlation. Radiographics 14:1291–1307, 1994.

MORTELE KJ, ROS PR: Cystic focal liver lesions in the adult: Differential CT and MR imaging features. Radiographics 21:895–910, 2001.

MORTELE KJ, SEGATTO E, ROS PR: The infected liver: Radiologic-pathologic correlation. Radiographics 24:937–955, 2004.

PARVEY HR, RAVAL B, SANDLER CM: Portal vein thrombosis: imaging findings. AJR Am J Roentgenol 162:77–81, 1994.

PEDROSA I, SAIZ A, ARRAZOLA J, et al: Hydatid disease: Radiologic and pathologic features and complications. Radiographics 20:795–817, 2000.

QUIROGA S, SEBASTIA C, PALLISA E, et al: Improved diagnosis of hepatic perfusion disorders: Value of hepatic arterial phase imaging during helical CT. Radiographics 21:65–81, 2001.

SICA GT, JI H, ROS PR: CT and MR imaging of hepatic metastases. AJR Am J Roentgenol 174:691–698, 2000.

SOYER P, BLUEMKE DA, BLISS DF, et al: Surgical segmental anatomy of the liver: Demonstration with spiral CT during arterial portography and mulitplanar reconstruction. AJR Am J Roentgenol 163:99–103, 1994.

SZKLARUK J, SILVERMAN PM, CHARNSANGAVEJ C: Imaging in the diagnosis, staging, treatment, and surveillance of hepatocellular carcinoma. AJR Am J Roentgenol 180:441–454, 2003.

VILGRAIN M, BOULOS L, VULLIERME M-P, et al: Imaging of atypical hemangiomas of the liver with pathologic correlation. Radiographics 20:379–397, 2000.

WINTER TC III, NGHEIM HV, FREENY PC, et al: Hepatic arterial anatomy: Demonstration of normal supply and vascular variants with three-dimensional CT angiography. Radiographics 15:771–780, 1995.

YOSHIMITSU K, HONDA H, KUROIWA T, et al: Unusual hemodynamics and pseudolesions of the noncirrhosis liver at CT. Radiographics 21:S81–S96, 2001.

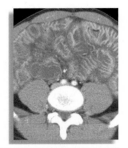

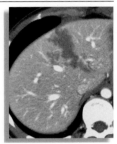

12

Biliary Tree and Gallbladder

William E. Brant, M.D.

☐ BILIARY TREE

Anatomy

The bile ducts arise as biliary capillaries between hepatocytes. Bile capillaries coalesce to form intrahepatic bile ducts. Intrahepatic ducts branch in a predictable manner corresponding to the segments of the liver. Interlobular bile ducts combine to form two main trunks from the right and left lobes of the liver. The 3- to 4-cm-long common hepatic duct is formed in the porta hepatis by the junction of the main right and left bile ducts. The cystic duct runs posteriorly and inferiorly from the gallbladder neck to join the common hepatic duct and form the common bile duct (CBD). The 6- to 7-cm-long CBD courses ventral to the portal vein and to the right of the hepatic artery, descending from the porta hepatis along the free right border of the hepatoduodenal ligament to behind the duodenal bulb. Its distal third turns directly caudad, descending in the groove between the descending duodenum and the head of the pancreas just ventral to the inferior vena cava. The CBD tapers distally as it ends in the sphincter of Oddi, which protrudes into the duodenum as the ampulla of Vater. The CBD and the pancreatic duct share a common orifice in 60% of patients and have separate orifices in the remainder. In any case, they are in such close proximity that tumors of the ampullary region will generally obstruct both ducts.

Normal-sized intrahepatic bile ducts are not usually visible on routine abdominal CT. However, with thin collimation (3–5 mm) and dynamic bolus intravenous contrast medium enhancement, normal intrahepatic ducts may be visualized in up to 40% of patients. Normal intrahepatic ducts are 2 mm in diameter in the central liver and taper progressively toward the periphery. The common hepatic duct is usually seen in the porta hepatis, and the CBD is routinely visualized descending adjacent to the descending duodenum. It is fair to use the generic term *common duct* to refer to both the common hepatic and the common bile ducts because the cystic duct junction marking their anatomic partition is not routinely visualized on CT. The normal common duct does not exceed 6 mm in diameter in most adult patients. In elderly patients, the normal common duct diameter increases about 1 mm per decade (i.e., 7 mm is normal for patients in their 70s, and 8 mm is normal for those in their 80s). Contrast medium enhancement improves identification of both normal and dilated bile ducts by enhancing blood vessels and the surrounding parenchyma. Bile ducts are seen as lucent branching tubular structures. The bile ducts may be difficult to differentiate from blood vessels without contrast agent administration.

Technique

Evaluation for biliary obstruction is the most common reason to perform CT of the bile ducts. Water is preferred as an oral contrast agent in this clinical setting because high-density contrast in the duodenum may cause streaks and obscure stones in the adjacent CBD.

- The patient drinks 300 mL water over 15 to 20 minutes just before CT examination.
- Thin sections (1–2.5 mm) using multidetector CT provide high resolution of the bile ducts.
- Multiphase imaging is commonly used. Stones may be seen best on noncontrast images. Scanning during arterial phase demonstrates pancreatic lesions best. Delayed imaging at 15 to 20 minutes after intravenous contrast administration shows the delayed enhancement characteristic of cholangiocarcinomas.

Biliary Obstruction

CT is about 96% accurate in determining the presence of biliary obstruction, 90% accurate in determining its level, and 70% accurate in determining its cause. The major causes of biliary obstruction are gallstones, tumor, stricture, and pancreatitis (Table 12-1). A rare but interesting cause of biliary obstruction is Mirizzi syndrome. A gallbladder stone impacted in the cystic duct induces cholangitis or erodes into the common duct to cause obstructive jaundice. Tumors include cholangiocarcinoma, pancreatic carcinoma, ampullary carcinoma, and benign tumors of the bile duct such as biliary cystadenomas and granular cell tumors.

CT diagnosis of biliary obstruction depends on the demonstration of dilated bile ducts. The biliary tree dilates proximal to the point of obstruction, whereas bile ducts below the obstruction remain normal or are reduced in size. When cirrhosis, cholangitis, or periductal fibrosis prohibits dilatation of the bile ducts in obstructive jaundice, there will be false-negative CT results. The CT findings of biliary obstruction are:

TABLE 12-1

Causes of Obstructive Jaundice in Adults

Gallstone impacted in bile duct
Bile duct stricture
  Traumatic/surgery/instrumentation
  Chronic pancreatitis
  Sclerosing cholangitis
  Oriental cholangiohepatitis
  Acquired immunodeficiency syndrome–associated cholangitis
Malignancy
  Pancreas carcinoma
  Duodenal/ampullary carcinoma
  Cholangiocarcinoma
  Metastases
Parasites (Ascaris, Clonorchis)
Choledochal cyst

- Multiple branching, round or oval, low-density tubular structures, representing dilated intrahepatic biliary ducts, coursing toward the porta hepatis (Fig. 12-1)
- Dilatation of the common duct in the porta hepatis seen as a tubular or oval, fluid density tube greater than 7 mm in diameter
- Dilatation of the CBD in the pancreatic head seen as a round fluid density tube larger than 7 mm
- Enlargement of the gallbladder to greater than 5 cm diameter, when the obstruction is distal to the cystic duct

Clues to the cause of biliary obstruction are shown in Figure 12-2 and are as follows:

- Abrupt termination of a dilated CBD, which is characteristic of a malignant process even in absence of a visible mass; common tumors causing biliary obstruction are pancreatic carcinoma, ampullary carcinoma, and cholangiocarcinoma; a mass is often visible on CT at the point of biliary obstruction
- Gradual tapering of a dilated duct seen most commonly with benign disease such as inflammatory stricture or pancreatitis (Fig. 12-3); calcifications in the pancreas are a clue to the presence of chronic pancreatitis
- Evidence of choledocholithiasis

Choledocholithiasis

Choledocholithiasis is a common cause of pancreatitis, jaundice, biliary colic, or cholangitis.

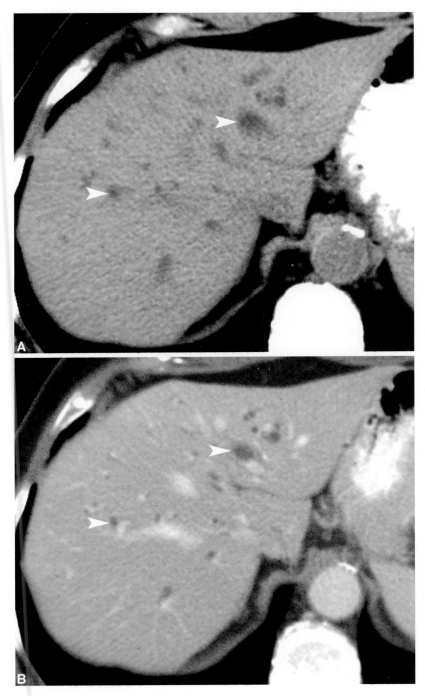

FIGURE 12-1 **Dilated bile ducts.** *A,* On noncontrast CT, dilated bile ducts *(arrowheads)* are seen as ill-defined low densities. The vascular structures are not well defined. *B,* After intravenous contrast administration, the dilated bile ducts *(arrowheads)* are much better defined, and the blood vessels are now well seen.

Continued

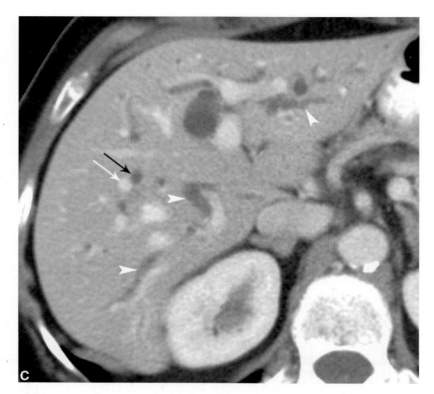

FIGURE 12-1 **Cont'd** *C*, Postcontrast image at a lower level shows the dilated bile ducts as tortuous tubes *(arrowheads)*. Note that in cross section the dilated bile duct *(black arrow)* is slightly larger in diameter than the adjacent portal vein *(white arrow)*.

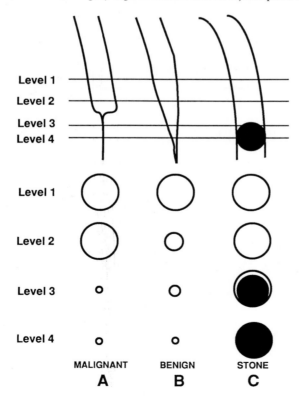

FIGURE 12-2 **Clues to the cause of biliary obstruction.** (A) Malignant tumors cause abrupt termination of the distal common bile duct. (B) Inflammatory strictures and pancreatitis cause progressive tapering of the distal common bile duct. (C) Impacted gallstones may be seen as rounded structures in the distal common bile duct. The CT density of gallstones varies from calcific density to fat density.

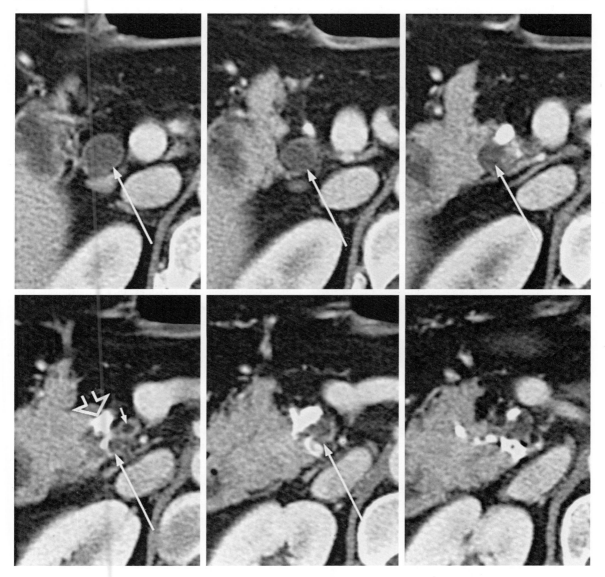

FIGURE 12-3 **Benign stricture of common bile duct caused by chronic pancreatitis.** Serial CT images demonstrate progressive tapering of the distal common bile duct *(long arrows)* as it passes through the head of the pancreas. The pancreatic head is deformed, and multiple calcifications *(open arrow)* and cystic changes *(short arrow)* indicate chronic pancreatitis.

However, stones in the bile ducts may also be asymptomatic. Most (95%) stones in the bile form in the gallbladder, although stones may also develop primarily within the bile ducts. CT demonstrates approximately 75% of stones in the CBD. CT findings include:

- Gallstones in the bile ducts are seen as calcific (calcium bilirubinate stones), soft-tissue (mixed stones), or fat (cholesterol stones) density structures (Fig. 12-4). Stones may be isodense with bile and not visualized by CT (15–25% of gallstones).

- The stone may appear as a central density surrounded by a rim or crescent of lower density bile—the target or crescent sign.
- Low-attenuation stones may be defined by a higher attenuation outer rim—the rim sign.
- Abrupt termination of the CBD proximal to the ampulla is suggestive of a stone in the CBD.

Cholangiocarcinoma

Cholangiocarcinoma is a slow-growing adeno-carcinoma arising from the epithelium of the

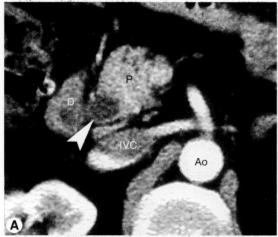

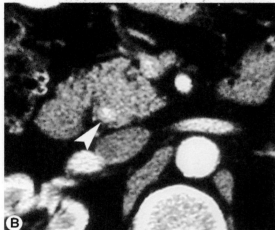

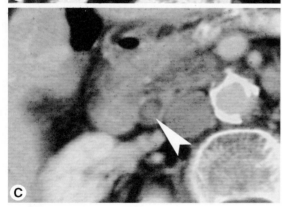

FIGURE 12-4 **Stone in common bile duct.** *A,* Postcontrast CT image through the head of the pancreas (P) shows a dilated distal common bile duct *(arrowhead)* adjacent to the descending duodenum (D). The inferior vena cava (IVC) and abdominal aorta (Ao) are identified. *B,* CT image slightly more caudad shows a high-density gallstone *(arrowhead)* obstructing the common bile duct. *C,* In a different patient, a stone *(arrowhead)* in the distal common bile duct has the attenuation of soft tissue.

bile ducts. It occurs as a complication of choledochal cyst, primary sclerosing cholangitis (PSC), Caroli's disease, intrahepatic stone disease, or clonorchiasis. The growth patterns of cholangiocarcinoma are mass forming, periductal infiltrating, and intraductal growing. Tumors occur in the periphery of the liver (10%), in the hilum (25%), or in the extrahepatic bile ducts (65%). The tumors are hypovascular and markedly fibrotic, resulting in poor contrast enhancement and limited CT detection especially on early postcontrast scans. Delayed scans at 10 to 20 minutes after contrast injection are recommended for optimal tumor detection. CT indications of cholangiocarcinoma are:

- Intrahepatic mass-forming cholangiocarcinoma appears as a homogeneous tumor with irregular borders and remarkably low attenuation. The mass is highly fibrotic and often shows only weak peripheral enhancement on early postcontrast images (Fig. 12-5). Delayed images (up to several hours) may show central or diffuse enhancement. Bile ducts peripheral to the tumor are usually obstructed and dilated.
- Periductal infiltrating lesions grow along the bile ducts in an elongated, branching pattern. Irregular narrowing of the duct produces obstruction. Involved ducts are narrowed with thick walls, whereas peripheral ducts are dilated. Visible tumor mass is minimal (Fig. 12-6).
- Intraductal tumors are polypoid or sessile papillary lesions that extend superficially along the bile duct mucosa. Some of these tumors produce large amounts of mucin, which disproportionately dilates the biliary system.
- Extrahepatic cholangiocarcinomas may appear as a duct-obstructing tumor nodule 1 to 2 cm in diameter (Fig. 12-7), as an abrupt stricture with wall thickening up to 1 cm, or as single or multiple intraductal frondlike masses.

Sclerosing Cholangitis

Primary sclerosing cholangitis (PSC) is an idiopathic inflammatory condition characterized by progressive fibrosis of the bile ducts leading to obstruction, cholestasis, and biliary cirrhosis. PSC is strongly associated (70% of patients)

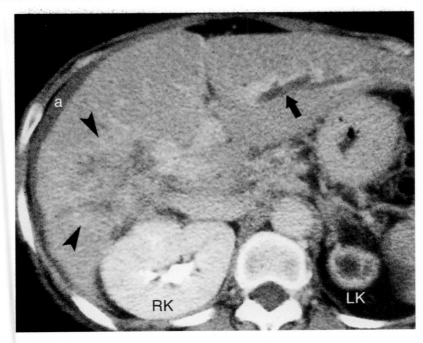

FIGURE 12-5 **Cholangiocarcinoma: intrahepatic.** Delayed postcontrast image (note the pyelogram phase of the right kidney [RK]) shows weak peripheral enhancement *(arrowheads)* of an intrahepatic cholangiocarcinoma. Intrahepatic bile ducts *(arrow)* are dilated. Ascites (a) is present. The left kidney (LK) is atrophic.

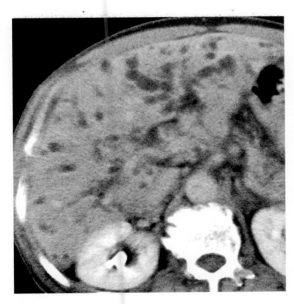

FIGURE 12-6 **Cholangiocarcinoma: infiltrating hilar.** An infiltrating cholangiocarcinoma at the junction of the right and left bile ducts (a Klatskin tumor) causes generalized dilatation of the intrahepatic biliary tree. The primary tumor is not visualized with CT.

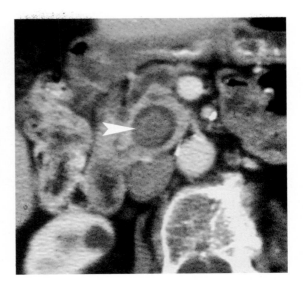

FIGURE 12-7 **Cholangiocarcinoma: intraductal polypoid.** A polypoid cholangiocarcinoma *(arrowhead)* causes obstructive jaundice with marked dilatation of the common bile duct. Note the similarity in appearance to the low-attenuation stone shown in Figure 12-4 C.

with ulcerative colitis and other inflammatory bowel diseases. CT findings of sclerosing cholangitis include:

- CT in PSC demonstrates multiple segmental strictures with thickening (2–5 mm) of the bile duct walls alternating with normal caliber or slightly dilated duct segments that produce a beaded appearance. Stones are seen in the ducts in 30% of patients.
- *Ascending cholangitis* occurs when bacteria contaminate an obstructed biliary system. Liver abscesses and sepsis may occur.
- *Oriental cholangiohepatitis* refers to recurrent pyogenic cholangitis associated with pigmented stones and multifocal biliary strictures and dilatations. Infestations with *Clonorchis sinensis* and *Ascaris lumbricoides*, malnutrition, and portal vein bacteremia all play a role in its cause. The condition is endemic in Southeast Asian and Chinese populations and is seen predominantly in immigrants in Western countries. Dilated bile ducts with enhancing walls are filled with stones and pus. Marked dilatation of the CBD is characteristic.
- *AIDS-related cholangitis* is associated with opportunistic infection with *Cryptosporidium* or cytomegalovirus. Intrahepatic bile ducts show focal narrowing and dilatation similar to PSC. Striking thickening of the walls of the bile ducts and gallbladder is often evident. The distal CBD is commonly strictured.

Choledochal Cyst

Choledochal cysts are congenital dilatations of the biliary tree that are usually discovered in childhood. Adult patients with undetected biliary cysts may present with pancreatitis, cholangitis, jaundice, or unexplained abdominal pain, nausea, or vomiting. Complications include gallstones and cholangiocarcinoma. CT demonstrates cystic structures in the course of the intrahepatic bile ducts or CBD and separate from the gallbladder. Todani classifies choledochal cysts into five types:

- Type I (~77%), classic choledochal cyst, is localized cystic dilatation of the CBD (Fig. 12-8). This may appear large and saccular or small and fusiform.

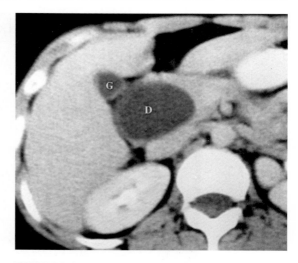

FIGURE 12-8 **Choledochal cyst.** The common bile duct (D) is massively enlarged. The neck of the gallbladder (G) is seen adjacent to the dilated common bile duct.

- Type II (~1.5%) is a diverticulum arising from the CBD or common hepatic duct. The remainder of the biliary system is normal.
- Type III (~1.5%), choledochocele, is rare bulbous dilatation of the intramural portion of the distal CBD that protrudes into the lumen of the duodenum. Choledochoceles are most commonly detected in adults. Stones are commonly present in the biliary tree.
- Type IV is divided into type IV A (~20%), cystic dilatation of the intrahepatic bile ducts associated with saccular dilatation of the CBD, and type IV B (extremely rare), multiple cystic dilatations of the extrahepatic bile ducts with normal intrahepatic bile ducts.
- Type V is Caroli's disease.

Caroli's Disease

Caroli's disease is a rare congenital anomaly of the biliary tract characterized by saccular dilatation of the intrahepatic biliary tree, cholangitis, and gallstone formation in the absence of cirrhosis or portal hypertension. Patients are at greatly increased risk for bile duct carcinoma (7% of patients). CT demonstrates cystic dilatation of the intrahepatic biliary tree with focal areas of tubular and saccular enlargement (Fig. 12-9).

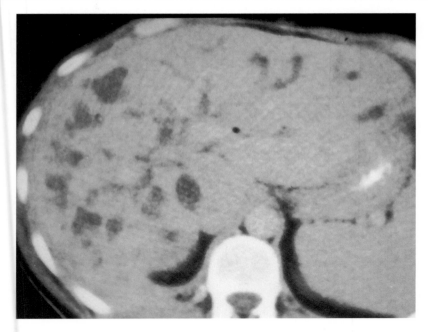

FIGURE 12-9 **Caroli's disease.** Abnormally dilated intrahepatic bile ducts are seen as tubular and rounded cystic lucency in the liver.

Gas or Contrast Material in Biliary Tree

Gas or contrast material in the biliary tree (Fig. 12-10) is an abnormal finding that must be explained. Most often the cause is iatrogenic. The differential diagnosis is listed in Table 12-2.

☐ GALLBLADDER

Anatomy

The gallbladder lies in the fossa formed by the junction of the right and left lobes of the liver. Although the position of the fundus varies, the neck and body of the gallbladder are invariably positioned in the porta hepatis and major interlobar fissure. The gallbladder is in close proximity to the duodenal bulb and hepatic flexure of the colon. The normal gallbladder is 3 to 5 cm in diameter and 10 cm in length and has a capacity of roughly 50 mL. Agenesis of the gallbladder is extremely rare (<0.02%), and duplication of the gallbladder occurs in about 1 in 4000 individuals. Folds in the gallbladder, producing a Phrygian cap deformity, are common (1% to 6% incidence rate) and are not significant clinically.

Ultrasonography, not CT, is the primary modality for imaging the gallbladder. However, significant gallbladder pathology may be diagnosed by CT, especially when screening the acutely ill patient. Normal bile is of fluid density (0–20 H)

on CT. Higher density bile suggests bile stasis (sludge), hemorrhage, or infection (pus). The gallbladder wall enhances avidly with bolus contrast agent administration.

Gallstones

Although gallstones may be detected by CT, the sensitivity of CT is only about 85%, which is much less than that of ultrasonography or oral cholecystography. Gallstones vary in CT density from negative numbers, indicating fat density of cholesterol stones, to high positive numbers of calcified stones (Fig. 12-11). Fissured stones may contain linear streaks of air. Some gallstones may not be seen on CT because they are isodense with bile or because they are too small. Contrast agents in adjacent bowel loops may obscure, or mimic, gallstones.

Acute Cholecystitis

Acute cholecystitis is usually diagnosed clinically or by ultrasonography or radionuclide hepatobiliary scan. Cases are studied with CT usually because they are atypical or suspected to be complicated. Gangrenous cholecystitis may lead to perforation, abscess, fistula, or peritonitis. Acalculous cholecystitis occurs most commonly in critically ill patients, especially after

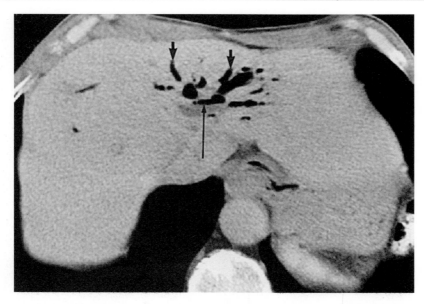

FIGURE 12-10 **Air in the biliary tree.** Air is seen in the bile ducts *(short arrows)* of the left lobe of the liver in this patient with a choledochojejunostomy performed as part of a Whipple procedure. Air fills the left hepatic bile ducts in a supine patient and the right hepatic bile ducts in a prone patient. Note the air–bile level *(long arrow).*

surgery, trauma, or burns or in patients on hyperalimentation. Acalculous cholecystitis is induced by biliary stasis, ischemia, and bacteremia. Emphysematous cholecystitis is a severe form of cholecystitis that tends to occur in elderly patients and in patients with diabetes. It may produce deceptively mild symptoms but carries high morbidity and mortality rates. The CT findings in acute cholecystitis are as follows:

- Gallstones are shown by CT to be present in the gallbladder in 75% of patients (Fig. 12-12).

TABLE 12-2

Reflux of Gas or Bowel Contrast into Biliary Tree

Iatrogenic
  Sphincterotomy
  Choledochojejunostomy
Gallstone fistula
  Cholecystoduodenal fistula
Perforated ulcer
  Choledochoduodenal fistula
Carcinoma
  Choledochoenteric fistula

- The gallbladder is usually distended to 4 to 5 cm in diameter.
- The gallbladder wall is thickened (>3 mm) and appears indistinct. It commonly enhances brightly, but this finding is not diagnostic.
- Transient, early-phase, increased attenuation of the liver adjacent to the gallbladder is strong evidence of hyperuremia and inflammation.
- Halo of subserosal edema in the gallbladder wall and stranding in the pericholecystic tissues is evident.
- Pericholecystic fluid collection is associated with perforation and abscess.
- Increase in bile density (>20 H) is caused by biliary stasis, intraluminal pus, hemorrhage, or cellular debris.
- The CT findings of acalculous cholecystitis are identical except that stones are absent. This condition occurs only in patients with the predisposing conditions listed.
- Air in the gallbladder wall or lumen is seen with *emphysematous cholecystitis,* a severe form of acute cholecystitis caused by gas-forming organisms and associated with a high mortality rate (Fig. 12-13).

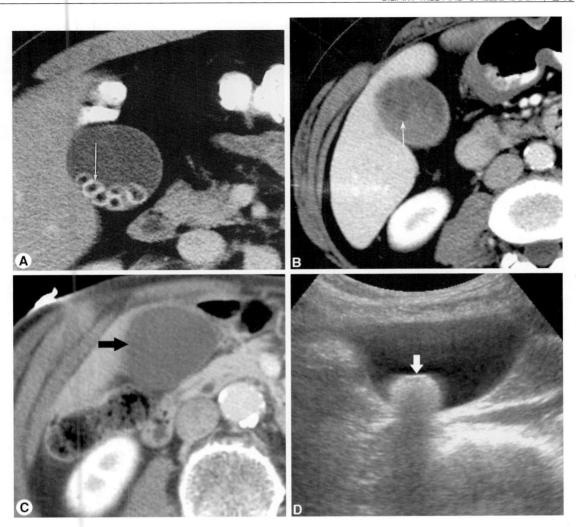

FIGURE 12-11 **Gallstones.** *A,* Gallstones *(arrow)* settle dependently in the gallbladder. These stones demonstrate low-density centers of high-cholesterol content and calcified outer margins. *B,* Low-attenuation cholesterol gallstones float within the gallbladder lumen. *C,* No gallstone was seen in the gallbladder *(arrow)* on this CT. *D,* However, an ultrasound performed on the same patient shows a large gallstone *(arrow).* Some gallstones are not visualized on CT because their attenuation is isodense with surrounding bile.

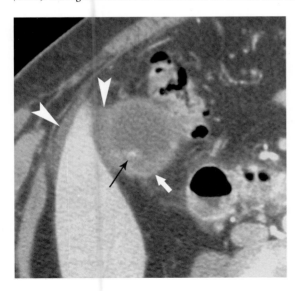

FIGURE 12-12 **Acute cholecystitis.** The gallbladder is distended and its wall *(white arrow)* is shaggy and poorly defined. Fluid *(arrowheads)* is seen adjacent to the gallbladder and around the edge of the liver. Numerous gallstones *(black arrow)* were present within the gallbladder. Surgery confirmed acute cholecystitis with a focal gallbladder perforation.

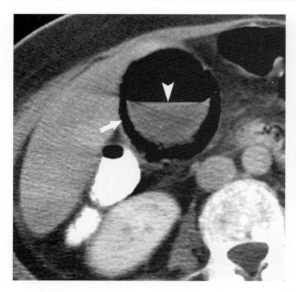

FIGURE 12-13 **Emphysematous cholecystitis.** Gas infiltrates the wall *(arrow)* of the gallbladder and forms an air–fluid level *(arrowhead)* with bile in the gallbladder lumen.

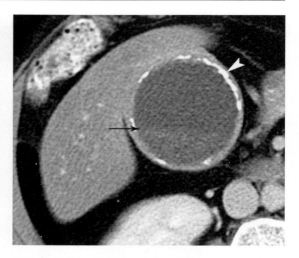

FIGURE 12-14 **Porcelain gallbladder.** The wall of the gallbladder *(arrowhead)* is thickened and calcified. A faint fluid level *(black arrow)* is seen in the gallbladder lumen because of chronic bile stasis.

Porcelain Gallbladder

Calcification of the gallbladder wall (Fig. 12-14), in association with chronic cholecystitis, is termed *porcelain gallbladder.* The calcification may be broad and continuous or multiple and punctate. Gallstones are nearly always present. Gallbladder carcinoma may develop in 25% of patients with porcelain gallbladder. Cholecystectomy is advocated even when the patient is asymptomatic.

Gallbladder Carcinoma

Gallbladder carcinoma is the most common malignancy of the biliary system. Most patients are 50 years and older. Clinical and imaging evalua-tion commonly overlooks early disease. Chronic cholelithiasis is the major risk factor for this tumor. CT demonstrates three major patterns of disease:

- A polypoid soft-tissue mass within the gallbladder lumen (Fig. 12-15)
- Focal or diffuse thickening of the gallbladder wall
- A mass containing gallstones replaces the gallbladder and invades the adjacent liver

Associated findings include gallstones; biliary dilatation; metastases in the liver; invasion of liver (Fig. 12-16), bowel, and adjacent structures; and calcification of the gallbladder wall.

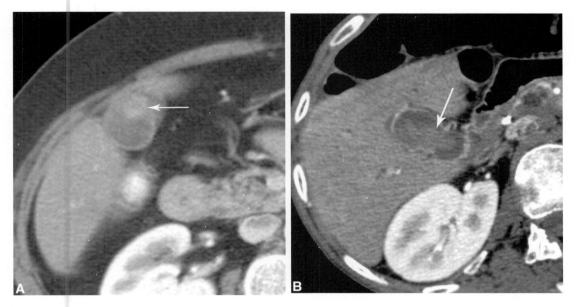

FIGURE 12-15 **Gallbladder carcinoma and gallbladder sludge.** *A,* A gallbladder carcinoma *(arrow)* is seen as a poorly defined, polypoid, soft-tissue density mass in the nondependent portion of the gallbladder. *B,* In another patient, sludge *(arrow)* within the gallbladder has a similar appearance. Sludge is concentrated bile that thickens to toothpaste consistency. It occurs primarily in acutely ill patients who are not eating, and therefore do not empty their gallbladder. Findings that may be used to differentiate the two conditions include contrast enhancement of carcinoma (or lack of contrast enhancement with sludge) or demonstration of movement of sludge with change in patient position. Doppler ultrasound may also be used to document blood flow within tumor.

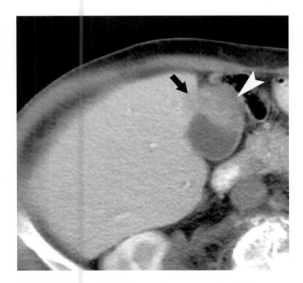

FIGURE 12-16 **Gallbladder carcinoma invades the liver.**
A carcinoma *(arrowhead)* arising within the gallbladder extends directly into the liver *(arrow)*.

▨ SUGGESTED READING

BENNETT GL, RUSINEK H, LISI V, et al: CT findings in acute gangrenous cholecystitis. AJR Am J Roentgenol 178:275–281, 2002.

BORTOFF GA, CHEN MYM, OTT DJ, et al: Gallbladder stones: Imaging and intervention. Radiographics 20:751–766, 2000.

GRAND D, HORTON KM, FISHMAN E: CT of the gallbladder: Spectrum of disease. AJR Am J Roentgenol 183:163–170, 2004.

HAN JK, CHOI BI, KIM AY, et al: Cholangiocarcinoma: Pictorial essay of CT and cholangiographic findings. Radiographics 22:173–187, 2002.

HANBIDGE AE, BUCKLER PM, O'MALLEY ME, WILSON SR: Imaging evaluation for pain in the right upper quadrant. Radiographics 24:1117–1135, 2004.

KEOGAN MT, SEABOURN JT, PAULSON EK, et al: Contrast-enhanced CT of intrahepatic and hilar cholangiocarcinoma: Delay time for optimal imaging. AJR Am J Roentgenol 169:1493–1499, 1997.

KIM OH, CHUNG HJ, CHOI BG: Imaging of choledochal cyst. Radiographics 15:69–88, 1995.

LEE W, LIM HK, JANG KM, et al: Radiologic spectrum of cholangiocarcinoma: Emphasis on unusual manifestations and differential diagnosis. Radiographics 21:S97–S116, 2001.

LEVY AD, MURAKATA LA, ABBOTT RM, ROHRMANN CA Jr: Benign tumors and tumorlike lesions of the gallbladder and extrahepatic bile ducts: Radiologic-pathologic correlation. Radiographics 22: 387–413, 2002.

LEVY AD, MURAKATA LA, ROHRMANN CA Jr: Gallbladder carcinoma: Radiologic-pathologic correlation. Radiographics 21:295–314, 2001.

LEVY AD, ROHRMANN CA Jr, MURAKATA LA, LONERGAN GJ: Caroli's disease: Radiologic spectrum with pathologic correlation. AJR Am J Roentgenol 179:1053–1057, 2002.

LIM JH: Oriental cholangiohepatitis: Pathologic, clinical, and radiologic features. AJR Am J Roentgenol 157:1–8, 1991.

LIM JH: Cholangiocarcinoma: Morphologic classification according to growth pattern and imaging findings. AJR Am J Roentgenol 181:819–827, 2003.

LIM JH, YOON K-H, KIM SH, et al: Intraductal papillary mucinous tumor of the bile ducts. Radiographics 24:53–67, 2004.

MILLER FH, HWANG CM, GABRIEL H, et al: Contrast-enhanced helical CT of choledocholithiasis. AJR Am J Roentgenol 181:125–130, 2003.

MILLER WJ, SECHTIN AG, CAMPBELL WL, PIETERS PC: Imaging findings in Caroli's disease. AJR Am J Roentgenol 165:333–337, 1995.

PAULSON EK: Acute cholecystitis: CT findings. Sem Ultrasound CT MRI 21:56–63, 2000.

RIZZO RJ, SZUCS RA, TURNER MA: Congenital abnormalities of the pancreas and biliary tree in adults. Radiographics 15:49–68, 1995.

ROOHOLAMINI SA, TEHRANI NS, RAZAVI MK, et al: Imaging of gallbladder carcinoma. Radiographics 14:291–306, 1994.

SOYER P, GOUHIN M, BROCHEIOU-SPELLE I, et al: Carcinoma of the gallbladder: Imaging features with surgical correlation. AJR Am J Roentgenol 169:169–181, 1997.

VITELLAS KM, KEOGAN MT, FREED KS, et al: Radiologic manifestations of sclerosing cholangitis with emphasis on MR cholangiopancreatography. Radiographics 20:959–975, 2000.

YAMASHITA K, JIN MJ, HIROSE Y, et al: CT finding of transient focal increase attenuation of the liver adjacent to the gallbladder in acute cholecystitis. AJR Am J Roentgenol 164:343–346, 1995.

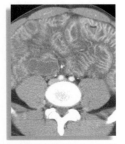

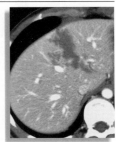

Pancreas

William E. Brant, M.D.

CT is the imaging method of choice for the pancreas for most indications. Multi-detector CT (MDCT) has improved pancreatic imaging by providing the ability to obtain thinner slices to improve spatial resolution and shorter acquisition times to improve assessment of contrast enhancement.

☐ CT TECHNIQUE

Optimal CT technique is based on thin sections (≤3–5 mm) obtained dynamically during intravenous contrast enhancement. MDCT offers great advantage through its capability of obtaining many scans within a short period. Water is preferred as an oral contrast agent because dense contrast may obscure small stones near the ampulla and detail in the pancreatic head. Dual-phase scans during arterial and venous enhancement are routine. A preliminary non-contrast scan is obtained through the abdomen. A power injector is used to administer 120 to 150 mL intravenous contrast at 3 to 5 mL/second. The "arterial" phase scan is obtained at 30 to 35 seconds after onset of injection. With MDCT, these scans may be acquired using 1- to 2.5-mm collimations and a field of view reduced

to the size of the pancreas for high-resolution images. Thin slices allow for detailed three-dimensional reconstruction of CT angiograms. The "venous" phase scan is obtained at 65 to 70 seconds after initiation of contrast injection. This scan routinely encompasses the entire abdomen and may be extended to include the pelvis.

☐ ANATOMY OF THE PANCREAS

The pancreas lies within the anterior pararenal compartment of the retroperitoneal space, behind the left lobe of the liver and the stomach, and in front of the spine and great vessels (Fig. 13-1). The peritoneum-lined lesser sac forms a potential space between the stomach and pancreas. The pancreas somewhat resembles a question mark turned on its left side with the hook portion formed by the pancreatic head and uncinate process as they lie cradled in the duodenal loop. The portal vein fills the center of the hook. The uncinate process cradles the superior mesenteric vein and tapers to a sharpened point beneath it. The body and tail taper as they extend toward the splenic hilum. The pancreas is usually directed upward

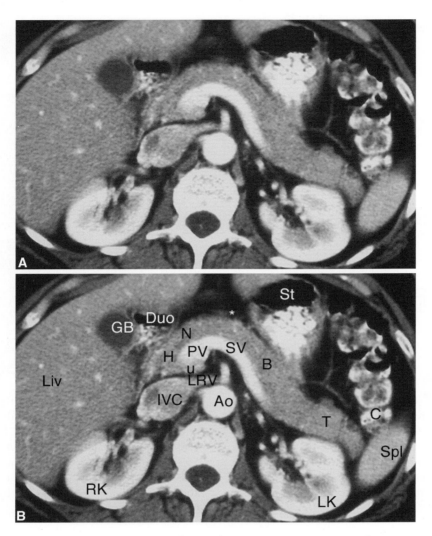

FIGURE 13-1 **Normal pancreas anatomy.** *A,* CT image of a normal pancreas. *B,* Same image as A with anatomic structures labeled.

Continued

and to the left, although it may form an inverted *U* shape with the tail directed caudad. Sequential CT slices must be mentally summated to assess the shape and size of the pancreas. The gland is 12 to 15 cm in length. Maximum dimensions for width are 3.0 cm for the head, 2.5 cm for the body, and 2.0 cm for the tail. The gland is larger in young patients and progressively decreases in size with age. The CT attenuation is uniform and approximately equal to muscle. In young patients, the pancreas resembles a slab of meat. Progressive infiltration of fat between the lobules of the pancreas gives it a feathery appearance with advancing age. The pancreatic duct is best visualized with thin slices (<5 mm). It measures a maximum of 3 to 4 mm in diameter in the head and tapers smoothly to the tail.

The complex vascular anatomy about the pancreas must be understood to correctly interpret pancreatic CT. The splenic vein runs a relatively straight course in the dorsum of the pancreas from the splenic hilum to its junction with the superior mesenteric vein just posterior to the neck of the pancreas. The plane of fat between the splenic vein and pancreas must not be mistaken for the pancreatic duct. The splenic artery runs an undulating course through the pancreas from the celiac axis to the spleen. Atherosclerotic calcifications are common in the splenic artery and are easily mistaken for pancreatic calcifications. The superior mesenteric artery arises from the aorta dorsal to the pancreas and courses caudally surrounded by a collar of fat. The superior mesenteric vein courses crani-

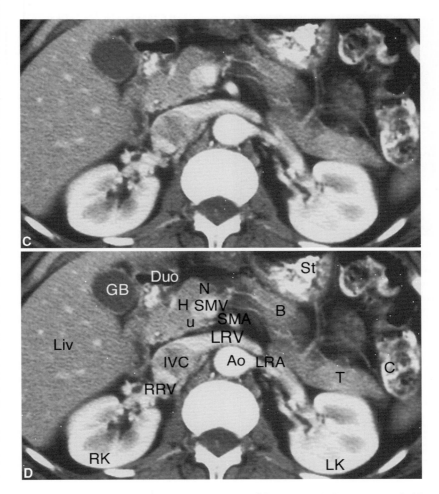

FIGURE 13-1 **Cont'd** *C*, CT image of normal head and uncinate process of the pancreas. *D*, Same image as *C* with anatomic structures labeled. *Asterisk* indicates location of lesser sac. Ao, aorta; B, body of pancreas; C, colon; Duo, duodenum; GB, gallbladder; H, head of pancreas; IVC, inferior vena cava; Liv, liver, LK, left kidney; LRV, left renal vein; N, neck of pancreas; PV, commencement of portal vein RK, right kidney; RRV, right renal vein; SMA, superior mesenteric artery; SMV, superior mesenteric vein; Spl, spleen; St, stomach; SV, splenic vein; T, tail of pancreas; u, uncinate process of pancreatic head.

ally, just to the right of the superior mesenteric artery, until it joins the splenic vein to form the portal vein. The pancreatic head entirely surrounds this junction with the uncinate process extending beneath the superior mesenteric vein. The portal vein courses upward and rightward with the hepatic artery and common bile duct to the porta hepatis.

☐ FATTY INFILTRATION OF THE PANCREAS

Fatty infiltration of the pancreas occurs commonly with aging and obesity without affecting the function of the pancreas. In advanced cystic fibrosis, the pancreatic parenchyma is atrophic and is diffusely replaced by fat, whereas exocrine function of the pancreas is severely impaired. CT findings indicating fatty infiltration include:

- Because the gland is not encapsulated, fatty infiltration between the lobules in older patients gives the pancreas a delicate, feathery appearance resembling a dust mop (Fig. 13-2).
- Fatty replacement may be diffuse or distributed unevenly through the pancreas. Common areas of focal sparing of fat infiltration are the head and uncinate process. In some patients, the head and uncinate process are involved and the remainder of the pancreas is spared.

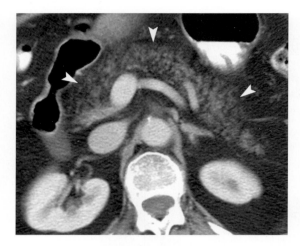

FIGURE 13-2 **Fatty infiltration of the pancreas.** The pancreas *(arrowheads)* shows fat infiltrating between the atrophic lobules of parenchyma. Despite diffuse atrophy and fatty infiltration, the exocrine and endocrine functions of the pancreas were normal in this patient.

☐ ACUTE PANCREATITIS

Inflammation of the pancreas damages acinar tissue and leads to focal disruption of small ducts, resulting in leakage of pancreatic juice. The absence of a capsule around the pancreas allows easy access of pancreatic secretions to surrounding tissues. Pancreatic enzymes digest through fascial layers to spread to multiple anatomic compartments. Acute pancreatitis in adults is most often caused by passage of a gallstone or by alcohol abuse (Table 13-1). The diagnosis of pancreatitis is made clinically. CT may be normal in mild cases. The role of CT is to document the presence and severity of complications. Severity of CT findings correlates with prognosis.

- *Pancreatic changes* include focal or diffuse enlargement of the pancreas, decrease in density of pancreatic parenchyma because of edema, and blurring of the margins of the gland by inflammation.
- *Peripancreatic changes* include stranding densities in fat and blurring of fat planes

TABLE 13-1

Causes of Pancreatitis

Alcohol abuse—most common cause of chronic pancreatitis
Gallstone passage/impaction—most common cause of acute pancreatitis
Metabolic disorders
   Hereditary pancreatitis—autosomal dominant
   Hypercalcemia
   Hyperlipidemia—types I and V
   Malnutrition
Trauma
   Blunt abdominal trauma
   Surgery
   Endoscopic retrograde cholangiopancreatography
Penetrating ulcer
Malignancy
   Pancreatic adenocarcinoma
   Lymphoma
Drugs—corticosteroids, tetracycline, furosemide, many others
Infection
   Viral—mumps, hepatitis, infectious mononucleosis, acquired immunodeficiency syndrome
   Parasitic—ascariasis, clonorchiasis
Structural
   Choledochocele
   Pancreas divisum
Idiopathic—20% of cases of acute pancreatitis

with thickening of involved retroperitoneal fascia.

Complications related to acute pancreatitis include:

- *Fluid collections* are nonencapsulated homogeneous aggregations of fluid in the pancreatic bed, retroperitoneum, and often widespread throughout the abdomen (Figs. 13-3 and 13-4).
- *Pseudocysts* are well-defined round or oval collections of fluid with a clearly identifiable fibrous capsule. The fluid collection must remain present for approximately 6 weeks for the fibrous capsule to form and for the fluid collection to qualify being identified as a pancreatic pseudocyst (Fig. 13-5).
- *Necrosis* is liquefaction of portions of the gland, which are identified by lack of contrast enhancement during bolus contrast administration (Fig. 13-6). Necrotic tissue is highly susceptible to infection. Accurate diagnosis requires bolus contrast administration and scanning during the arterial phase of enhancement. The presence of necrosis establishes the diagnosis of necrotizing pancreatitis, which is associated with increased severity of disease and increased risk for death.

- *Phlegmon* is a mass of edema and inflammation seen as ill-defined, heterogeneous, soft-tissue and fluid densities (20–40 H) in and around the pancreas.
- *Abscess* refers to foci of bacterial growth within necrotic tissues seen as loculated fluid collections that may contain gas (Fig. 13-7). CT- or ultrasonography-guided percutaneous aspiration is needed to confirm diagnosis.
- *Hemorrhage* is caused by erosion of blood vessels or bowel. It is seen as high-attenuating fluid in retroperitoneum or peritoneal cavity. Hemorrhage commonly accompanies necrosis, resulting in the interchangeable terms *hemorrhagic pancreatitis* or *necrotizing pancreatitis.*
- *Pseudoaneurysms* are encapsulations of arterial hemorrhage with continued communication with eroded artery. Swirling and "to and fro" blood flow continue within the pseudoaneurysm. Risk for massive hemorrhage is high. A pseudoaneurysm must be excluded before percutaneous puncture of pancreatic fluid collections (Fig. 13-8).
- *Thrombosis* of splenic vein and other peripancreatic vessels occurs as a result of the inflammatory process. The thrombosed

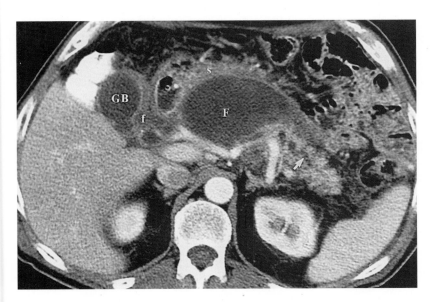

FIGURE 13-3 **Acute pancreatitis: fluid collections.** Fluid collections (f) resulting from acute pancreatitis extend from the necrotic pancreas into the lesser sac (F) compressing the stomach (s) and are evident around the gallbladder (GB). The distal pancreatic duct *(arrow)* is dilated.

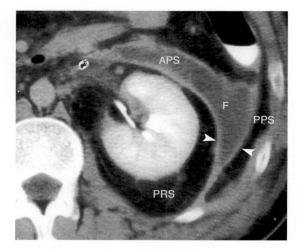

FIGURE 13-4 **Acute pancreatitis: fluid collection.** Pancreatic fluid (F) and inflammation extend from the pancreas in the anterior pararenal space (APS) partially around the left kidney between the leaves of the posterior renal fascia *(arrowheads)*. Note that the perirenal space (PRS) and the posterior pararenal space (PPS) are spared.

veins are distended with low-attenuation thrombus and fail to enhance on venous phase scans.
- *Pancreatic ascites* is caused by leakage of pancreatic juice into the peritoneal cavity inducing secretion of fluid from peritoneal membranes. Pancreatic ascites contains a high level of amylase.

☐ CHRONIC PANCREATITIS

Chronic pancreatitis is a chronic inflammatory disease of the pancreas characterized by progressive pancreatic damage with irreversible fibrosis. This process results in major structural abnormalities in varying combination, including parenchymal atrophy, calcifications, stricture and dilatation of the pancreatic duct, fluid collections, pseudomass formation, and alteration of peripancreatic fat. Although many patients with chronic pancreatitis have recurrent episodes of acute pancreatitis, chronic pancreatitis appears to be a separate entity. Patients with chronic pancreatitis are an average of 13 years younger than patients with acute pancreatitis. Acute pancreatitis seldom results in the development of chronic pancreatitis. Causes of chronic pancreatitis include alcoholism (70%), autoimmune disease, tropical pancreatitis, and nonalcoholic duct-destructive pancreatitis. CT indications of chronic pancreatitis include:

- Calcifications are commonly present (50% of patients) in focal areas or are spread diffusely throughout the pancreas (Fig. 13-9). Calcifications vary in appearance from finely stippled to coarse. Pancreatic calcifications occur most frequently in hereditary pancreatitis and in chronic pancreatitis caused by alcoholism.

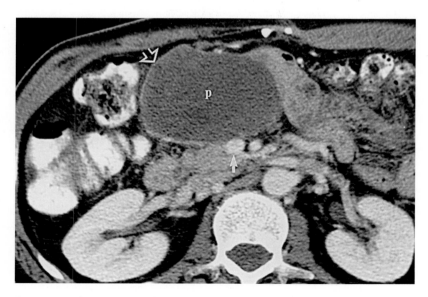

FIGURE 13-5 **Pseudocyst.** A pseudocyst (p) with a thin capsule *(open arrow)* persists 8 weeks after an episode of acute pancreatitis. The pseudocyst compressed the superior mesenteric vein *(small arrow)* and portal vein, resulting in dilatation of portosystemic collateral vessels.

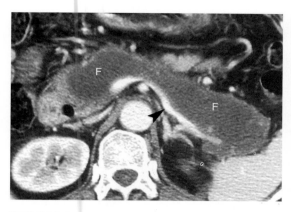

FIGURE 13-6 **Necrotizing pancreatitis.** Liquefaction necrosis has completely destroyed the pancreas replacing it with a loculated collection of fluid (F) in the pancreatic bed anterior to the splenic vein *(arrowhead).*

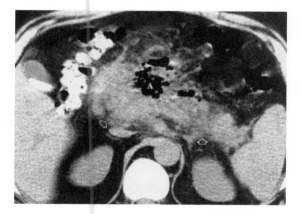

FIGURE 13-7 **Pancreatic abscess.** A penetrating duodenal ulcer resulted in pancreatitis, pancreatic abscess, and pancreaticoduodenal fistula. An extensive gas collection (A) occupies the pancreatic bed. The margins of the pancreas are blurred by the inflammatory process *(open arrows).*

- The gland is focally or diffusely atrophic (54%; Fig. 13-10). Atrophy may result in exocrine insufficiency and diabetes mellitus.
- The pancreatic duct has focal strictures and dilated segments (68%). This "beaded" dilatation is characteristic (see Fig. 13-10).
- Focal areas of pancreatic enlargement caused by focal inflammation are common (30%) and must be distinguished from tumors (Fig. 13-11). The presence of calcifications within the mass strongly favors pancreatitis over tumor. Percutaneous biopsy, guided by ultrasonography or CT, is commonly needed to make an accurate diagnosis.
- Bile ducts may be dilated because of inflammatory stricture of the common bile

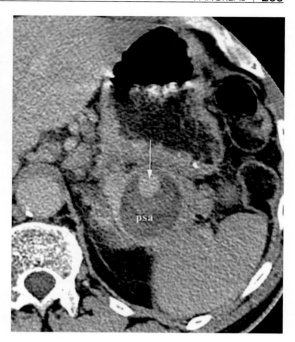

FIGURE 13-8 **Pseudoaneurysm.** A pseudoaneurysm (psa) of the splenic artery, developing as a complication of recurrent pancreatitis, is identified by a nodule of enhancement *(arrow).* The remainder of the pseudoaneurysm was low in density, indicating thrombus.

duct as it passes through the pancreas (see Fig. 13-9).
- Fluid collections are caused by superimposed acute pancreatitis (30%).
- Pancreatic pseudocysts are found in 25% to 40% of patients.
- Peripancreatic tissues show inflammatory change with fascial thickening and stranding densities in peripancreatic fat. These changes result in poor definition of the pancreatic margins.

☐ ADENOCARCINOMA OF THE PANCREAS

Pancreatic carcinoma is an aggressive and usually fatal tumor. Only 3% of afflicted patients survive 5 years. The only realistic hope for cure is early detection and aggressive surgery (Whipple procedure). CT plays a pivotal role in preoperative staging, separating those patients who are obviously *unresectable* from the 10% to 15% who are *potentially resectable*. CT angiography is helpful in determining vascular involvement by tumor. Unfortunately, most of those who

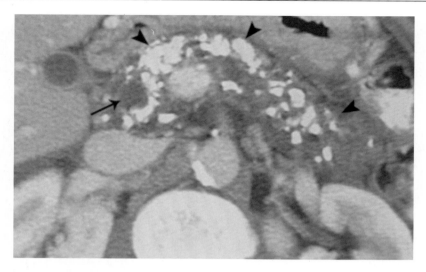

FIGURE 13-9 **Chronic pancreatitis: calcifications.** Numerous coarse calcifications are seen throughout the pancreas *(arrowheads)* in this patient with recurrent alcoholic pancreatitis. The common bile duct *(arrow)* is mildly dilated because of benign stricture in the pancreatic head.

undergo aggressive resection still eventually die of their disease. CT findings of adenocarcinoma include:

- The tumor appears as a hypodense mass (96% of patients), which enhances minimally compared with normal pancreatic parenchyma. Because focal chronic pancreatitis may closely simulate malignancy in the pancreas, biopsy is frequently needed to confirm the diagnosis. Calcifications are rarely associated with adenocarcinoma. Tumors are localized in the head (60%), body (15%), tail (5%), and are diffuse throughout the pancreas in 20% of patients.

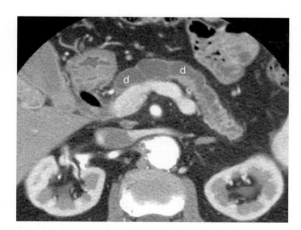

FIGURE 13-10 **Chronic pancreatitis: dilated pancreatic duct.** The pancreatic duct (d) shows marked beaded dilatation. The pancreatic parenchyma is severely atrophied.

- The tumor may be subtle, appearing as focal enlargement of the pancreas with loss of surface lobulation.
- The pancreatic or common bile duct, or both ducts, are commonly dilated proximal to the tumor.
- Atrophy of pancreatic tissue may occur proximal to the tumor.
- Signs of acute or chronic pancreatitis may be simultaneously present.

Signs of potential resectability include:

- Isolated pancreatic mass with or without dilatation of the bile and pancreatic ducts (Fig. 13-12)
- Combined bile-pancreatic duct dilatation without an identifiable pancreatic mass (pancreatic duct > 5 mm in head or > 3 mm in tail; common bile duct > 9 mm)
- Detectable regional lymph nodes may or may not be involved with tumor; size of nodes is not a reliable criterion for tumor involvement; the presence of enlarged lymph nodes (>10 mm) does not preclude resectability

Signs of unresectability include:

- Involvement of major arteries, or long segment involvement or occlusion of major veins makes the tumor unresectable (Fig. 13-13)
- Extension of tumor beyond the margins of the pancreas

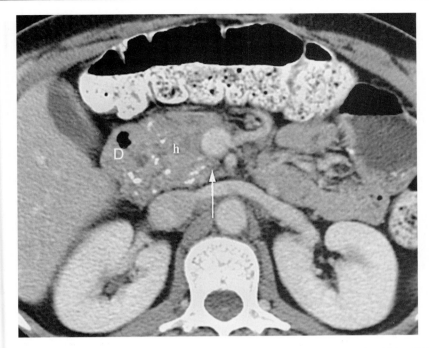

FIGURE 13-11 **Chronic pancreatitis: mass.** Chronic pancreatitis causes enlargement of the pancreatic head (h) and blunting of the tip of the uncinate process *(arrow)*. The mass partially encases the duodenum (D). A benign causative factor is suggested by the presence of calcifications, which are common with chronic pancreatitis and rare with pancreatic carcinoma. Compare with Figures 13-12 and 13-13.

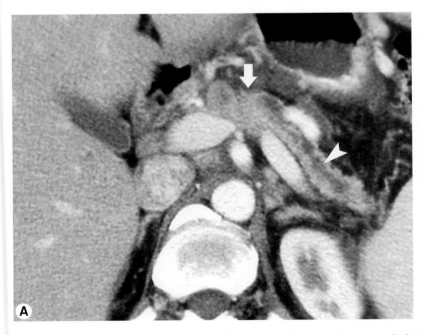

FIGURE 13-12 **Potentially resectable pancreatic carcinomas.** *A,* A subtle carcinoma *(arrow)* in the pancreatic body is detectable because it causes dilatation of the pancreatic duct *(arrowhead)* and atrophy of the pancreatic tail.

Continued

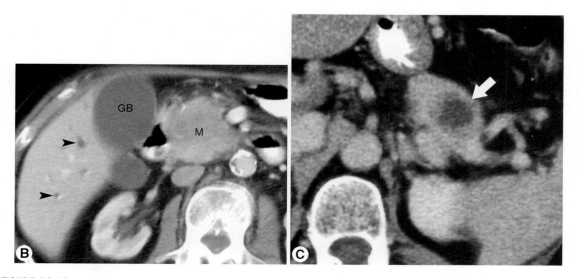

FIGURE 13-12 *Cont'd* *B,* A mass (M) in the pancreatic head causes dilatation of the bile ducts *(arrowheads).* The gallbladder (GB) is distended. *C,* An isolated mass *(arrow)* in the pancreatic tail showed no additional findings. All three lesions were resectable at surgery.

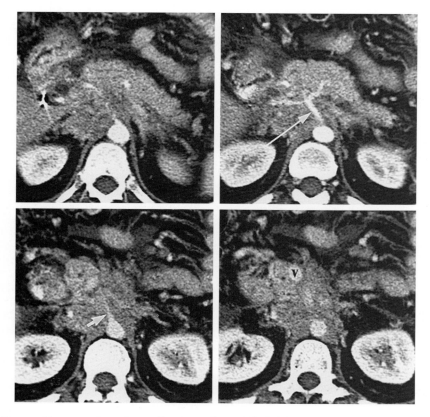

FIGURE 13-13 **Unresectable pancreatic carcinoma.** Four images from a helical CT examination demonstrate tumor encasement of the celiac axis *(long arrow)* and its branches, the superior mesenteric artery *(short arrow)* and the superior mesenteric vein (V). Tumor extensively infiltrates the retroperitoneal fat and partially encases the aorta.

- Tumor tissue invasion of adjacent organs (spleen, stomach, and duodenum)
- Involvement of celiac axis; superior mesenteric artery; or portal, splenic, or superior mesenteric veins; involvement includes the following signs:
  - Thickening of the vessel walls
  - Soft tissue obscuring the normally sharp definition of the vessel by perivascular fat; this finding may also be caused by pancreatitis
  - Deformity of the vessel by adjacent tumor
  - Enlargement of collateral vessels
  - Absence of vessels enhancement
- Metastases to the liver (usually hypodense and poorly enhancing)
- Ascites, which is presumptive evidence of peritoneal carcinomatosis

☐ ISLET CELL TUMOR

Functioning islet cell tumors produce distinct clinical syndromes and usually present while the tumors are small. Nonfunctioning islet cell tumors are clinically silent until they present with symptoms of a large, growing mass. Functioning tumors vary in malignant potential from 10% for insulinoma to 60% for gastrinoma and 80% for glucagonoma. Up to 80% of nonfunctioning tumors are malignant. CT findings for islet cell tumors include:

- Small tumors (<4 cm) are homogeneous and usually isodense with the unenhanced pancreas. They enhance brightly and usually uniformly during arterial phase of contrast administration (Fig. 13-14). Hormone-producing tumors are usually small.
- Large tumors (6–20 cm) are usually heterogeneous with calcification, cystic degeneration, necrosis, vascular invasion, and direct tumor extension into adjacent structures (Fig. 13-15). Nonfunctioning tumors are commonly large.
- Metastases occur to the liver and to distant organs.

☐ PANCREATIC LYMPHOMA

Lymphoma must be differentiated from adenocarcinoma because the diagnosis and treatment are radically different. Lymphoma involves the

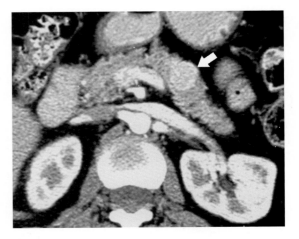

FIGURE 13-14 **Insulinoma.** A small insulin-producing islet cell tumor *(arrow)* shows early enhancement during an arterial phase CT image. The patient presented with episodes of hypoglycemia.

pancreas most commonly by direct extension from peripancreatic lymphadenopathy. The pancreas may be involved in 30% of patients with non–Hodgkin's lymphoma, especially in patients with AIDS-related lymphoma. Primary pancreatic lymphoma is rare. CT findings of pancreatic lymphoma include:

- Focal tumor that is well circumscribed with homogeneous attenuation less than muscle and that enhances weakly but uniformly is characteristic.
- Diffuse infiltration of the pancreas resembles pancreatitis but without clinical evidence of pancreatitis.

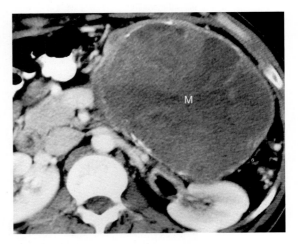

FIGURE 13-15 **Malignant nonfunctioning islet cell tumor.** Huge heterogeneous solid mass (M) arising from the body and tail of the pancreas displaces bowel and compresses the left kidney.

- Peripancreatic lymphadenopathy that extends into and displaces the pancreas is characteristic of secondary pancreatic lymphoma (Fig. 13-16).
- A bulky mass with no or minimal dilatation of the pancreatic duct strongly favors lymphoma over adenocarcinoma.
- Lymphadenopathy below the level of the renal veins is seen with lymphoma but not with pancreatic adenocarcinoma.

☐ METASTASES TO THE PANCREAS

Metastases to the pancreas are unusual and are present in only 3% to 12% of patients with advanced malignancy. The most common primary tumors are melanoma and carcinomas of the kidney, lung, or breast. Pancreatic metastases have the following characteristics:

- Most tumors are round or ovoid with smooth, discrete margins.
- Metastases are found with equal frequency in all portions of the pancreas.
- Most (75%) demonstrate heterogeneous contrast enhancement.
- Tumors are commonly solitary (50–79%) and simulate primary pancreatic adenocarcinoma.
- Diffuse involvement (5–44%) causes generalized pancreatic enlargement.

- Multiple nodules are found in 5% to 17% of patients.
- Involvement of pancreatic blood vessels is rare.
- Lesions in the head and neck may obstruct the main pancreatic duct (37%) or common bile duct.
- Metastases in other organs and at other sites are usually present.

☐ INTRADUCTAL PAPILLARY MUCINOUS NEOPLASM

An intraductal papillary mucinous neoplasm secretes an excessive volume of mucin into the pancreatic ducts, producing progressive dilation of the main pancreatic duct and cystic ectasia of the branch pancreatic ducts. Intraductal, mucin-producing tumors are best considered a separate entity from mucinous-cystic tumors of the pancreas. Intraductal tumors arise from the epithelium lining the pancreatic ducts. Histology ranges from hyperplasia to adenocarcinoma. CT findings include:

- Tumors arising in the main pancreatic duct produce marked diffuse or segmental enlargement of the pancreatic duct associated with atrophy of the pancreatic

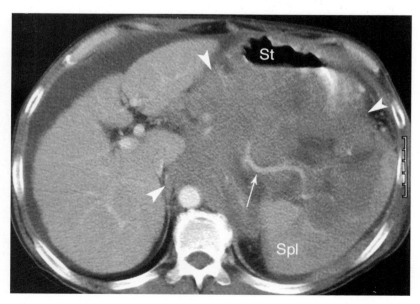

FIGURE 13-16 **Lymphoma.** Massive confluent adenopathy *(arrowheads)* envelopes the pancreas, invades the spleen (Spl), and displaces the stomach (St). Only the splenic artery *(arrow)* is clearly visible within the mass of tumor.

parenchyma (Fig. 13-17). Amorphous calcification may be evident within the dilated duct.

- Cystic ectasia of branch ducts produces a "bunch-of-grapes" appearance that bulges the contour of the pancreas.
- Intraductal papillary solid masses are seen within the dilated pancreatic ducts and may bulge into the lumen of the duodenum at the papilla.
- Tumors arising in the branch ducts produce a multicystic mass. This lesion is markedly predisposed to occur in the uncinate process (see Fig. 13-17).
- Endoscopic retrograde cholangiopancreatography shows characteristic communication between the dilated main pancreatic duct and the multicystic dilatation of the branch pancreatic ducts.

☐ CYSTIC LESIONS

Cystic lesions of the pancreas are notoriously difficult to diagnose accurately by CT. Cystic tumors of the pancreas represent only 10% of all pancreatic cysts and 1% of all pancreatic neoplasms. Accurate diagnosis is important because: (a) mucinous cystadenomas are malignant and deserve surgical resection; (b) serous cystadenomas are benign and can be observed; and (c) pseudocysts, resulting from pancreatitis, are the most common lesions and frequently require drainage. CT is sensitive in the detection of cystic lesions, but other techniques such as endoscopic ultrasound with aspiration-biopsy are usually used to provide definitive diagnosis.

Pseudocysts

By far the most common cystic lesion in and around the pancreas, pseudocysts are collections of pancreatic fluid that have become encapsulated within fibrous walls. They result from episodes of acute pancreatitis. Although most patients with pancreatitis have abdominal pain, some do not. Pseudocyst must always be included in the differential diagnosis of cystic pancreatic lesions. Fluid aspirated from pseudocysts has high levels of amylase. CT findings of pseudocysts include:

- Pseudocysts appear as low-density collections of fluid, cellular debris, or blood (see Fig. 13-5).
- Distinct walls are well defined and of variable thickness. Calcifications are occasionally present in the cyst wall.
- Most are unilocular. Some contain a few septa.
- Signs of pancreatitis are usually present.

Mucinous Cystic Neoplasm

Mucinous cystic neoplasms are rare primary tumors of the pancreas found most commonly in middle-aged women (95% of patients). All are low-grade mucinous cystadenocarcinomas.

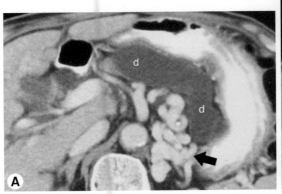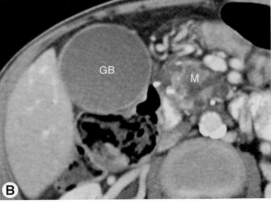

FIGURE 13-17 **Intraductal papillary mucinous tumor.** *A,* The pancreatic duct (d) is massively dilated and little pancreatic parenchyma is visible. Huge portosystemic collateral vessels *(arrow)* are caused by splenic vein thrombosis. *B,* The head of the pancreas is replaced by a heterogeneous solid mass (M) with cystic areas representing dilated branch pancreatic ducts. The gallbladder (GB) is markedly dilated. Biopsy confirmed mucin-secreting papillary adenocarcinomas. The marked dilatation of the pancreatic duct caused by a combination of ductal obstruction and excessive mucin secretion.

They have an excellent prognosis with surgical resection. CT findings include:

- Tumors appear as multiloculated cysts with thin (<2 mm) septa (Fig. 13-18). Six or less cysts larger than 2 cm are considered typical of the lesion. CT may not demonstrate the thin septa on unenhanced images, but the septa usually enhance and are seen well after contrast administration.
- Attenuation of fluid within the cyst varies with content (water to mucoid to hemorrhagic).
- Calcifications are seen in the capsule or septa in 10% of lesions. Peripheral calcifications are characteristic of mucinous cystic tumors, whereas serous cystadenomas have only central calcifications.
- Lesions range in size from 2 to 36 cm with an average size of 6 to 10 cm.
- Tumors are most common in the tail of the pancreas.
- These tumors do not communicate with the ductal system of the pancreas.
- Metastases may be evident (Fig. 13-19).

Serous Cystadenoma

Serous cystadenomas are benign pancreatic tumors with no malignant potential. Serous cysts contain clear fluid. Endoscopic ultrasound-guided aspiration that yields clear rather than

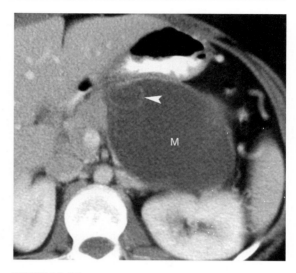

FIGURE 13-18 **Mucinous cystic neoplasm.** A large cystic mass (M) arises from the body of the pancreas. A thin enhancing septation *(arrowhead)* is evident. Differential diagnosis would include pseudocyst and the macrocystic form of serous cystadenoma.

mucinous fluid helps confirm the diagnosis. These lesions occur in two morphologic forms:

- The classic appearance is a well-circumscribed mass of innumerable small cysts. When the cysts are tiny, the mass appears solid and characteristically has a central stellate scar, often with central calcification (Fig. 13-20). When the cysts are larger (up to 2 cm), the mass assumes a honeycomb appearance (Fig. 13-21).

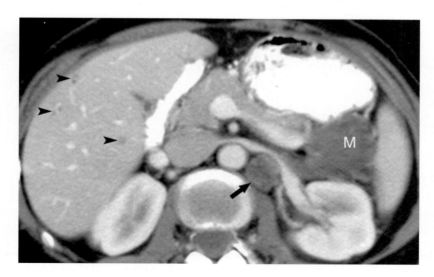

FIGURE 13-19 **Mucinous cystic neoplasm: metastases.** A low-attenuation cystic mass is evident at the tail of the pancreas. Small, low-density lesions *(arrowheads)* in the liver and an enlarged lymph node *(arrow)* behind the left renal vein represent metastatic spread of the malignant tumor.

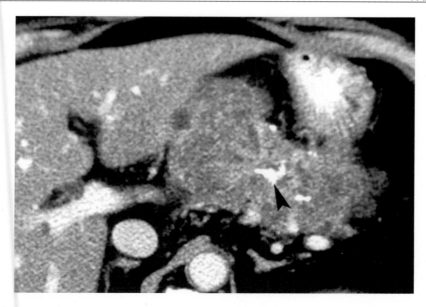

FIGURE 13-20 **Serous cystadenoma: microcystic tumor.** Although it consists of innumerable tiny cysts, this tumor resembles a solid mass. The central calcification *(arrowhead)* within a stellate scar is characteristic. This is a benign tumor arising from the neck of the pancreas.

- The unilocular form is 2 to 6 cm in size and may be indistinguishable from mucinous cystic neoplasms. Lobulated contour, absence of wall enhancement, and location in the pancreatic head favor serous cystadenoma.

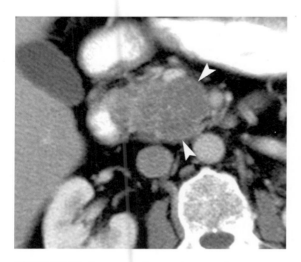

FIGURE 13-21 **Serous cystadenoma: honeycomb appearance.** This cystic lesion *(arrowheads)* arising in the pancreatic head has somewhat larger cysts, creating a honeycomb appearance. The location and appearance is characteristic of serous cystadenoma.

True Pancreatic Cysts

True pancreatic cysts are rare and are seen far less frequently than pancreatic pseudocysts. Congenital epithelial-lined cysts are usually solitary. Multiple pancreatic cysts are seen with von Hippel–Lindau syndrome (50% of patients) and autosomal dominant polycystic disease (5% of patients). Rarely, epithelial-lined cysts are seen in patients with cystic fibrosis. CT findings include:

- Cysts appear as well-defined, fluid-filled masses of various sizes with walls of variable thickness (Fig. 13-22).
- In von Hippel–Lindau syndrome, the pancreas is also involved with serous cystadenomas (12%) and neuroendocrine tumors (7% to 12%). A small number of the neuroendocrine tumors are malignant. The cystic lesions in the pancreas are benign.

Duodenal Diverticulum

Duodenal diverticula are common lesions that may be entirely fluid filled and mimic a cystic neoplasm of the pancreas.

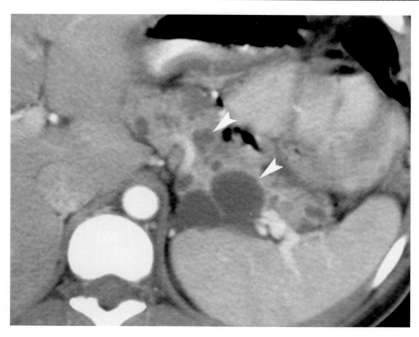

FIGURE 13-22 **von Hippel–Lindau syndrome.** Multilocular and unilocular cysts *(arrowheads)* are seen throughout the pancreas in this patient with von Hippel–Lindau syndrome.

☐ SUGGESTED READING

BALTHAZAR EJ: Acute pancreatitis: Assessment of severity with clinical and CT evaluation. Radiology 223:603–613, 2002.

BUETOW PC, MILLER DL, PARRINO TV, BUCK JL: Islet cell tumors of the pancreas: Clinical, radiologic, and pathologic correlation in diagnosis and localization. Radiographics 17:453–472, 1997.

BUETOW PC, RAO P, THOMPSON LDR: Mucinous cystic neoplasms of the pancreas: Radiologic-pathologic correlation. Radiographics 18:433–449, 1998.

CASAS JD, DIAZ R, VALDERAS G, et al: Prognostic value of CT in the early assessment of patients with acute pancreatitis. AJR Am J Roentgenol 182:569–574, 2004.

COHEN-SCALI F, VILGRAIN V, BRANCATELLI G, et al: Discrimination of unilocular macrocystic serous cystadenoma from pancreatic pseudocyst and mucinous cystadenoma with CT: Initial observations. Radiology 228:727–733, 2003.

CURRY CA, ENG J, HORTON KM, et al: CT of primary cystic pancreatic neoplasms: Can CT be used for patient triage and treatment? AJR Am J Roentgenol 175:99–103, 2000.

DEMOS TC, POSNIAK HV, HARMATH C, et al: Cystic lesions of the pancreas. AJR Am J Roentgenol 179:1375–1388, 2002.

GROGAN JR, SAEIAN K, TAYLOR AJ, et al: Making sense of mucin-producing pancreatic tumors. AJR Am J Roentgenol 176:921–929, 2001.

HORTON KM, FISHMAN EJ: Multidetector CT angiography of pancreatic carcinoma: Part 1, evaluation of arterial involvement. AJR Am J Roentgenol 178:827–831, 2002.

HORTON KM, FISHMAN EJ: Multidetector CT angiography of pancreatic carcinoma: Part 2, evaluation of venous involvement. AJR Am J Roentgenol 178:833–836, 2002.

KATZ DS, HINES J, MATH KR, et al: Using CT to reveal fat-containing abnormalities of the pancreas. AJR Am J Roentgenol 172:393–396, 1999.

KIM T, MURAKAMI T, TAKAMURA M, et al: Pancreatic mass due to chronic pancreatitis: Correlation of CT and MR imaging features with pathologic findings. AJR Am J Roentgenol 177:367–371, 2001.

KLIEN KA, STEPHENS DH, WELCH TJ: CT characteristics of metastatic disease of the pancreas. Radiographics 18:369–378, 1998.

LESNIAK RJ, HOHENWALTER MD, TAYLOR A: Spectrum of causes of pancreatic calcifications. AJR Am J Roentgenol 178:79–86, 2002.

LIM JH, LEE G, OH YL: Radiologic spectrum of intraductal papillary mucinous tumor of the pancreas. Radiographics 21:323–340, 2001.

MACARI M, LAZARUS D, ISREAL G, MEGIBOW A: Duodenal diverticula mimicking cystic neoplasms of the pancreas: CT and MR imaging findings in seven patients. AJR Am J Roentgenol 180:195–199, 2003.

MERKLE EM, BENDER GN, BRAMBS H-J: Imaging findings in pancreatic lymphoma: Differential aspects. AJR Am J Roentgenol 174:671–675, 2000.

O'MALLEY ME, BOLAND GWL, WOOD BJ, et al: Adenocarcinoma of the head of the pancreas: Determination of surgical unresectability with thin-section pancreatic-phase helical CT. AJR Am J Roentgenol 173:1513–1518, 1999.

PATEL BK, CHENOWETH JL, GARVIN PJ, et al: Role of imaging in the diagnosis of chronic pancreatitis and differentiation from carcinoma of the pancreas. Radiologist 5:245–255, 1998.

PAULSON EK, VITELLAS KM, KEOGAN MT, et al: Acute pancreatitis complicated by gland necrosis: Spectrum of findings on contrast-enhanced CT. AJR Am J Roentgenol 172:609–613, 1999.

PROCACCI C, MEGIBOW A, CARBOGNIN G, et al: Intraductal papillary mucinous tumor of the pancreas: A pictorial essay. Radiographics 19:1447–1463, 1999.

PROKESCH RW, CHOW LC, BEAULIEU CF, et al: Isoattenuating pancreatic adenocarcinoma at multidetector row CT: Secondary signs. Radiology 224: 764–768, 2002.

ROCHE CJ, HUGHES ML, GARVEY CJ, et al: CT and pathologic assessment of prospective nodal staging in patients with ductal adenocarcinoma of the head of the pancreas. AJR Am J Roentgenol 180:475–480, 2003.

SCATARIGE JC, HORTON KM, SHETH S, FISHMAN EK: Pancreatic parenchymal metastases: Observations on helical CT. AJR Am J Roentgenol 176:695–699, 2001.

STONE EE, BRANT WE, SMITH GB: Computed tomography of duodenal diverticula. J Comput Assist Tomogr 13:61–63, 1989.

TAMM EP, SILVERMAN PM, CHARNSANGAVEJ C, EVANS DB: Diagnosis, staging, and surveillance of pancreatic cancer. AJR Am J Roentgenol 180: 1311–1323, 2003.

TAOULI B, GHOUADNI M, CORREAS J, et al: Spectrum of abdominal imaging findings in von Hippel-Lindau disease. AJR Am J Roentgenol 181: 1049–1054, 2003.

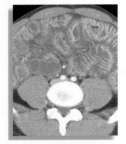

14

Spleen

William E. Brant, M.D.

☐ ANATOMY

The spleen occupies a relatively constant position in the left upper quadrant of the abdomen. It is a soft and pliable organ that conforms to the shape of adjacent structures. The diaphragmatic surface is smooth and convex, conforming to the dome of the diaphragm, whereas the visceral surface has concavities for the stomach, kidney, and colon. The splenic artery and vein course in close relation with the pancreas to the splenic hilum where each vessel divides into multiple branches. The normal spleen has lobulations, notches, and clefts that may be mistaken for abnormalities (Fig. 14-1). Lobulations in the splenic contour can generally be identified on serial slices as part of the spleen.

The CT density of the normal spleen is less than, or equal to, the CT density of the normal liver. Normal spleen attenuation unenhanced is 40 to 60 H, which is 5 to 10 H less than the normal unenhanced liver. Most splenic lesions are seen best on contrast-enhanced CT scans. The spleen enhances irregularly in the early phase after bolus injection of contrast agents, creating transient pseudomasses caused by variable rates of blood flow through its pulp (Fig. 14-2).

☐ TECHNICAL CONSIDERATIONS

The spleen is included on every CT of the abdomen. Typically, images are viewed at 5-mm thickness. Contrast is administered at 2 to 3 mL/ second for a total dose of 120 to 150 mL. Scans are obtained at 60 to 70 seconds after contrast injection.

☐ ANOMALIES

Accessory Spleen

Accessory spleens, or splenules, are nodules of normal splenic tissue that are formed separately from the main spleen. They are present in 10% to 30% of individuals and may be solitary or multiple. Accessory spleens have the following characteristics:

- Splenules appear as round or oval masses up to 2 to 3 cm in diameter, most commonly located in the hilum of the spleen (Fig. 14-3).
- They have the same CT density and tissue texture as the main spleen.
- Accessory spleens may hypertrophy after splenic resection.

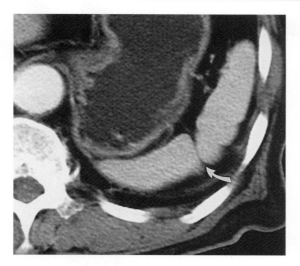

FIGURE 14-1 **Normal cleft.** A prominent, but normal, cleft *(arrow)* is evident in the spleen of a 72-year-old man.

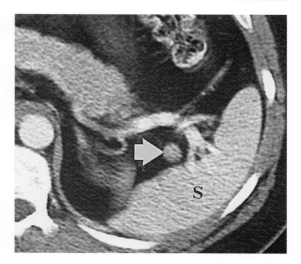

FIGURE 14-3 **Accessory spleen.** An accessory spleen *(arrow)* is evident near the hilum of the spleen (S) adjacent to the splenic vein.

Wandering Spleen

Wandering spleen refers to a normal spleen that is found outside the left upper quadrant of the abdomen. Congenital laxity of the ligaments, often associated with anomalies of intestinal fixation, causes the spleen to be freely mobile and to be located anywhere in the abdomen.

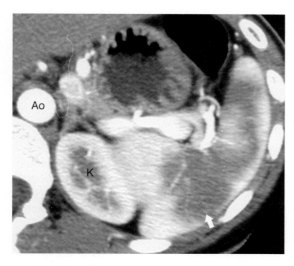

FIGURE 14-2 **Transient pseudomass.** Inhomogeneous enhancement of the spleen produces pseudomass effect *(arrow)* during the early stage of intravenous contrast medium administration using a power injector. The bright enhancement of the aorta (Ao) and enhancement of only the cortex of the kidney (K) indicate early arterial stage of contrast enhancement. Images obtained a few minutes later (not shown) demonstrated uniform density of the spleen.

Wandering spleens are usually asymptomatic, but they may be a cause of a palpable abdominal mass and are more susceptible to traumatic injury and torsion. Diagnosis is made by noting the absence of a normal spleen in its typical location and recognizing that the ectopic mass is supplied by splenic vessels.

Splenic Regeneration

Accessory spleens or remnants of splenic tissue after splenic injury may hypertrophy after splenectomy, resulting in single or multiple left upper abdominal masses. The diagnosis is suggested clinically when a patient, with a history of splenectomy, has no Howell–Jolly bodies on peripheral blood smear. Howell–Jolly bodies are remnants of nuclear material in red blood cells that are usually removed from the circulating blood by the spleen.

Regenerative splenic remnants have the CT appearance of abnormally shaped but otherwise normal-appearing splenic tissue (Fig. 14-4). The presence of splenic tissue is confirmed by technetium–99m sulfur colloid radionuclide imaging.

Splenomegaly

Spleen size varies with age, body habitus, state of hydration, and nutrition. The spleen normally decreases in size with age. The causes of splenomegaly are exhaustive but can be classified into

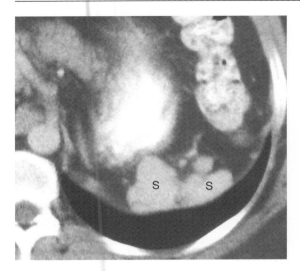

FIGURE 14-4 **Splenic regeneration.** This patient underwent splenectomy for a shattered spleen 8 years before this CT scan. Retained remnants of the spleen (S) have regenerated into multiple nodules of functioning splenic tissue.

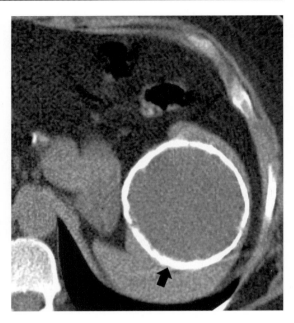

FIGURE 14-5 **Post-traumatic cyst.** Liquefaction of an old hematoma resulted in formation of this cystic mass *(arrow)* with a densely calcified wall.

myeloproliferative, infectious, congestive, and infiltrative categories. Most conditions do not affect CT density of the spleen, thus differentiation is based on other CT findings or clinical evaluation. Size greater than 14 cm in any dimension is a primary sign of splenomegaly in adults.

☐ FOCAL LESIONS

Cysts

Cystic lesions of the spleen have a variety of causes. An accurate diagnosis can usually be made by correlating CT findings with the medical history and clinical findings.

- *Posttraumatic cyst* is the most common splenic cyst accounting for 80% of all splenic cystic lesions. These cysts result from previous hemorrhage, infarction, or infection, and basically represent the end stage of an intrasplenic hematoma. The wall is fibrous tissue of variable thickness (Fig. 14-5). Internal debris, fluid levels, and milk of calcium are common features. Calcification is found in the wall in 30% to 40% of cases.
- *Congenital epidermoid cysts* are true cysts with epithelial-lined walls. They are well defined, spherical, and usually unilocular with thin walls (Fig. 14-6). Internal debris is sometimes present. No contrast enhance-

ment occurs. Calcification is found in the walls in about 5% of cases.
- *Echinococcal cysts* may be indistinguishable from traumatic and epidermoid cysts but are rare in the United States. Patients have abdominal pain, fever, and splenomegaly.

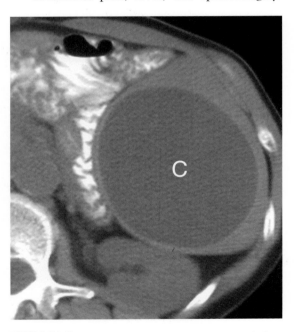

FIGURE 14-6 **Epidermoid cyst.** A large cyst (C) expands the spleen compressing the left kidney and displacing bowel on this noncontrast CT image.

The lesion consists of a larger mother cyst containing smaller daughter cysts near the periphery. Ringlike calcification of the walls of the mother cyst and the internal daughter cysts is common. Hydatid sand appears as internal debris of higher density than the cyst fluid. Less than 2% of patients with hydatid disease have splenic involvement.

- *Pancreatic pseudocysts* result from pancreatitis with fluid gaining access to the splenic parenchyma from the pancreas by dissection through the splenic hilum (Fig. 14-7). CT demonstrates findings of pancreatitis in association with subcapsular splenic fluid.

Infarction

Splenic infarctions may be asymptomatic or present with left upper quadrant pain. Causes include involvement of splenic vessels by atherosclerosis, arteritis, tumor, or pancreatitis. Additional causes include systemic emboli and sickle disease. Splenomegaly is a predisposing factor to infarction. Infarcts easily become infected if bacteremia develops in the patient. CT findings of infarction include:

- The classic appearance is wedge-shaped, low-attenuation defect that extends to the splenic capsule.
- Many infarcts are not classic in appearance. Any nonenhancing area of the spleen that extends right up to the splenic capsule is likely to be an infarction (Fig. 14-8).
- Infarctions will atrophy over time, resulting in depressed areas and notching of the splenic contour.

Bacterial Abscesses

Bacterial abscesses occur uncommonly but have a high mortality rate when untreated. Signs and symptoms may be vague. Diseased spleens are particularly susceptible to abscess formation when organisms are delivered hematogenously from distant foci of infection. Abscesses may also result from spread of infection from adjacent organs or from suppuration in a traumatic hematoma. Abscesses appear as single or multiple low-density areas with ill-defined walls, which may be thickened and enhance with contrast medium. Internal attenuation is 20 to 40 H. Abscesses may contain gas or demonstrate fluid levels. Diagnosis is confirmed by percutaneous aspiration. Treatment is catheter drainage or splenectomy.

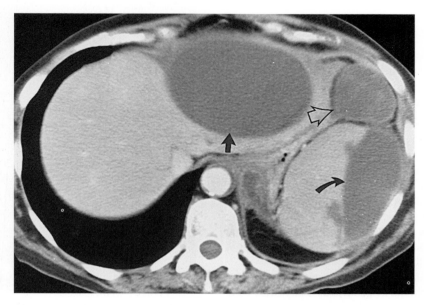

FIGURE 14-7 **Pancreatic pseudocysts.** Subcapsular fluid collections associated with acute pancreatitis are evident in the spleen *(curved arrow)* and liver *(straight arrow)*. Loculated fluid is also seen in a recess of the lesser sac *(open arrow)*. High amylase content of the fluid was confirmed by CT-guided aspiration and drainage.

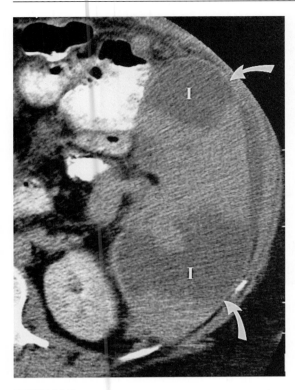

FIGURE 14-8 **Infarction.** Splenic infarctions (I) are seen as low-density lesions extending to the splenic capsule *(arrows)* in this patient with massive splenomegaly.

Microabscesses

Patients who are immunocompromised because of AIDS, chemotherapy, lymphoma, leukemia, or organ transplantation may experience development of microabscesses caused by opportunistic infections. Causes include fungi (*Candida, Aspergillus, Cryptococcus, Histoplasma*), tuberculosis, *Pneumocystis carinii*, and cytomegalovirus. CT findings of microabscesses include:

- Multiple low-density defects in the spleen are 2 to 10 mm in size (Fig. 14-9).
- Differential diagnosis of multiple, small, low-density splenic defects includes lymphoma, Kaposi's sarcoma, sarcoidosis, and metastases.

Lymphoma

The spleen is the largest lymphoid organ in the body, thus it is not surprising that involvement by lymphoma is common. Approximately one third of all patients with lymphoma have involve-

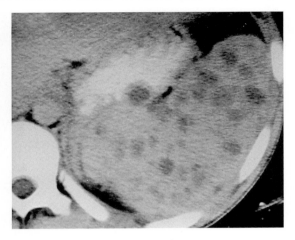

FIGURE 14-9 **Microabscesses.** Many low-density lesions are seen in the spleen in this patient with acute myelogenous leukemia. The lesions were caused by *Candida albicans* sepsis.

ment of the spleen. CT is not reliable in the detection of lymphomatous involvement. The spleen may be normal yet involved, or it may be enlarged and not involved. Focal lesions are a reliable sign of disease. CT findings of lymphoma include:

- Diffuse infiltration may result in homogeneous enlargement without masses.
- Multiple lesions are the most characteristic. They vary from miliary pattern of tiny lesions up to 2 to 10 cm in size. Lesions do not enhance with intravenous contrast administration.
- A solitary large mass represents a confluent deposit of lymphomatous tissue (Fig. 14-10).
- Enlarged nodes may be seen in the splenic hilum, along the splenic vessels, and elsewhere in the abdomen.

Metastases

Melanoma and lung, breast, and ovarian carcinomas are the most common sources of splenic metastases. Metastases are surprisingly uncommon and are seen in only 7% of patients with widespread malignancy. Melanoma is the source of 50% of the splenic metastases detected radiographically. Lesions appear late in the course of the disease:

- Most appear as ill-defined, low-density nodules with some degree of peripheral enhancement (Fig. 14-11).
- Melanoma commonly causes well-defined cystic metastases.

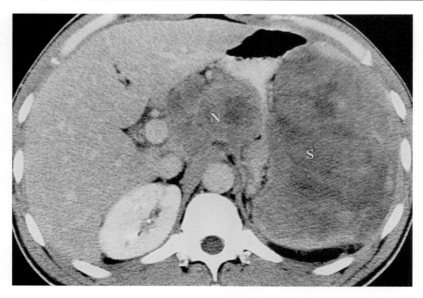

FIGURE 14-10 **Lymphoma.** The spleen (S) is greatly enlarged and the parenchyma is mostly replaced by a diffuse, mottled, low-density lesion representing non–Hodgkin's lymphoma. A mass of adenopathy (N) compresses the stomach and abuts the portal vein.

Hemangioma

Although unusual, hemangioma is the most common neoplasm of the spleen. As in the liver, the lesion consists of endothelial-lined, blood-filled spaces of varying size. Most are asymptomatic, but large hemangiomas may cause pain and splenomegaly. CT findings of hemangioma include:

- Lesions may appear cystic or solid on unenhanced CT. They may be solitary or multiple.
- After contrast administration, splenic hemangiomas demonstrate nodular enhancement from the periphery similar to the enhancement pattern of liver hemangiomas (Fig. 14-12).
- Central punctate or peripheral curvilinear calcifications may be present.

Angiosarcoma

Angiosarcoma is a rare primary malignancy of the spleen. The tumor is aggressive, usually presenting with widespread metastases, especially to the liver. The tumor may spontaneously rupture and hemorrhage into the peritoneal cavity. CT findings include:

- Multiple, well-defined, enhancing nodules are the most common CT appearance.
- Angiosarcoma may also appear as a complex mass of cystic and solid components that enhance irregularly (Fig. 14-13).

Splenic Calcifications

Splenic calcifications are a frequent CT finding. CT findings include:

- Multiple small focal calcifications (Fig. 14-14) in an otherwise normal-appearing spleen are the result of previous infection with histoplasmosis or tuberculosis.
- Larger, coarser calcifications result from previous infarction, infection, or trauma.

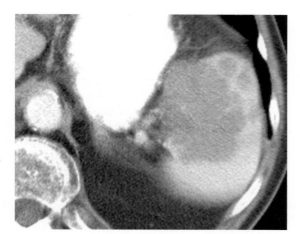

FIGURE 14-11 **Metastases.** Metastases from malignant melanoma cause multiple homogeneous low-attenuation lesions in the spleen.

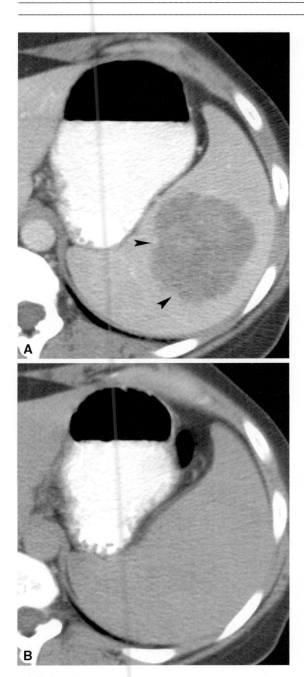

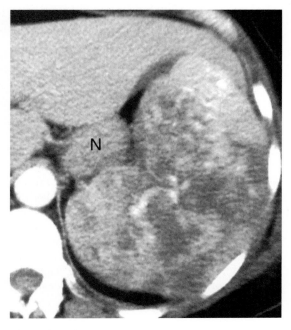

FIGURE 14-13 **Angiosarcoma.** A complex mass of low- and high-density components with tangled enhancing vessels replaces most of the splenic parenchyma. Metastatic tumor causes enlargement of a lymph node (N) in the splenic hilum.

FIGURE 14-12 **Hemangioma.** *A,* Relatively early postcontrast image shows small nodules of peripheral enhancement *(arrowheads)*. *B,* Delayed postcontrast scan shows that the lesion has become isodense with the splenic parenchyma and is no longer evident.

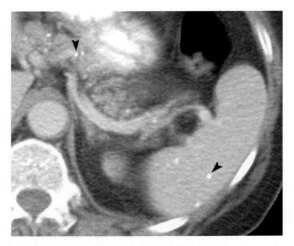

FIGURE 14-14 **Calcified granulomas.** Calcified granulomas *(arrowheads)* without associated mass are seen in the spleen and pancreas. These were most likely caused by histoplasmosis.

- Sickle hemoglobinopathy alone or in combination with thalassemia or hemoglobin C disease can result in calcification of the entire spleen, which commonly atrophies and becomes functionless.

SUGGESTED READING

ABBOTT RM, LEVY AD, AGUILERA NS, et al: Primary vascular neoplasms of the spleen: Radiologic-pathologic correlation. Radiographics 24:1137–1163, 2004.

BRANT WE, JAIN KA: Current imaging of the spleen. Radiologist 3:185–192, 1996.

DODDS WJ, TAYLOR AJ, ERICKSON SJ, et al: Radiologic imaging of splenic anomalies. AJR Am J Roentgenol 155:805–810, 1990.

FERROZZI F, BOVA D, DRAGHI F, GARLASCHI G: CT findings in primary vascular tumors of the spleen. AJR Am J Roentgenol 166:1097–1101, 1996.

FREEMAN JL, JAFRI SZH, ROBERTS JL, et al: CT of congenital and acquired abnormalities of the spleen. Radiographics 13:597–610, 1993.

PATERSON A, FRUSH DP, DONNELLY LF, et al: A pattern-oriented approach to splenic imaging in infants and children. Radiographics 19:1465–1485, 1999.

RABUSHKA LS, KAWASHIMA A, FISHMAN EK: Imaging of the spleen: CT with supplemental MR examination. Radiographics 14:307–332, 1994.

TAYLOR AJ, DODDS WJ, ERICKSON SJ, STEWART ET: CT of acquired abnormalities of the spleen. AJR Am J Roentgenol 157:1213–1219, 1991.

URBAN BA, FISHMAN EK: Helical CT of the spleen. AJR Am J Roentgenol 170:997–1003, 1998.

URRITIA M, MERGO PJ, ROS LH, et al: Cystic lesions of the spleen: Radiologic-pathologic correlation. Radiographics 16:107–129, 1996.

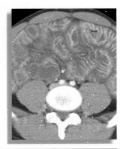

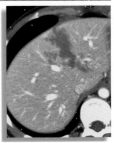

15

Kidneys and Ureters

William E. Brant, M.D.

☐ KIDNEYS

Anatomy of the Retroperitoneal Space

Detailed understanding of the retroperitoneal fascial planes and compartments is a prerequisite for accurate interpretation of abdominal CT. The retroperitoneal space between the diaphragm and the pelvic brim is divided into anterior pararenal, perirenal, and posterior pararenal compartments by the anterior and posterior renal fascia (Fig. 15-1).

The *anterior pararenal space* extends between the posterior parietal peritoneum and the anterior renal fascia. It is bounded laterally by the lateroconal fascia, which is the continuation of the posterior layer of the posterior renal fascia. The pancreas, duodenal loop, and ascending and descending portions of the colon are within the anterior pararenal space.

The anterior and posterior renal fascia encompass the kidney, renal pelvis, proximal ureter, adrenal gland, and perirenal fat within the *perirenal space.* The anterior renal fascia is thin and consists of one layer of connective tissue. The posterior renal fascia is thicker and consists of two layers of connective tissue. The anterior layer of the posterior renal fascia is continuous with the anterior renal fascia. The

posterior layer of the posterior renal fascia is continuous with the lateroconal fascia forming the lateral boundary of the anterior pararenal space. The anterior and posterior layers of the posterior renal fascia may be separated by inflammatory processes, such as pancreatitis, extending from the anterior pararenal space. The perirenal space is discontinuous across the midline because of fusion of the renal fascial layers with connective tissues surrounding the aorta and inferior vena cava. The perirenal compartment narrows as it extends inferiorly to form an inverted cone shape. The ureter passes through the apex of the cone.

The *posterior pararenal space* is a potential space, usually occupied only by fat, extending from the posterior renal fascia to the transversalis fascia. The posterior pararenal fat continues into the flank as the properitoneal fat stripe seen on plain films of the abdomen. This compartment is limited medially by the lateral edge of the psoas and quadratus lumborum muscles.

The kidneys are covered by a tight, fibrous capsule that produces a sharp margin defined by perirenal fat on CT. Subcapsular collections of fluid or blood will compress and distort the renal parenchyma, often without affecting the perirenal fat. The perirenal fat extends into the renal sinus outlining blood vessels and the renal

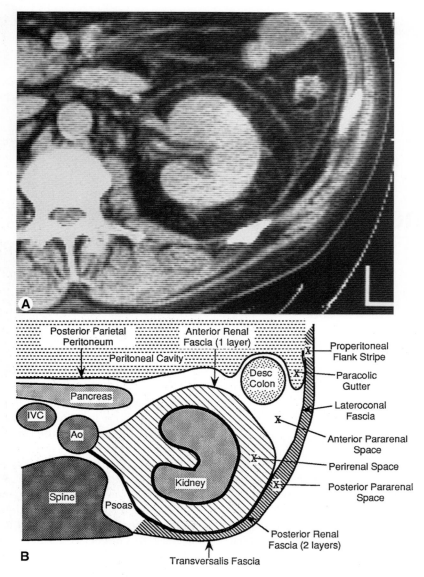

FIGURE 15-1 **Retroperitoneal anatomy.** CT image of the left kidney *(A)* and a diagram *(B)* demonstrate the fascial planes and compartments of the retroperitoneum. Ao, aorta; IVC, inferior vena cava.

collecting system. Connective tissue septa extend between the kidney and the renal fascia. These septa may be seen as prominent stranding densities in the perirenal fat when they are thickened by inflammation, hemorrhage, or ischemia. The renal arteries and veins can be identified from the great vessels to the kidneys. The right renal artery courses behind the vena cava. The left renal vein crosses between the aorta and the superior mesenteric artery.

Technical Considerations

Because the kidneys actively concentrate contrast medium within the parenchyma, most renal abnormalities are best seen on CT after intravenous (IV) contrast medium administration. Unenhanced CT is performed to demonstrate calcifications and calculi that may be obscured by contrast agent. Multidetector helical CT (MDCT) is optimal for renal evaluation and is the current technique of choice. Sensitivity for detection of renal masses varies considerably with imaging modality: 67% for excretory urography, 79% for sonography, 94% for conventional nonhelical CT, and at least 95% for MDCT.

CT for Renal Masses

To evaluate for renal mass on spiral CT, we use MDCT with contiguous thin slices with a single breath hold at identical locations before and after bolus contrast administration. CT procedures include:

- Most protocols use 5 mm or thinner collimation and a single breath hold of 20 to 30 seconds. Thinner slices can be obtained with a multidetector scanner. Images obtained at 2.5-mm collimation or smaller are usually fused and viewed at 5-mm thickness. For problematic lesions, the 5-mm slices can be unfused and viewed as the thinner slices originally obtained.
- A *precontrast scan* is performed through both kidneys (Fig. 15-2*A*).
- A total of 150 mL of 60% iodine nonionic contrast is given intravenously by power injector at 2.5 mL/second.
- A *corticomedullary phase scan* is obtained using a 70-second scan delay (see Fig. 15-2*B*). This scan extends from the dome of the diaphragm through the bottom of the kidneys. Scanning during this phase is to evaluate other abdominal organs for metastatic disease and to evaluate the renal arteries and veins.
- A *nephrogram phase scan* is obtained at 100 to 120 seconds after contrast (see Fig. 15-2*C*). Scan extent includes only the kidneys from top to bottom.
- A *pyelogram phase scan* is added at 3 to 5 minutes after injection. This scan repeats images of the kidneys at 5-mm collimation.
- The scan may be continued through the pelvis to evaluate the retroperitoneum, ureters, and bladder.

Corticomedullary Phase Scans

When scanning the abdomen for reasons other than renal mass characterization, renal images are commonly obtained with contrast enhancement limited to the renal cortex (see Fig. 15-2*B*). The corticomedullary phase is usually seen at about 70 seconds after contrast injection into an arm vein. This phase is of limited use for detection of renal masses because only the renal cortex is enhanced and the medullary portions of the kidney remain unenhanced. The corticomedullary phase defines the renal artery and vein better than the nephrogram phase.

CT-Urogram

The CT-urogram (CT-IVP) has evolved as the imaging method of choice to provide the most comprehensive evaluation of the urinary tract, often used in the setting of hematuria. A noncontrast CT scan is obtained from the kidneys through the bladder to document the presence of calculi or parenchymal calcifications. The renal parenchyma is evaluated in nephrogram phase. The collecting system and ureters are documented by either post-CT radiographs or by MDCT with thin collimation and coronal reformation of the ureters. CT urogram procedures include:

- No bowel preparation is used.
- A precontrast (stone protocol) CT from the top of the kidneys through the base of the bladder is obtained.
- A total of 150 mL of 60% iodine nonionic contrast is injected intravenously at 2.5 mL/ second.
- CT of the kidneys is obtained at 100-second scan delay using 5-mm or thinner collimation and a single breath hold.
- Immediately after renal CT, the patient is moved to a radiography room for the 5-minute anteroposterior abdominal film and bilateral full-abdomen obliques of the ureters and bladder. Additional delayed radiographs of the ureters and bladder are taken if needed. Postvoid erect radiographs of the bladder complete the study.
- Alternatively, MDCT is now being used by many to complete the study in the CT suite. Thin slices (1–3 mm) are obtained at 3 to 5 minutes after IV contrast through the full length of the ureters and are reformatted using three-dimensional protocols (Fig. 15-3).

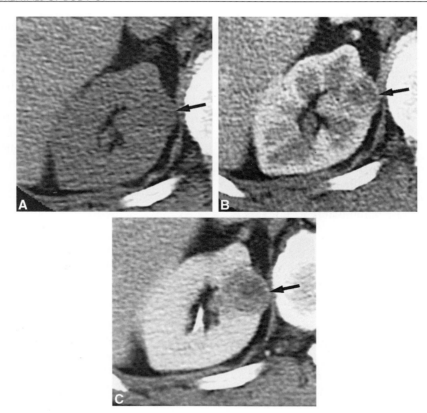

FIGURE 15-2 **Renal cell carcinoma.** Noncontrast *(A)*, corticomedullary phase *(B)*, and nephrogram phase *(C)* images from a helical CT study demonstrate a small renal carcinoma *(arrows)* arising from the right kidney. The tumor is near isointense with the renal parenchyma on the noncontrast study. Early arterial enhancement of the tumor coincides with enhancement of the renal cortex on *B*. The tumor is hypointense compared with the renal parenchyma during nephrogram phase.

Stone Protocol CT

Renal stone CT (sometimes called CT-KUB) is a noncontrast helical CT of the urinary tract used to diagnose the presence of urinary tract calculi and to detect acute urinary obstruction caused by stones:

- No oral or IV contrast is administered.
- Data acquisition is continuous from top of kidneys through base of bladder (mid-T-12 level through the symphysis pubis) using 2.5- to 3-mm collimation. Images may be viewed at 2.5- to 5-mm slice thickness.
- MDCT technique allows retrospective 1- to 3-mm slices to be reconstructed. Thin slices allow identification of small stones that may be overlooked with thicker slices.
- Turning the patient to prone position will allow differentiation of stones impacted at the ureterovesical junction from stones that have already passed into the bladder.

- Whenever the noncontrast renal stone CT is equivocal, IV contrast may be given to clarify the diagnosis. The pyelogram phase of contrast excretion with filling of the ureters is of most interest. An IV injection of 100 mL of 60% contrast is given. Power injection is not needed. The renal stone protocol outlined above is repeated with a scan delay of 3 to 5 minutes after completion of contrast injection. This prolonged scan delay usually results in filling of both collecting systems and ureters.

Congenital Anomalies

Horseshoe Kidney

Congenital fusion of the lower poles of the kidneys is a relatively common (1–4/1000) congenital anomaly. CT findings of horseshoe kidney include:

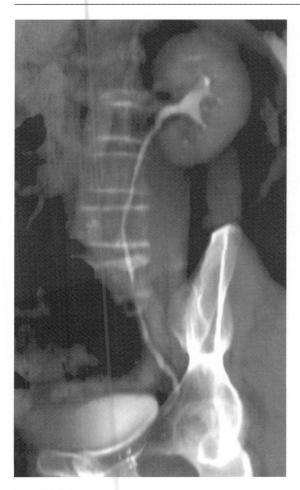

FIGURE 15-3 CT-intravenous pyelogram. This oblique view of the left ureter, collecting system, and kidney was created from a series of thin-slice axial CT images. It nicely demonstrates the course and size of the ureter but lacks the high resolution of a standard radiographic image.

- The isthmus extends across the aorta at the level of the inferior mesenteric artery, which prevents the normal ascent of the kidneys to the renal beds (Fig. 15-4).
- The fused kidneys are low in position and malrotated with the renal pelvis directed anteriorly. Malposition commonly causes urinary stasis, stone formation, and recurrent infection.
- Transitional cell carcinoma (TCC) is three to four times more common in horseshoe kidneys compared with the general population.

Renal Masses

Features that must be evaluated to characterize a renal mass are presence and type of calcifica-tion, attenuation of the mass before and after contrast administration, margin of the mass with the kidney and with surrounding tissues, presence and thickness of septa, and thickness of the wall of cystic masses. Artifactual pseu-doenhancement, related to beam hardening effect from iodinated contrast, may increase attenuation of lesions by up to 10 H. Attenuation must increase by a *minimum of 10 to 15 H* after bolus IV contrast to be considered enhanced.

Renal Cell Carcinoma

Renal cell carcinoma (RCC) accounts for 90% of solid tumors of the kidney. Most large lesions can be easily diagnosed by CT. Small lesions are commonly indeterminate. CT findings include:

- Large tumors (>3 cm) are heterogeneous and multilobulated. Internal hemorrhage and cystic necrosis are common (Fig. 15-5). Calcifications are common and are usually coarse and irregular.
- Enhancement is usually evident with an increase in attenuation in the range of 10 to 25 H. Most lesions are hypervascular and enhance inhomogeneously (see Figs. 15-2 and 15-6).
- About 5% of RCCs are predominantly cystic. Most appear as a multicystic mass with noncommunicating cystic spaces of varying size. Cysts are filled with variable amounts of new and old blood. Cystic and complex multicystic variants are identified by thick-ened enhancing walls and septa, or by the presence of a solid tumor nodule. Septa con-tain malignant cells and usually enhance.
- Small solid lesions (<3 cm) overlap some benign lesions in appearance.

CT Staging of Renal Cell Carcinoma

RCC responds poorly to all types of radiation therapy and chemotherapy despite many new and innovative therapy attempts. The only effec-tive therapy remains surgical excision of all of the tumor. CT is highly accurate in assisting the urologist in planning surgery (Table 15-1):

- Extension of tumor through the renal cap-sule into the perinephric fat is not accu-rately demonstrated by CT. However, this differentiation does not affect the surgical approach to the lesion.
- Tumor may grow into the main renal vein (30%) and inferior vena cava (10%). Venous

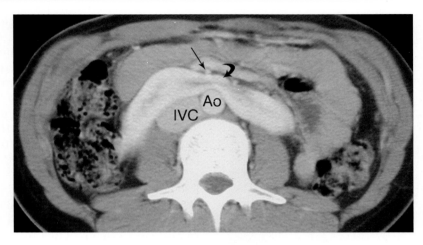

FIGURE 15-4 **Horseshoe kidney.** The isthmus *(curved arrow)* of the horseshoe kidney crosses the midline between the inferior vena cava (IVC) and aorta (Ao) and the inferior mesenteric artery *(arrow)*. In this case, the isthmus consists of enhancing functioning renal parenchyma. In some cases, the isthmus consists of a fibrous band.

invasion is indicated by visualization of tissue plug within the renal vein or inferior vena cava. Venous invasion consists of tumor growing within the vein often associated with variable amount of bland thrombus. Involved veins are usually enlarged. Tumor thrombus is seen as nodular low density within the vein (Fig. 15-7). Enhancement of the thrombus within the vein is evidence that the thrombus consists of growing tumor. Determining the presence or absence of venous involvement is essential to surgical planning. CT is 95% accurate in the determination of venous involvement.

- Lymph nodes larger than 2 cm in short axis nearly always contain metastatic tumor. Involved lymph nodes are most common in renal hilum, pericaval, and periaortic regions.
- Lymph nodes 1 to 2 cm in short axis are indeterminate, hyperplastic versus metastatic, and should always be removed at sur-

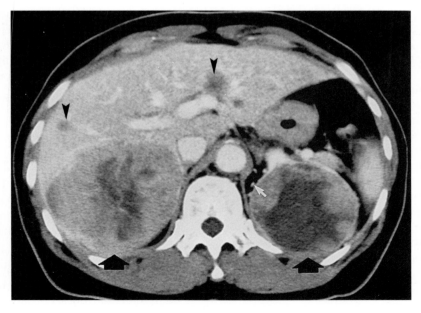

FIGURE 15-5 **Bilateral renal cell carcinoma.** Renal cell carcinomas *(black arrows)* arise from the upper poles of both kidneys. The low-density regions within the tumors are areas of necrosis and hemorrhage. Enhancing tumor vessels *(white arrow)* are seen in the perirenal fat. Metastases are seen in the liver *(black arrowheads)*.

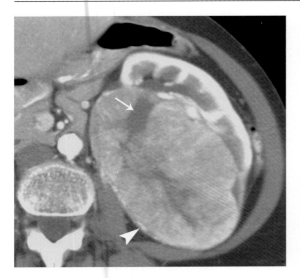

FIGURE 15-6 **Large renal cell carcinoma.** A large, lobulated, solid mass extends from the left kidney on this cortical phase image. Enhancing tumor vessels *(arrowhead)* are seen in the periphery of the lesion. Areas of necrosis and hemorrhage *(arrow)* appear as low-density regions within the mass.

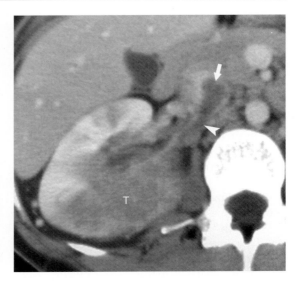

FIGURE 15-7 **Invasion of right renal vein and inferior vena cava (IVC).** An infiltrative renal cell carcinoma (T) replaces parenchyma in the right kidney and tumor thrombus extends into the right renal vein *(arrowhead)* and IVC *(arrow).*

gery to determine prognosis. Lymphadenectomy does not improve prognosis.

- Lymph nodes smaller than 1 cm in short axis are usually benign.
- Hematogenous metastases are most common in lung, liver, and bone.
- Adrenalectomy is optional if the adrenal gland appears normal on CT.

Recurrence of Renal Cell Carcinoma

CT is highly accurate for surveillance for recurrent disease after surgery. Recurrence of RCC usually occurs within the first 6 years after surgery. Median time for appearance of detectable recurrent disease is 15 to 18 months after nephrectomy. Risk for recurrence increases with the stage of the tumor at the time of the initial surgery. Occasionally, the tumor will recur after

the patient has been apparently free of disease for 10 years or longer. CT findings for recurrence of RCC include:

- Local recurrence in the renal fossa occurs in 5% of patients. Recurrent tumor appears as an irregularly enhancing mass that commonly involves the psoas or quadratus lumborum muscles. Adjacent structures are displaced.
- Lymphatic recurrence usually occurs in lymph nodes close to the renal vascular pedicle.
- Distant metastases develop in 20% to 30% of patients. The most common sites are the lungs (50% to 60%), mediastinum, bone, liver, contralateral kidney or adrenal gland, and brain.
- Late metastases (>10 years after surgery) are most common to lung, pancreas, bone,

TABLE 15-1

Staging of Renal Cell Carcinoma (Robson)

Stage I	Tumor confined to the kidney
Stage II	Tumor growth through the capsule into the perirenal space
Stage IIIA	Tumor involves main renal vein
Stage IIIB	Tumor involves regional lymph nodes
Stage IIIC	Tumor involves main renal vein and regional lymph nodes
Stage IVA	Tumor extends through renal fascia into adjacent organs
Stage IVB	Hematogenous or lymphatic metastases to distant sites

skeletal muscle, and bowel. Surgical resection of isolated late metastases may be curative.

Oncocytoma

Oncocytoma is a benign solid tumor that arises from the proximal renal tubule. Most are seen in men in their 60s. Unfortunately, no imaging test can reliably differentiate these benign tumors from RCC. Treatment is surgical. Exploration with limited tumor excision may be attempted if CT findings suggest the possibility of oncocytoma.

"Classic" CT features of oncocytoma, which unfortunately can also be seen with RCC, are homogeneous attenuation after contrast and a central, sharply marginated, stellate, low-attenuation scar. Features more characteristic of RCC, such as heterogeneous attenuation, necrosis, and hemorrhage, may also be seen with oncocytoma.

Angiomyolipoma

Angiomyolipoma (AML) is a benign tumor composed of blood vessels *(angio)*, smooth muscle *(myo)*, and fat *(lipoma)*. Arteries have thicker than normal, but abnormally weak, vessel walls and are predisposed to aneurysm formation. Larger tumors and larger aneurysms have a greater rate of rupture, making hemorrhage the most common complication. AML occurs in two distinct clinical settings. The sporadic and usually solitary tumor (80% to 90%) is most common in middle-aged women (female:male ratio, 4:1; average age, 43 years). Multifocal and bilateral tumors occur in association with tuberous sclerosis. Many tumors are discovered incidentally during CT or ultrasound imaging for other reasons. The presence of distinct pockets of fat allows a specific CT diagnosis of AML. CT findings include:

- The proportion of each tissue element present within the tumor determines imaging appearance.
- CT shows a well-marginated predominantly fat lesion arising from the cortex. Most tumors are smaller than 5 cm. Vascular and smooth muscle portions of the tumor enhance with contrast administration.
- The diagnostic feature of AML on CT is presence of fat (CT density < -20 H; Fig. 15-8). Soft-tissue density elements are often dispersed through a background of distinctly

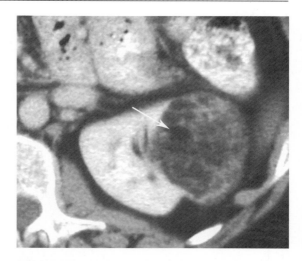

FIGURE 15-8 Solitary angiomyolipoma. Foci of distinct fat density *(arrow)* define this renal mass as an angiomyolipoma. Compare the fat density within the lesion to the fat surrounding the kidney. Areas of soft-tissue density, representing smooth muscle, are also evident within the mass.

fatty tissue. At other times, soft-tissue density predominates and diagnosis is made by the presence of small discrete pockets of fat. Thin-section CT (<5-mm collimation) is recommended for confident diagnosis. Use of IV contrast is not necessary to confirm the presence of fat within the lesion.

- Sonography characteristically demonstrates AML as small (<3 cm), well-defined echogenic tumors. Unfortunately, up to 32% of small (<3 cm) RCC also appear as echogenic masses. Therefore, CT characterization of all small echogenic renal mass lesions is recommended.
- Hemorrhage is common with AML because of the characteristically weak wall of the tumor blood vessels. Hemorrhage commonly extends into the perirenal space, may obscure fat density within the tumor, and often makes tumor margins indistinct. Risk for hemorrhage is increased when tumors exceed 4 cm.
- Approximately 5% of AML show no areas of distinct fat attenuation on CT. These tumors are indistinguishable from RCC. However, AML is suggested if the lesions are homogeneous high attenuation on unenhanced CT and show homogeneous increased density on enhanced CT.
- In patients with tuberous sclerosis, multiple cysts and AMLs are usually found in both kidneys (80% of patients). Lesions are

often large, and the risk for hemorrhage is increased (Fig. 15-9).

- Tumors may grow extensively into the perirenal space. Tumor margins are commonly indistinguishable from perirenal fat.
- A few cases of fat-containing RCC have been reported. In each case the presence of fat has been attributed to osseous metaplasia of stromal portions of the tumor with growth of fatty marrow. Calcifications are usually present in association with these fat deposits. Intratumoral calcifications are virtually never present with AML. Fat-containing RCCs show other signs of malignancy.

Transitional Cell Carcinoma

TCCs may arise anywhere along the uroepithelial lining the collecting system, renal pelvis, ureter, or bladder. Most tumors (90%) arise in the bladder with only 5% to 10% arising within the renal pelvis or ureter. A characteristic of TCC is that additional TCC may be present synchronously or may arise subsequently elsewhere in the uroepithelial. CT has been increasingly used for detection and staging. Four patterns of disease have been described. CT findings of TCC include:

- On unenhanced CT, TCC is isodense to renal parenchyma. With contrast, TCC shows variable, but usually poor, enhancement.
- *Single or multiple filling defects (35%) in the renal pelvis* have a smooth surface or a stippled papillary pattern (Fig. 15-10) with tracking of contrast into the interstices of the tumor.
- *Filling defects are seen within dilated calyces* obstructed at the infundibulum (26%). A "phantom" calyx fails to opacify and may be associated with a focal delayed or increasingly dense lobar nephrogram.
- *Absent or decreased contrast excretion (13%)* is caused by long-standing obstruction at the ureteropelvic junction.
- *Diffuse hydronephrosis with renal enlargement (6%)* is seen with tumor obstruction at the ureteropelvic junction.
- Large tumors invade the renal sinus fat and infiltrate into the parenchyma. Differentiation from RCC may be difficult.
- Advanced disease shows extrarenal extension, regional lymph node involvement, and distant metastases to lungs and bone. TCC may rarely invade the renal vein and inferior vena cava.

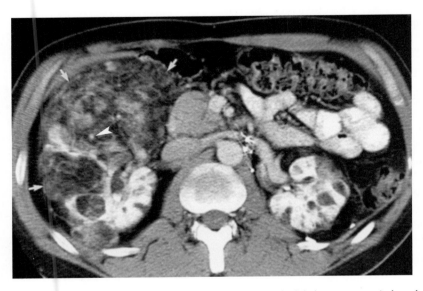

FIGURE 15-9 **Bilateral angiomyolipomas.** In this patient with tuberous sclerosis, both kidneys are extensively replaced by angiomyolipomas. The tumor *(arrows)* arising from the right kidney extends all the way to the anterior abdominal wall. Low-density areas within the tumor are nearly identical in density to subcutaneous and intra-abdominal fat, confirming the diagnosis of angiomyolipoma. Soft-tissue density nodules and strands correspond to smooth muscle components of the tumor. Bright dots *(arrowhead)* represent blood vessels within the highly vascular tumor. Functioning renal parenchyma enhances brightly with contrast medium.

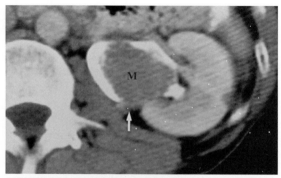

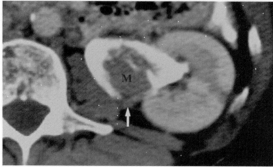

FIGURE 15-10 **Transitional cell carcinoma: renal pelvis.** Two sequential images of the left kidney demonstrate a transitional cell carcinoma appearing as a low-density mass (M) surrounded by high-density contrast within the renal pelvis. The tumor extends through the wall of the renal pelvis into the perirenal fat *(arrows)*.

- Calcification occurs in up to 5% of tumors. It may appear coarse, punctate, linear, granular, or stippled and indistinct.

Renal Lymphoma

Renal involvement with lymphoma almost always occurs in the setting of systemic disease. Whereas autopsy studies show the kidneys are involved in 34% to 68% of patients with lymphoma, CT shows renal involvement in only 3% to 8%. Involvement of the kidneys is more common with non–Hodgkin's lymphoma as compared with Hodgkin's lymphoma. Five characteristic patterns of involvement have been described. Atypical patterns of involvement present a diagnostic challenge. CT findings of renal lymphoma include:

- On unenhanced CT, lymphoma is homogeneous and may be isodense or slightly hyperdense compared with renal parenchyma. Margins with the renal parenchyma are usually indistinct.
- After contrast enhancement, lymphoma remains homogeneous and is always hypodense compared with enhanced renal parenchyma.
- *Multiple bilateral renal masses* are the most common (60%) CT appearance of lymphoma (Fig. 15-11). Occasionally, the multiple masses may affect only one kidney. Size of the lesions is typically 1 to 3 cm. Necrosis and calcification is rare. Retroperitoneal adenopathy accompanies only 50% of cases.
- *Contiguous invasion from the retroperitoneum* is seen in 35% to 60% of patients. Bulky retroperitoneal adenopathy extends along the renal vessels into the renal sinus and then into the renal parenchyma (Fig. 15-12). Tumor encasement of the renal artery and vein rarely results in thrombosis. This finding is highly characteristic of lymphoma.
- A *solitary mass* (10% to 20%) may highly resemble RCC. However, the mass is routinely homogeneous and shows minimal enhancement (Fig. 15-13). Tumor invasion of the renal vein is exceedingly rare.
- *Perirenal lymphoma* most often accompanies contiguous invasion from the retroperitoneum. Bulky disease surrounds the kidney but usually does not compress the parenchyma or interfere with its function. Disease patterns include multiple perirenal masses, soft-tissue nodules and plaques, curvilinear soft-tissue mass separate from the kidney (Fig. 15-14), and thickened renal fascia.
- *Diffuse infiltration* (~20%) enlarges the kidney without altering its reniform shape.

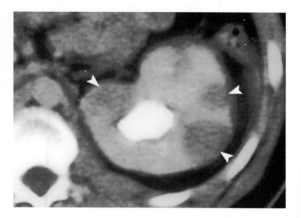

FIGURE 15-11 **Renal lymphoma: multiple masses.** The left kidney of a 16-year-old boy shows the multiple renal mass *(arrowheads)* pattern of renal lymphoma. Note the poorly defined interface between the lymphoma masses and the enhanced renal parenchyma.

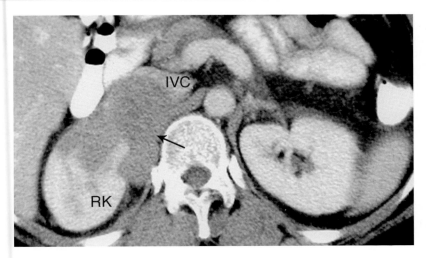

FIGURE 15-12 **Renal lymphoma: contiguous invasion.** A homogeneous, minimally enhancing mass *(arrow)* invades the right kidney (RK) and distorts the inferior vena cava (IVC), whereas displacing it anteriorly.

Nearly all cases involve both kidneys. Contrast enhancement is typically limited, patchy, and associated with poor contrast excretion.

- Absence of involvement of retroperitoneal nodes is relatively common (up to 43% of all cases) and does exclude lymphoma as a cause of renal mass.
- Atypical manifestations include spontaneous hemorrhage, necrosis, heterogeneous attenuation, cystic change, and calcification. Atypical findings are most common after treatment. Usually with successful therapy, the CT appearance of the kidney eventually returns to normal.

Renal Medullary Carcinoma

Renal medullary carcinoma is an aggressive infiltrative tumor that arises from the collecting tubules of the renal medulla. It is also called collecting duct carcinoma of the kidney. In distinction, RCC arises from the convoluted tubules of the renal cortex. CT findings of renal medullary carcinoma include:

- The mass appears infiltrative replacing renal parenchyma and showing ill-defined, nonencapsulated margins.

FIGURE 15-13 **Renal lymphoma: solitary mass.** Lymphoma replaces parenchyma in the mid-portion of the left kidney appearing as a large mass (M) with ill-defined borders. An enlarged lymph node *(arrow)* is seen posterior to the left renal vein *(arrowhead)*. Note that the renal vein is uninvolved. Renal cell carcinoma commonly invades the renal vein, whereas renal lymphoma rarely does. Compare with Figure 15-7.

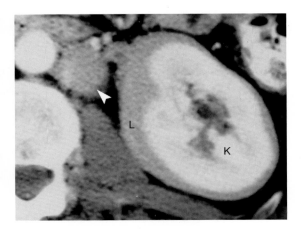

FIGURE 15-14 **Renal lymphoma: perirenal.** The enhancing parenchyma of the left kidney (K) is completely encased by nonenhancing, homogenous, soft tissue representing lymphomatous tissue. An enlarged lymph node *(arrowhead)* is seen between the kidney and the aorta.

- The tumor arises from the medulla extending into the renal sinus replacing sinus fat and protruding into the collecting system. It commonly spreads to involve the cortex and may have an exophytic component.
- The reniform contour of the kidney is preserved when the tumor is small.
- Large tumors often become expansile and are indistinguishable from RCC.

Renal Metastases

Renal metastases are present in 7% to 13% of cases with extrarenal cancers on autopsy series. Most common primaries are lung, breast, and gastrointestinal adenocarcinomas. Lesions are identified on CT usually only in patients with advanced widespread metastatic disease. CT findings include:

- Multiple, bilateral, low-attenuation renal nodules are the most common CT pattern (Fig. 15-15).
- Solitary exophytic masses may be seen with colon cancer and melanoma.
- Diffusely infiltrative metastases are uncommon.

Cystic Renal Masses

Cystic renal masses are an extremely common finding on abdominal CT. The challenge is to separate the ubiquitous simple cyst and other benign cysts from a host of potentially malignant cystic lesions.

Simple renal cysts are benign, non-neoplastic, fluid-filled masses that are present in half the population older than 55 years old. Small cysts are asymptomatic incidental findings. Large cysts (>4 cm) occasionally cause hypertension, hematuria, pain, or ureteral obstruction. Multiple and bilateral cysts are common. Strict criteria that allow confident CT diagnosis of a renal mass as a simple cyst (Fig. 15-16) are:

- Sharp margination with the renal parenchyma
- No perceptible wall
- Homogeneous attenuation near water density (−10 to +20 H)
- No enhancement after IV contrast medium administration
- Simple cysts commonly slowly increase in size (~6% per year) on follow-up

Complex cystic masses appear cystic but do not meet the criteria for simple cyst. The following lesions should be considered: complicated simple cyst, renal abscess, multicystic renal cell carcinoma, multilocular cystic renal tumor, and localized renal cystic disease.

Complicated Simple Cyst. Simple cysts may be complicated by hemorrhage, infection, or calcification within the wall. Some may have internal septa. Multiple simple cysts adjacent to each other may appear as a complex mass. If septa are thin, smooth, and regular, a diagnosis of benign cyst can be made (Fig. 15-17A). Thin

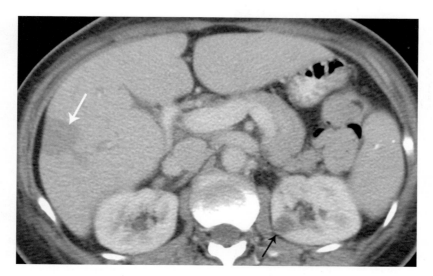

FIGURE 15-15 **Metastasis to the kidney.** Low-density masses are shown in the left kidney *(black arrow)* and in the liver *(white arrow)*. The full CT demonstrated multiple low-attenuation masses in the liver and both kidneys. Biopsy confirmed metastatic melanoma.

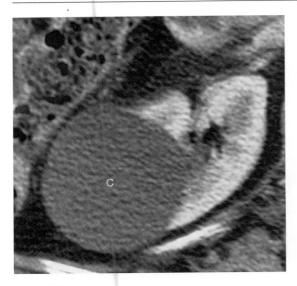

FIGURE 15-16 **Simple renal cyst: Bosniak Category I.** A large cyst (C) arising from the left kidney demonstrates the classic CT features of a simple renal cyst. No further evaluation or follow-up is necessary.

calcification of the wall of a cyst, or of a septa, is still compatible with benign cyst (see Fig. 15-17B). Small cysts (<3 cm), which are uniformly hyperdense (25–90 H) on noncontrast CT, may also be considered benign when they have other CT characteristics of simple cyst (see Fig. 15-17C and D).

Renal Abscess. Pyelonephritis complicated by suppuration and liquefaction may result in formation of an abscess requiring drainage. Alternatively, preexisting cysts may become infected. On CT, abscesses appear as thick-walled, low-density fluid collections within the renal parenchyma. Gas is sometimes seen within the pus collection. The wall commonly enhances with contrast medium administration. Extension of infection into the perirenal space is common.

Multicystic Renal Cell Carcinoma. Some renal carcinomas are composed of multiple fluid-filled noncommunicating cystic spaces (see Fig. 15-20). Malignant tumor cells line the loculations. Rarely, renal carcinoma may arise within or adjacent to a simple renal cyst.

Multilocular Cystic Renal Tumor. Multilocular cystic nephroma is an uncommon benign renal neoplasm composed of cysts of varying size separated by connective tissue septa. Two thirds of these tumors occur in male infants between 2 months and 3 years old. The remainder occurs in women aged 40 to 60 years. Treatment is surgical excision. CT findings include:

- The mass is solitary, unilateral, and most commonly arises from the upper pole.
- The multiple fluid-filled locules range from a few millimeters to 2.5 cm in size.
- The septa enhance moderately but less than RCC.
- Small locules and high-density fluid with the locules may make portions of the mass appear solid.
- Calcification, hemorrhage, and necrosis are rare.

Localized Renal Cystic Disease. Localized cystic disease is a benign condition that resembles multilocular cystic nephroma. The lesion consists of multiple cysts of varying size separated by normal or atrophic renal parenchyma (Fig. 15-18). The disease is not hereditary and is not associated with renal insufficiency. CT findings include:

- Multiple cysts of varying size are separated by normally enhancing renal parenchyma.
- No discrete encapsulation is present.
- Other, clearly separate, benign cysts are often found nearby.
- The lesion most commonly affects a portion of one kidney.
- Occasionally, one entire kidney is affected and resembles unilateral autosomal dominant polycystic kidney disease.
- Localized renal cystic disease is not associated with the presence of cysts in other organs.

Bosniak Classification of Cystic Renal Masses

In 1986, Morton Bosniak described a classification system for cystic renal masses that now is widely used. The classification scheme was modified in 1993. Cystic lesion classification is based on CT findings:

- *Bosniak Category I: Benign Simple Cyst.* CT shows homogeneous internal attenuation of water density; hairline thin wall; no enhancement with IV contrast; and no septa, calcifications, or solid components (see Fig. 15-16).

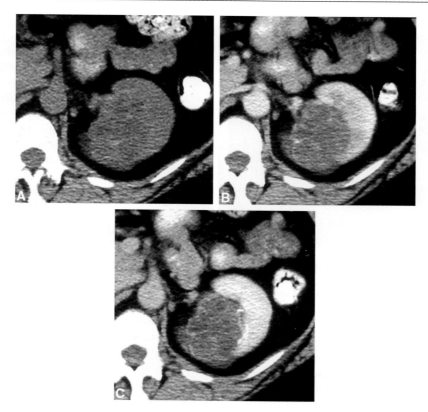

FIGURE 15-20 **Cystic mass: marked enhancement, Bosniak Category IV.** Noncontrast *(A)*, postcontrast corticomedullary phase *(B)*, and nephrogram phase *(C)* images demonstrate striking enhancement of septations in this cystic renal mass. Nephrectomy confirmed multicystic renal cell carcinoma.

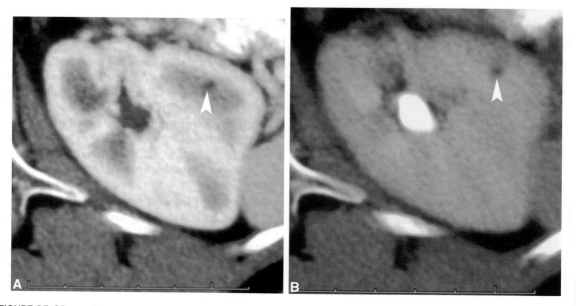

FIGURE 15-21 **Small indeterminate renal mass.** Postcontrast corticomedullary phase *(A)* and pyelogram phase *(B)* images show a tiny, nonenhancing, low-attenuation renal mass. This most likely represents a tiny renal cyst.

grow slowly (mean, 0.36 cm/year) and are not an immediate threat to the patient's life. Evidence of lesion growth or the appearance of more aggressive features is indicative of RCC.

- Image-guided biopsy of a renal mass is rarely indicated. Percutaneous biopsy of a small renal mass is less accurate than imaging diagnosis. Core biopsy histology specimens obtained at surgery had only an 81% sensitivity and a 67% specificity. The false-positive rate was 34%, and the false-negative rate was 20%. In patients with suspected RCC believed to be metastatic, biopsy of a suspected metastasis is usually more fruitful than biopsy of the renal mass.

Multiple Renal Cysts

When multiple renal cysts are encountered, the following conditions should be considered: multiple simple cysts, autosomal dominant polycystic disease, multicystic dysplastic kidney, von Hippel–Lindau disease, tuberous sclerosis, and acquired renal cystic disease.

Multiple Simple Cysts. Simple cysts increase in frequency with age and are commonly multiple and bilateral (Fig. 15-22). Patients older than age 50 with no cysts in other organs and who have no family history of renal cystic disease are most likely to have multiple simple cysts.

Autosomal Dominant Polycystic Disease. The cortex and medulla of both kidneys are progressively replaced by multiple noncommunicating cysts of varying size in autosomal dominant polycystic disease, which is a common hereditary disorder. Although this disease may be detected in childhood, most patients present clinically with hypertension and renal failure at ages 30 to 50 years. The renal cysts are commonly complicated by bleeding or infection, which causes thickening of the cyst walls and an increase in density of cyst fluid. Berry aneurysms are present in the circle of Willis in 10% to 15% of patients. CT findings become more pronounced as the disease progresses. Autosomal dominant ("adult") polycystic disease is differentiated from other conditions by the presence of cysts in other organs, positive family history, and the presence of renal failure and hypertension. Diagnostic CT findings include:

- Progressive replacement of renal parenchyma with cysts of varying size associated with progressive bilateral increase in renal volume.
- Cysts are present in other organs, most commonly the liver (30% to 50%) and pancreas (10%).
- Cysts in the kidneys may have calcified walls and high internal attenuation caused by previous hemorrhage (Fig. 15-23).
- Renal stones are common (20% to 40% of patients).

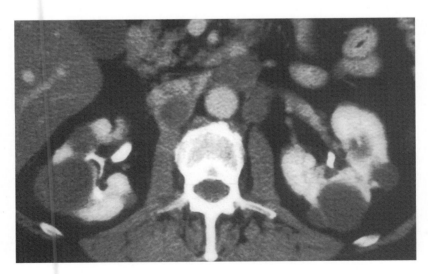

FIGURE 15-22 **Multiple simple cysts.** CT demonstrates multiple simple cysts of various sizes throughout both kidneys. These are incidental findings.

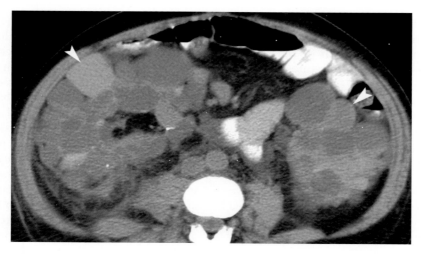

FIGURE 15-23 **Autosomal dominant polycystic kidney disease.** Noncontrast CT shows that both kidneys are massively enlarged and that cysts of varying size and attenuation replace the renal parenchyma. High-attenuation cysts *(arrowheads)* are caused by hemorrhage into the cyst.

Multicystic Dysplastic Kidney. Multicystic dysplastic kidney is a nonhereditary renal dysplasia in which the kidney consists of multiple thin-walled cysts held together by connective tissue. The involved kidney is functionless. At birth, the involved kidney is greatly enlarged. With advancing age the kidney progressively shrinks and often becomes calcified. Rarely, only a portion of one kidney may be involved. Bilateral multicystic dysplastic kidneys occur but are fatal at birth. The opposite kidney is affected by ureteropelvic junction obstruction or another anomaly in 30% of patients.

von Hippel–Lindau Disease. von Hippel–Lindau disease is an autosomal dominant disorder characterized by cerebellar, spinal cord, and retinal hemangioblastomas; renal and pancreatic cysts; RCC; and pheochromocytoma. CT findings include:

- Multiple bilateral renal cysts are present in 50% to 75% of patients (Fig. 15-24).
- RCC occurs in 28% to 45% of patients. Tumors are most often solid, multicentric, and bilateral. Some appear as complex cysts with enhancing septa.
- Pheochromocytoma is seen in 30% of patients; they are bilateral in 50% and malignant in 10% to 15%.

Tuberous Sclerosis. Tuberous sclerosis is an autosomal dominant syndrome that combines multiple renal cysts and multiple and bilat-

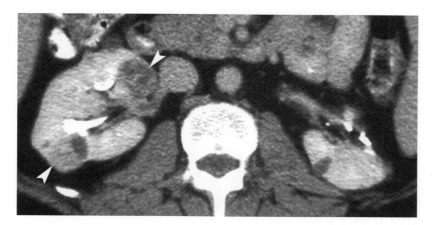

FIGURE 15-24 **von Hippel–Lindau disease.** Two partially cystic renal cell carcinomas *(arrowheads)* are seen in the right kidney. A partial nephrectomy has been performed on the left to remove a renal cell carcinoma. The complete CT scan showed numerous cysts in both kidneys.

eral renal AMLs (see Fig. 15-9) with cutaneous, retinal, and cerebral hamartomas. The renal lesions are commonly detected in infancy and childhood.

Acquired Renal Cystic Disease. Patients on chronic hemodialysis commonly develop innumerable cysts in their native kidneys. More than 90% of patients who are on dialysis for 5 to 10 years are affected. Many of the cysts are lined by hyperplastic and dysplastic epithelium. The condition is complicated by hemorrhage from the cysts and the development of RCC. CT findings include:

- The renal parenchyma is progressively replaced by myriad tiny cysts (<6 mm; Fig. 15-25). Some cysts are up to 2 cm in size. The kidney slowly enlarges over time as cysts develop. Calcification of the wall of cysts is common.
- The cysts usually regress within months of renal transplantation.

Infection

CT is indicated when complications of renal infection are suspected. Predisposing conditions, including urinary calculi, neurogenic bladder, immune system compromise, diabetes, IV drug abuse, or chronic debilitating disease, increase the risk for complications that require intervention. Most urinary tract infections are caused by gram-negative bacilli, but the incidence of fungal and tuberculous infections is increasing.

Acute Pyelonephritis

Acute pyelonephritis is a multifocal infection of one or both kidneys. All symptoms usually resolve in patients with uncomplicated pyelonephritis within 72 hours of institution of appropriate antibiotic therapy. Patients who fail to improve should be imaged to detect complications. CT signs of acute bacterial infection of the kidneys include:

- Wedge-shaped areas of mottled decreased parenchymal enhancement are seen (Fig. 15-26). The CT appearance is similar to renal infarction. Decreased enhancement is the result of decreased blood flow caused by edema and inflammation within the parenchyma confined by the renal capsule.
- A striated pattern of linear alternating increased and decreased densities on enhanced scans is particularly characteristic.
- High-density areas of parenchyma on unenhanced scans indicate parenchyma hemorrhage caused by inflammation and ischemia.
- Stranding densities in the perirenal fat and thickening of the renal fascia occur as a result of inflammation and edema in the perirenal space.
- Severe localized infection (focal pyelonephritis, acute focal bacterial nephritis, lobar nephronia) produces a poorly defined, mottled, low-density mass without distinct liquefaction. These phlegmons may resolve

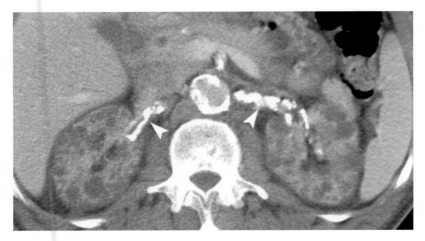

FIGURE 15-25 **Acquired renal cystic disease.** CT scan of a patient with a 15-year history of hemodialysis showed numerous small cysts in both kidneys. The kidneys are of low normal size. No solid masses were detected. Note the severe atherosclerosis involving both renal arteries *(arrowheads)* and the aorta.

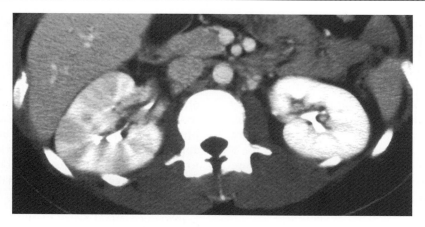

FIGURE 15-26 Acute pyelonephritis. The right kidney shows the wedge-shaped areas of decreased parenchymal enhancement characteristic of acute pyelonephritis. Severe edema in affected regions of the kidney results in diminished blood flow producing the enhancement defects. The left kidney is normal.

completely, result in a scar, or evolve into an abscess.

- *Emphysematous pyelonephritis* is a severe type of diffuse pyelonephritis that occurs in patients with diabetes and patients with urinary obstruction. Gas is produced by metabolism of glucose by gram-negative bacteria. CT shows gas in the renal parenchyma and the additional signs of renal inflammation. Emergency nephrectomy is usually the treatment of choice.

- *Emphysematous pyelitis* refers to gas confined to the renal pelvis and calyces. This finding may be found with infection, trauma, instrumentation, or fistula and lacks the dire implications of gas within the renal parenchyma.

- *Abscess* refers to a collection of pus and liquefied tissue within the kidney or with spread into the perirenal space (Fig. 15-27). CT demonstrates a fluid collection (10–30 H) with an enhancing rim. Gas may be present within the collection, especially in patients with diabetes. Large abscesses require catheter or surgical drainage.

Pyonephrosis

Pyonephrosis is acute infection with pus within an obstructed collecting system. Renal destruction is rapid, and urgent drainage is required. Characteristics of pyonephrosis include:

- The collecting system is dilated and the contained fluid is high in density with layering sometimes evident.

- The wall of the collecting system is thickened.
- The renal parenchyma is often thinned. Intraparenchymal abscesses may be present.

Renal Tuberculosis

Tuberculosis remains the number one cause of death from infectious disease in the world. The urinary tract is affected in 15% to 20% of

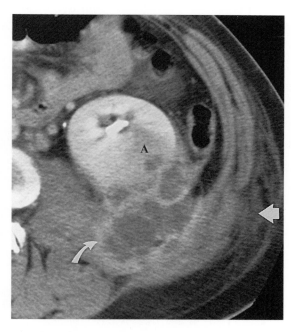

FIGURE 15-27 Renal and perirenal abscess. A bacterial abscess (A) complicating acute pyelonephritis has spread through the renal capsule into the perirenal space *(curved arrow)*. Edema and inflammation also involve the muscles and subcutaneous tissues *(large arrow)* of the flank.

patients. Multiple caseous granulomas form in the cortex because of its favorable blood supply. These may remain dormant or reactivate, spreading organisms to the tubules resulting in papillary necrosis. Progressive infection will eventually destroy the kidney. CT findings of renal tuberculosis include:

- Disease is often unilateral with a predilection for the poles of the kidney.
- Calcifications are a hallmark of disease shown by CT in 50% of cases. Calcifications are typically within the renal parenchyma and may be coarse, globular, curvilinear, or granular. Extensive calcification of a nonfunctioning kidney (putty kidney) is characteristic of end-stage renal tuberculosis.
- Fibrotic strictures of the infundibula, pelvis, and ureter are characteristic.
- Calyces are often dilated because of fibrosis and strictures of the collecting system. The dilated calyces are filled with clear fluid, debris, or calculi.
- Cortical thinning, caused by focal or diffuse parenchymal scarring, is usually present.

Xanthogranulomatous Pyelonephritis

Xanthogranulomatous pyelonephritis results from a combination of chronic renal obstruction and chronic infection. The renal parenchyma is progressively destroyed and replaced by lipid-filled macrophages. A staghorn calculus results in involvement of the entire kidney. Solitary calculus or infundibular stricture often results in focal involvement. CT findings include:

- CT shows low-density enlargement of the entire kidney or the affected area with multiple low-density masses representing dilated calyces (Fig. 15-28).
- The obstructing calculus is seen within the renal pelvis or calyces.
- Extension of the infective process into the perirenal tissues is common.

▢ URETER

Anatomy

The ureter is a muscular tube approximately 30 cm in length that lies on the psoas muscle. At the pelvic brim it courses medially to the

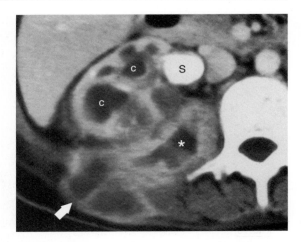

FIGURE 15-28 Xanthogranulomatous pyelonephritis. A large stone (s) fills the renal pelvis and causes obstruction, resulting in dilatation of the collecting system (c). The chronic infective process extends from the kidney through the perirenal space *(asterisk)* and into the subcutaneous soft tissues *(arrow).* A nephrectomy was performed and yielded *Proteus* organisms on bacterial culture.

sacroiliac joint, then laterally near the ischial spine before it turns medially to enter the bladder through a submucosal tunnel (the uterovesical junction). The ureter is lined by transitional epithelial, has a muscular wall consisting of circular and longitudinal muscle bundles, and has an outer adventitia that is continuous with the renal capsule and adventitia of the bladder. On unenhanced CT, 3 mm is the upper limit of normal diameter.

Ureteral Duplication

Duplication of the ureters is the most common anomaly of the urinary tract. Complete duplication is associated with ectopic insertion of the ureter, ectopic ureteroceles, and vesicoureteral reflux, and it is more common in female patients. Characteristics of ureteral duplication include:

- The ureter draining the upper pole of the kidney typically has fewer calyces, inserts into the bladder medially and inferiorly to the lower pole ureter (Weigert–Meyer rule), and is more likely to be ectopic, obstructed, and end in a ureterocele. With high-grade obstruction, the upper pole of the kidney is atrophic and is replaced by a cyst representing the dilated upper pole pelvis (Fig. 15-29).

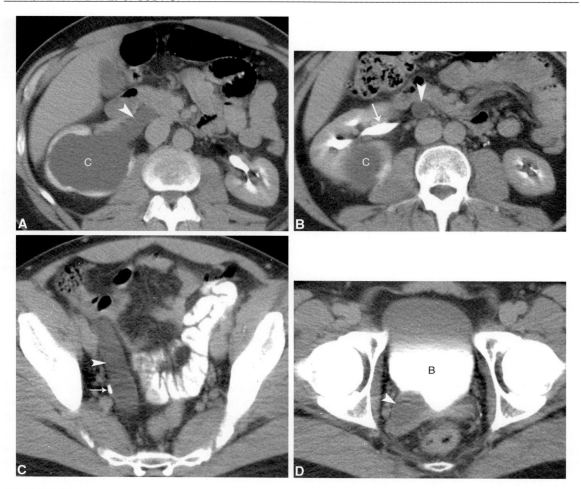

FIGURE 15-29 **Obstructed ureteral duplication.** *A,* A cystic structure (C) at the upper pole of the right kidney communicates with a dilated pelvis *(arrowhead).* The cystic structure represents the obstructed collecting system of the upper pole of the kidney. Absence of contrast excretion into the obstructed collecting system is evidence of absent renal function of the upper pole. *B,* CT image obtained below *A* shows the caudal portion of the obstructed upper pole system (C) and the functioning lower pole system excreting contrast into a separate renal pelvis *(arrow).* The dilated ureter *(arrowhead)* continuing from the upper pole system is also evident. *C,* Lower in the pelvis the greatly dilated upper pole ureter resembles a fluid-filled sausage. The normal lower pole ureter *(arrow)* is filled with contrast. *D,* The dilated ureter of the upper pole terminates in the bladder (B) as a bulging ectopic ureterocele *(arrowhead).*

- The ureter draining the lower pole of the kidney typically inserts into the bladder at a normal location. The lower pole system is prone to reflux if an ectopic ureterocele from the upper pole system distorts the lower pole uterovesical junction.
- An increased frequency of ureteropelvic junction obstruction is seen in the lower pole system.
- When duplication is incomplete, the ureters typically fuse at a variable distance from the kidney resulting in a single ureteral insertion into the bladder. Yo-yo reflux of urine occurs

between the two ureters induced by peristalsis of one ureter, then the other.

Transitional Cell Carcinoma of the Ureter

TCC accounts for 90% of ureteral tumors. About 75% occur in the distal ureter. More than 50% are associated with the presence or development of bladder TCC.

Tumors appear as a soft-tissue mass, lower in density than unopacified urine, expanding and obstructing the ureter. When contrast is present, the lesions appear as an irregular filling defect. Irregular thickening of the ureteral wall is seen with stricturing lesions (Fig. 15-30). Enhancement with IV contrast is minimal.

Renal Stone Disease

MDCT has forever changed the imaging of renal stone disease. CT is now the imaging method of choice to detect renal stones and to diagnose the complications of renal stone disease. Plain radiographs have a specificity for stones of only 77%. Noncontrast CT has been shown to be more effective than intravenous pyelograms in precisely identifying ureteral stones and is equally effective as intravenous pyelograms in determining the presence or absence of ureteral obstruction. Plain radiographs and intravenous pyelograms have been largely replaced by spiral CT. CT for stones requires no contrast and no patient preparation. With MDCT, the study is routinely completed in seconds. CT may also provide an alternate diagnosis for the patient's symptoms including other urinary pathology, acute appendicitis, diverticulitis, pancreatitis, adnexal masses, or leaking aneurysms.

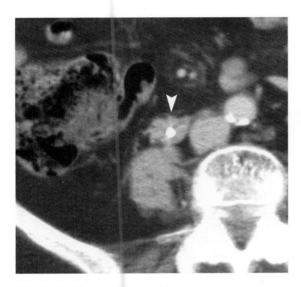

FIGURE 15-30 Transitional cell carcinoma: ureter. The ureter *(arrowhead)* is markedly and irregularly thickened with soft-tissue strands extending into the adjacent fat. CT-guided percutaneous biopsy confirmed transitional cell carcinoma. A stent, seen as a high-density structure, was placed because the ureter was severely strictured.

CT Appearance of Urinary Stones

Whereas only about 85% of urinary stones are seen as calcific densities on plain film radiographs, CT detects nearly all calculi. Calcium oxalate and calcium phosphate stones are most common (73%) and typically have a CT attenuation of 800 to 1000 H. Struvite stones (magnesium aluminum phosphate; 15% of renal stones) are seen with chronic infection. Struvite attenuation ranges from 300 to 900 H. Uric acid stones (8%), which are radiolucent on plain film, have an attenuation of 150 to 500 H. Cystine stones (1% to 4%) are moderately radiopaque because of their sulfur content. Calcium may be present in some cystine stones. Cystine stones have attenuation values of 200 to 880 H depending on calcium content. High CT attenuation makes stones easy to differentiate from other urinary tract lesions such as tumors, hematoma, fungus balls, or sloughed papilla. CT findings of urinary stones include:

- Virtually all stones, even those that are radiolucent on plain film radiographs, are identified as high-attenuation foci on CT images viewed on soft-tissue windows (Fig. 15-31). The threshold size for stone detection by CT is approximately 1 mm.

- Ureteral calculi are usually geometric or oval in shape (see Figs. 15-31 and 15-32). They are seldom completely round. This feature is useful in differentiating stones from phleboliths. The positive predictive value of geometric shape in identifying a calculus has been reported to be as high as 100%.

- The single exception to stones being high in density on CT is crystalline stones in the urine related to use of protease inhibitors (indinavir [Crixivan]) in the treatment of human immunodeficiency virus disease. These stones are nonopaque on CT scans but may cause ureteral obstruction. Contrast-enhanced CT demonstrates these stones as tiny filling defects in the collecting system or ureter.

- The burden of stones in the kidneys is easily determined by CT. Stones are seen in the region of the minor calices or medullary pyramids. The stone burden is defined as the number and size of stones present. Stone burden is used to determine therapy such as lithotripsy.

- The tips of the renal pyramids are high attenuation when the patient is dehydrated

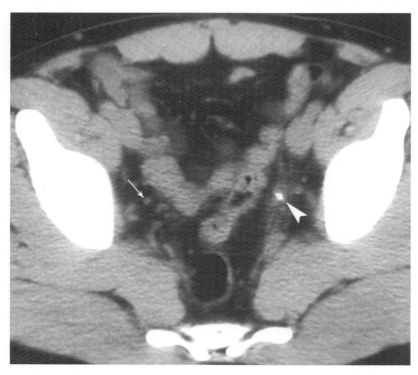

FIGURE 15-31 **Stone in ureter: tissue rim sign.** Noncontrast CT shows a stone impacted in the distal left ureter *(arrowhead)* seen as an irregularly shaped, high-attenuation focus. The wall of the ureter produces a rim of soft-tissue density around the stone (the "tissue rim sign"). The normal right ureter *(arrow)* is identified by scrolling through sequential CT images keeping track of the course of the ureter.

(see Fig. 15-34). This normal finding of "white pyramids" should not be interpreted as representing renal stones.

Acute Ureteral Obstruction

Noncontrast spiral CT has a reported sensitivity of 94% to 98% and specificity of 96% to 98% for acute ureteral obstruction caused by an impact-

ed stone. CT evidence of acute ureteral obstruction caused by stones includes:

- A stone is demonstrated in the ureter (see Figs. 15-31 and 15-32). The most common locations for stone impaction are at the ureteropelvic junction, where the ureter crosses the pelvic brim, and at the uter-

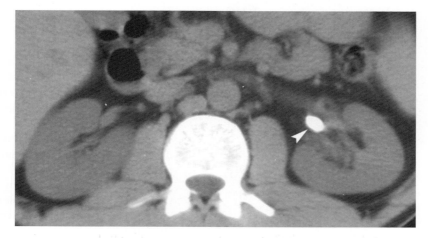

FIGURE 15-32 **Stone at ureteropelvic junction (UPJ).** A large stone is impacted at the left UPJ *(arrowhead)*. Bloom artifact from the high-attenuation stone obscures the tissue rim sign. The stone is confirmed to be located at the UPJ by careful inspection of serial CT images.

ovesical junction. The ureter is followed on consecutive slices until a stone is identified. Scrolling on the CT monitor is the easiest way to follow the course of the ureter. Knowledge of the anatomy of the course of the ureter and of adjacent vessels is crucial for accurate interpretation.

- The size of the stone is measured, and its location is precisely reported. The probability of spontaneous stone passage is related to size and location of the ureteral stone. Stones smaller than 4 mm nearly always pass spontaneously. Stones of 6 mm pass about half of the time. Stones larger than 8 mm rarely pass spontaneously. Size and location of the stone are important factors used to determine the treatment of stones that do not pass spontaneously. Stones larger than 5 mm and located in the proximal two thirds of the ureter are more likely to require lithotripsy or endoscopic removal.

- To confirm a stone in the ureter, look for a tissue rim sign (present in ~76% of patients). The *tissue rim sign* (see Fig. 15-31) describes a halo of soft tissue that surrounds stones in the ureter. The soft tissue rim is the wall of the ureter. The tissue rim sign may be absent because of bloom effect artifact or a thin ureteral wall.

- The CT scout scan is useful for detection of stones and other abnormalities. Examination of the scout scan should be included in every CT interpretation. If the stone is visible on the scout scan, then plain radiographs can be used to monitor its passage. Calculi not visible on plain radiographs can be followed, when necessary, with unenhanced CT.

- Secondary findings of urinary obstruction are common but often subtle (Fig. 15-33). Comparison with opposite side is highly useful in differentiating preexisting findings from acute obstruction. The presence of multiple secondary findings improves the confidence and accuracy of diagnosing acute obstruction. The frequency of visualization of secondary signs increases with the duration of symptoms.

- The obstructed kidney may be enlarged and slightly decreased in CT density because of edema. A 5-H attenuation decrease is significant as evidence of edema in an obstructed kidney.

- Periureteral and perinephric fat stranding occurs secondary to edema produced by acute obstruction. The amount of edema present correlates with the severity of obstruction.

- The pelvicaliceal system is at most mildly dilated with acute stone obstruction. Dilated calyces are best seen at the poles of the kidney as rounded, fluid-filled structures that displace renal sinus fat. Comparison with opposite kidney is always helpful. Profound dilatation of the collecting system is evidence of chronic, rather than acute, obstruction.

- Unilateral absence of "white pyramids" on the affected side has been described as a subtle sign of obstruction (Fig. 15-34).

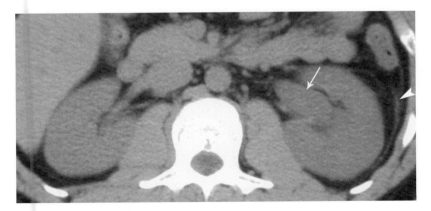

FIGURE 15-33 **Obstructed kidney.** CT image of a patient with left flank pain demonstrates subtle swelling and decreased density of the left kidney with mild dilatation of the left renal pelvis *(arrow)* and calyces. The margin of the left kidney with perirenal fat is indistinct. The left renal fascia *(arrowhead)* is mildly thickened. This constellation of subtle findings is suggestive of left ureteral obstruction. A stone impacted at the left uterovesical junction was seen on CT images through the pelvis.

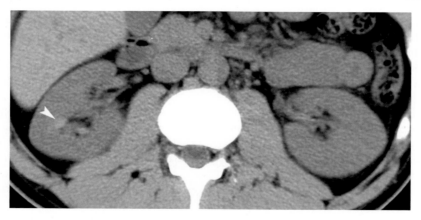

FIGURE 15-34 **Unilateral white pyramids.** The tips of the medullary pyramids in the right kidney show high attenuation *(arrowhead)*, indicating that this patient with left flank pain is dehydrated. On the symptomatic left side, no white pyramids are seen. The unilateral absence of white pyramids is a subtle sign of acute obstruction. A stone was demonstrated at the left ureterovesical junction.

Edema and swelling counteracts the urine concentration effect of systemic dehydration.

- The ureter is mildly dilated to the level of the stone. Normal ureteral peristalsis produces transient focal areas of dilatation and narrowing that must be differentiated from diffuse dilatation to the level of obstruction. The ureter below the obstructing calculus is not dilated.
- Focal perinephric fluid collections (Fig. 15-35) may occur secondary to fornical rupture caused by obstruction and high urine output.
- Axial plane CT images may be reformatted into coronal plane images that resemble intravenous pyelogram images in problematic cases. However, this procedure is time consuming and seldom necessary.

Pitfalls in Diagnosis of Stones in the Ureter

No imaging test is perfect. A wide variety of pitfalls complicate interpretation of renal stone CT. For example:

- An extrarenal pelvis may mimic pelviectasis.
- Peripelvic cysts may simulate hydronephrosis (Fig. 15-36).
- Many patients, especially older patients, have preexisting stranding in the peripelvic fat. Comparison with the opposite side is critical to detect asymmetric stranding.
- Preexisting postobstructive changes are difficult to differentiate from acute obstruction.

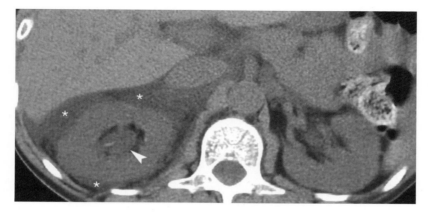

FIGURE 15-35 **Obstruction: ruptured calyx.** Noncontrast CT image shows dilatation of the calyx *(arrowhead)* at the upper pole of the right kidney. Fluid density *(asterisk)* in the perirenal space indicates rupture of a calyx induced by the increased pressures within the collecting system resulting from obstruction of the ureter and high urine output in this patient who had been forcing oral fluid intake. The left kidney is normal.

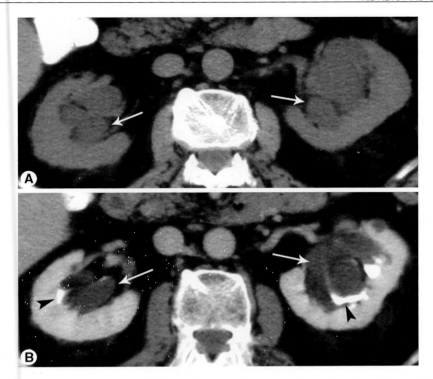

FIGURE 15-36 **Peripelvic cysts.** *A,* Noncontrast CT shows bilateral cystic structures *(arrows)* in the renal sinuses that resemble hydronephrosis. *B,* Postcontrast CT in the pyelogram phase shows no contrast filling of the cystic structures *(arrows),* indicating that they are peripelvic cysts. Contrast does opacify the collecting systems *(arrowheads),* which are compressed by the cysts within the renal sinuses of both kidneys. The clue to diagnosis is inspection of serial images that show no connection of the peripelvic cysts with a dilated renal pelvis.

- Phleboliths commonly mimic stones (Fig. 15-37). Phleboliths are calcifications that originate in thrombi within pelvic veins. Most phleboliths are found in perivesical veins, in periprostatic veins in men, and in periuterine and perivaginal veins in women. Occasionally, phleboliths are seen in gonadal veins that parallel the course of the ureters. Most phleboliths are round. They are seldom oval and are never geometric in shape. Visualization of a central lucency is highly characteristic of phleboliths but is less often evident on CT than on plain radiographs. The *tail sign* describes a tail of noncalcified vein extending from the phlebolith. A tail sign has been reported to be associated with 21% to 65% of phleboliths. Phleboliths are lower density than most stones with a mean attenuation value of 160 H and a range of 80 to 278 H. The probability that a calcification represented a phlebolith is 0.03% when mean attenuation is 311 H or more.

- Atherosclerotic calcifications may be mistaken for ureteral stones. Differentiation is made by carefully examining serial slices and determining if the calcification is vascular or ureteral.

- When signs of ureteral obstruction are present, yet no stone is evident, consider a recently passed stone, pyelonephritis, stricture or tumor, or protease inhibitor treatment-related stone.

- Stones passed from the ureter may be identified in the bladder or urethra or may not be seen.

- Always look for evidence of nonurinary causes of flank pain. Unenhanced CT has been reported to be 94% accurate in the diagnosis of appendicitis. Adnexal masses are usually easily detected.

- A subsequent contrast-enhanced CT may be needed in up to 20% of patients to provide an unequivocal diagnosis.

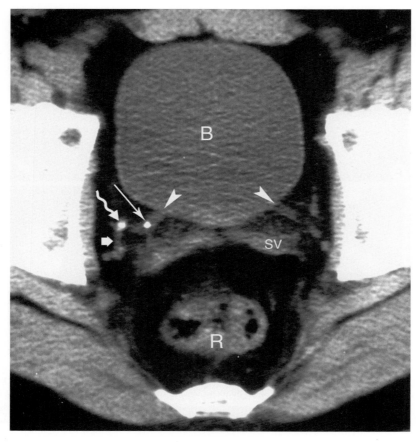

FIGURE 15-37 Phlebolith and stone. The seminal vesicles (SV) serve as an anatomic landmark for the level of the ureterovesical junctions *(arrowheads).* The right and left uterovesical junctions (UVJs) are located at same axial level on CT. A stone *(long straight arrow)* is impacted in the distal right ureter. An adjacent phlebolith *(squiggly arrow)* is identified by the tail sign, representing the thrombosed vein *(short wide arrow).* The bladder (B) is filled with urine making identification of the UVJs easier. The rectum (R) is seen posteriorly.

▇ SUGGESTED READING

ABRAMSON S, WALDERS N, APPLEGATE KE, et al: Impact in the emergency department of unenhanced CT on diagnostic confidence and therapeutic efficacy in patients with suspected renal colic: A prospective study. AJR Am J Roentgenol 175: 1689–1695, 2000.

AL-NAKSHABANDI NA: The soft-tissue rim sign. Radiology 229:239–240, 2003.

ASSI Z, PLATT JF, FRANCIS IR, et al: Sensitivity of CT scout radiography and abdominal radiography for revealing ureteral calculi on helical CT: Implications for radiologic follow-up. AJR Am J Roentgenol 175:333–337, 2000.

BAE KT, HEIKEN JP, SIEGEL CL, BENNETT HF: Renal cysts: Is attenuation artifactually increased on contrast-enhanced CT images? Radiology 216: 792–796, 2000.

BECHTOLD RB, CHEN MYM, DYER RB, ZAGORIA RJ: CT of the ureteral wall. AJR Am J Roentgenol 170:1283–1289, 1998.

BELL TV, FENLON HM, DAVISON BD, et al: Unenhanced helical CT criteria to differentiate distal ureteral calculi from pelvic phleboliths. Radiology 207:363–367, 1998.

BORIDY IC, NIKOLAIDIS P, KAWASHIMA A, et al: Ureterolithiasis: Value of the tail sign in differentiating phleboliths for ureteral calculi at nonenhanced helical CT. Radiology 211:619–621, 1999.

BOSNIAK MA: The current radiological approach to renal cysts. Radiology 158:1–10, 1986.

BOSNIAK MA: The small (<3.0 cm) renal parenchymal tumor: Detection, diagnosis, and controversies. Radiology 179:307–317, 1991.

BOSNIAK MA: Problems in the radiologic diagnosis of renal parenchymal tumors. Urol Clin North Am 20:217–230, 1993.

BRANT WE: Spiral CT replaces IVP and KUB for renal stone disease. Diag Imag 21:51–57, 2001.

COLL DM, VARANELLI MJ, SMITH RC: Relationship of spontaneous passage of ureteral calculi to stone size and location as revealed by unenhanced helical CT. AJR Am J Roentgenol 178:101–103, 2002.

COULAM CH, SHEAFOR DH, LEDER RA, et al: Evaluation of pseudoenhancement of renal cysts during contrast-enhanced CT. AJR Am J Roentgenol 174:493–498, 2000.

DALRYMPLE NC, CASFORD B, RAIKEN DP, et al: Pearls and pitfalls in the diagnosis of ureterolithiasis with unenhanced helical CT. Radiographics 20:439–447, 2000.

FERNBACH SK, FEINSTEIN KA, SPENCER K, LINDSTROM CA: Ureteral duplication and its complications. Radiographics 17:109–127, 1997.

GEORGIADES CS, MOORE CJ, SMITH DP: Differences of renal parenchymal attenuation for acutely obstructed and unobstructed kidneys on unenhanced helical CT: A useful sign? AJR Am J Roentgenol 176:965–968, 2001.

GIBSON M, PUCKETT M, SHELLY M: Renal tuberculosis. Radiographics 24:251–256, 2004.

GOLDMAN SM, FAINTUCH S, AJZEN SA, et al: Diagnostic value of attenuation measurements of the kidney on unenhanced helical CT of obstructive ureterolithiasis. AJR Am J Roentgenol 182:1251–1254, 2004.

GUEST AR, COHAN RH, KOROBKIN M, et al: Assessment of clinical utility of the rim and comet-tail signs in differentiating ureteral stones from phleboliths. AJR Am J Roentgenol 177:1285–1291, 2001.

HENEGHAN JP, DALRYMPLE NC, VERGA M, et al: Soft-tissue "rim" sign in the diagnosis of ureteral calculi with use of unenhanced helical CT. Radiology 202:709–711, 1997.

HOPKINS J, GILES H Jr, WYATT-ASHMEAD J, BIGLER SA: Cystic nephroma. Radiographics 24:589–593, 2004.

ISREAL GM, BOSNIAK MA: Follow-up CT of moderately complex cystic lesions of the kidney (Bosniak Category IIF). AJR Am J Roentgenol 181:627–633, 2003.

JAIN MK, SINGH R, KAROL I: Alternative pathologies on unenhanced helical CT scan in patients presenting with flank pain. Radiologist 10:55–59, 2003.

KAWASHIMA A, SANDLER CM, BORIDY IC, et al: Unenhanced helical CT of ureterolithiasis: Value of the tissue rim sign. AJR Am J Roentgenol 168:997–1000, 1997.

KAZEROONI NL, DUNNICK NR: Current diagnosis and treatment of urolithiasis. Radiologist 6:99–108, 1999.

KIM J, PARK S, SHON J, CHO K: Angiomyolipoma with minimal fat: Differentiation from renal cell carcinoma at biphasic helical CT. Radiology 230:677–684, 2004.

LEVINE JA, NEITLICH J, VERGA M, et al: Ureteral calculi in patients with flank pain: Correlation of plain radiography with unenhanced helical CT. Radiology 204:27–31, 1997.

MAKI DD, BIRNBAUM BA, CHAKRABORTY DP, et al: Renal cyst pseudoenhancement: Beam-hardening effects on CT numbers. Radiology 213:468–472, 1999.

MCNICHOLAS MMJ, RAPTOPOULOS VD, SCHWARTZ RK, et al: Excretory phase CT urography for opacification of the urinary collecting system. AJR Am J Roentgenol 170:1261–1267, 1998.

PICKHARDT PJ, LONERGAN GJ, DAVIS CJ Jr, et al: Infiltrative renal lesions: Radiologic-pathologic correlation. Radiographics 20:215–243, 2000.

SCATARIGE JC, SHETH S, CORL FM, FISHMAN EK: Patterns of recurrence of renal cell carcinoma: Manifestations on helical CT. AJR Am J Roentgenol 177:653–658, 2001.

SHEERAN SR, SUSSMAN SK: Renal lymphoma: Spectrum of CT findings and potential mimics. AJR Am J Roentgenol 171:1067–1072, 1998.

SOURTZIS S, THIBEAU JF, DAMRY N, et al: Radiologic investigation of renal colic: Unenhanced helical CT compared with excretory urography. AJR Am J Roentgenol 172:1491–1494, 1999.

TACK D, SOURTZIS S, DELPIERRE I, et al: Low-dose unenhanced multidetector CT of patients with suspected renal colic. AJR Am J Roentgenol 180:305–311, 2003.

TAMM EP, SILVERMAN PM, SHUMAN WP: Evaluation of the patient with flank pain and possible ureteral calculus. Radiology 228:319–329, 2003.

TAOULI B, GHOUADNI M, CORREAS J, et al: Spectrum of abdominal imaging findings in von Hippel–Lindau disease. AJR Am J Roentgenol 181:1049–1054, 2003.

TRAUBICI J, NEITLICH JD, SMITH RC: Distinguishing pelvic phleboliths from distal ureteral stones on routine unenhanced helical CT: Is there a radiolucent center? AJR Am J Roentgenol 172:13–17, 1999.

TUBLIN ME, TESSLER FN, MCCAULEY TR, KESACK CD: Effect of hydration on renal medulla attenuation on unenhanced CT scans. AJR Am J Roentgenol 168:257–259, 1996.

URBAN BA, FISHMAN EK: Renal lymphoma: CT patterns with emphasis on helical CT. Radiographics 20:197–212, 2000.

WARSHAUER DM, McCARTHY SM, STREET L, et al: Detection of renal masses: Sensitivities and specificities of excretory urography/linear tomography, US and CT. Radiology 169:363–365, 1988.

WONG-YOU-CHEONG JJ, WAGNER BJ, DAVIS CJ Jr: Transitional cell carcinoma of the urinary tract: Radiologic-pathologic correlation. Radiographics 18:123–142, 1998.

ZAGORIA RJ: Imaging of small renal masses: A medical success story. AJR Am J Roentgenol 175:945–955, 2000.

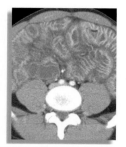

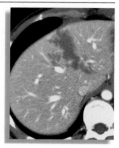

16

Adrenal Glands

William E. Brant, M.D.

The adrenal glands are imaged in three clinical circumstances. A patient may be referred because a clinical diagnosis of adrenal hormone hyperfunction has been made. CT is then used to identify and characterize the lesion. The adrenal glands are commonly imaged to detect suspected metastatic disease, especially when the primary tumor, such as lung carcinoma, commonly metastasizes to the adrenals. Adrenal lesions are frequently detected incidentally on imaging studies performed for other indications. The significance of the finding must be assessed radiographically and clinically. CT remains the imaging method of first choice for evaluation of the adrenal glands.

☐ NORMAL ADRENAL GLANDS

The adrenal glands have an outer cortex and an inner medulla that are functionally independent and anatomically distinct. The cortex secretes steroid hormones including cortisol, aldosterone, androgens, and estrogens. The medulla produces catecholamines. The adrenal glands lie in the perirenal space surrounded by fat. The glands are usually triangular, or inverted V- or Y-shaped. The right adrenal gland lies

above the right kidney posterior to the inferior vena cava between the right crus of the diaphragm and the right lobe of the liver (Fig. 16-1). The left adrenal gland lies adjacent to the upper pole of the left kidney posterior to the pancreas and splenic vessels and lateral to the left crus of the diaphragm (Fig. 16-2). The limbs of the adrenal gland are 4 to 5 cm in length and normally do not exceed 10 mm in thickness. Limb thickness is uniform, and the margins are straight or concave. Normal adrenal glands are about equal to muscle in CT attenuation.

☐ ADRENAL MASSES WITH A SPECIFIC IMAGING APPEARANCE

Myelolipoma

Myelolipoma is an uncommon benign adrenal tumor consisting of mature fat with interspersed hematopoietic bone marrow elements. Myelolipoma is most common in the adrenal gland but may be encountered in other sites, especially in the perirenal retroperitoneum or presacral region. The lesion is not associated with endocrine abnormalities. The tumor is most often discovered as an incidental finding. Occasionally, tumors present with acute spontaneous

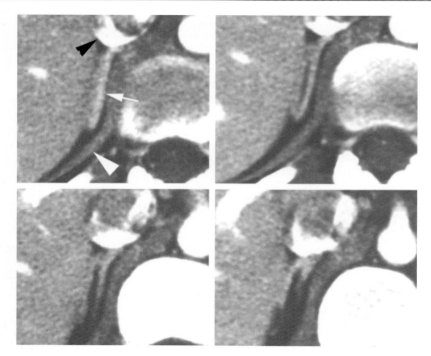

FIGURE 16-1 **Normal right adrenal gland.** A series of postcontrast CT images demonstrate the normal appearance of the right adrenal gland *(arrow)* extending posteriorly from the inferior vena cava *(black arrowhead)* between the right lobe of the liver and right crus of the diaphragm *(white arrowhead).*

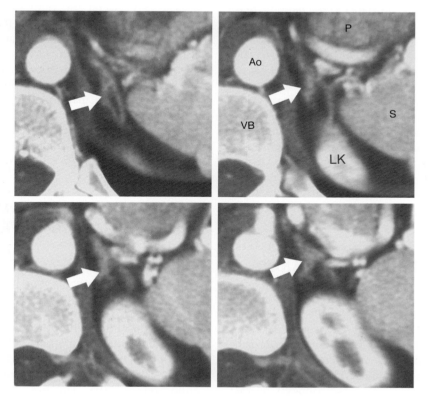

FIGURE 16-2 **Normal left adrenal gland.** Series of postcontrast CT images demonstrate the normal appearance of the left adrenal gland *(arrow)* in the space between the aorta (Ao), upper pole of the left kidney (LK), vertebral body (VB), pancreas (P), and spleen (S).

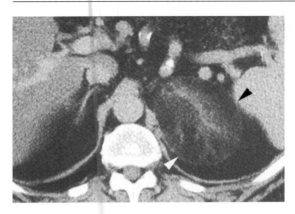

FIGURE 16-3 **Myelolipoma.** A fat-density tumor (between *arrowheads*) replaces the left adrenal gland. The streaks of soft-tissue density within the tumor represent hematopoietic bone marrow elements.

painful hemorrhage. CT findings of myelolipoma include:

- The presence of fat is characteristic. CT demonstrates large deposits of fat interspersed with higher density soft tissue (Fig. 16-3). The fat is near equal to subcutaneous fat in CT attenuation, typically −80 to −100 H. The soft-tissue components are relatively low in CT density (20–30 H), reflecting mixture of fat with the myeloid tissue.
- Small calcifications may be present.
- Hemorrhage is relatively common and alters the imaging appearance. CT shows acute hemorrhage as foci of high attenuation within the fatty mass.

Cysts

True cysts of the adrenal gland are lined with endothelium or epithelium. Most lesions are asymptomatic and are discovered incidentally. They may produce symptoms because of hemorrhage. CT findings of cysts include:

- Cysts are well-marginated, nonenhancing, homogeneous, fluid-containing masses (Fig. 16-4).
- The wall may have thin peripheral calcification if previous hemorrhage has occurred.
- Cyst contents have characteristics of simple fluid (<20 H) unless hemorrhage has occurred.

Pseudocysts

Pseudocysts account for about 40% of adrenal cysts. They occur as a sequela of previous adrenal hemorrhage. Pseudocysts have fibrous walls without cellular lining. CT findings of pseudocysts include:

- Pseudocyst appears as a hypodense mass with a thin or thick wall and, commonly, internal septations.
- Cyst contents are commonly higher density than simple fluid, but cyst contents do not enhance. Fluid–fluid levels may be present.
- Calcification in the wall is commonly present (56%; Fig. 16-5).

Adrenal Hemorrhage

Adrenal hemorrhage is common in the newborn and is caused by hypoxia, birth trauma, or septicemia. In adults and older children, hemorrhage is induced by trauma, coagulopathy, or underlying tumor. CT findings of adrenal hemorrhage include:

- On unenhanced CT adrenal hemorrhage appears round or oval and hyperdense (50–90 H; Fig. 16-6). Stranding is commonly present in the periadrenal fat.
- Post-traumatic adrenal hemorrhage has a marked predisposition to be unilateral on the right side.
- With evolution and liquefaction of the blood clot, the adrenal mass shrinks and decreases in density.

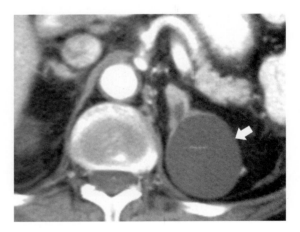

FIGURE 16-4 **Developmental adrenal cyst.** A purely cystic mass *(arrow)* replaces the left adrenal gland. No discernible cyst wall is evident. The internal density is homogeneously low and near water in attenuation.

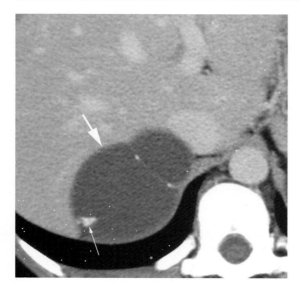

FIGURE 16-5 **Adrenal pseudocyst.** This cystic right adrenal mass *(large arrow)* has calcification in a thin septation and contains a coarse, dense calcium deposit *(small arrow).* This appearance is characteristic of a posthemorrhage adrenal pseudocyst.

- Chronic changes of hemorrhage may be difficult to differentiate from other adrenal masses.

Pseudotumors

A variety of nonadrenal structures may simulate adrenal masses. Differentiation is made by hav-

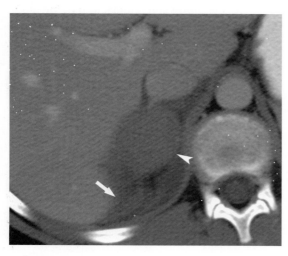

FIGURE 16-6 **Adrenal hemorrhage.** Postcontrast CT in a patient injured in a motor vehicle accident shows hemorrhage expanding the right adrenal gland *(arrowhead)* producing a homogeneous mass. Additional hemorrhage *(arrow)* is seen in the perirenal space. Follow-up CT 4 months later confirmed complete resolution of the adrenal hemorrhage.

ing a high index of suspicion and by performing appropriate correlative imaging tests. Accurate imaging diagnosis obviously should be made before performing adrenal biopsy. Pseudotumors are much more common on the left side because of the larger number of structures in the region of the left adrenal gland. Optimal CT technique makes confusion of pseudotumors with real adrenal lesions less likely. For example:

- Unopacified portions of the stomach or small bowel are differentiated from an adrenal mass by administering oral contrast and repeating the CT scan (Fig. 16-7).
- Tortuous blood vessels are identified by contrast-enhanced CT or Doppler ultrasonography.
- An accessory spleen or a splenic lobulation is recognized by its smooth margin and CT density and enhancement identical to splenic tissue.

Adrenocortical Carcinoma

Carcinoma of the adrenal gland is associated with adrenal hyperfunction in 50% of patients. Cushing's syndrome is most common. Most primary carcinomas are easily differentiated from adenomas. The tumor is aggressive and highly lethal with a strong propensity to invade blood vessels. CT findings of adrenocortical carcinoma include:

- The adrenal mass is usually large (>5 cm) and markedly heterogeneous (Fig. 16-8).
- Central necrosis is common, and irregular calcification (Fig. 16-9) is present in 30% of patients.
- Tumor thrombus in the renal vein or inferior vena cava is a frequent complication that carries a significant risk for pulmonary embolus.
- Direct invasion of adjacent structures and metastases to regional lymph nodes, liver, bone, and lung are common at presentation.
- Postcontrast CT shows nodular areas of enhancement, central hypoperfusion, and delayed contrast washout.
- Focal fat deposits are sometimes present in adrenal carcinomas. However, all fat-containing tumors reported have had other evidence of malignancy.
- Rarely, large degenerated benign adrenal adenomas have an appearance similar to adrenal carcinoma.

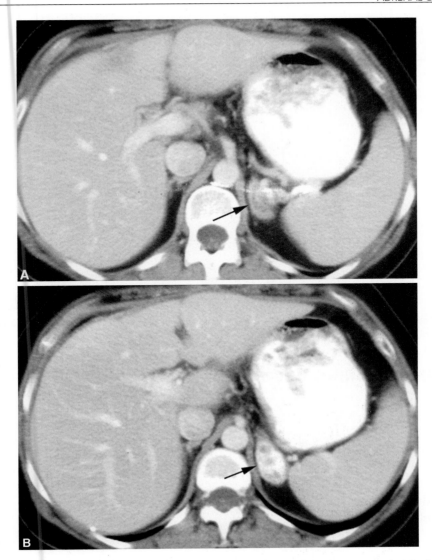

FIGURE 16-7 **Adrenal pseudotumor.** *A,* Initial CT scan shows an apparent mass *(arrow)* in the region of the left adrenal gland. *B,* Subsequent CT scan after administration of additional oral contrast shows contrast filling a gastric diverticulum *(arrow).*

Adrenal Calcifications

Most adrenal calcifications in both children and adults are sequelae of adrenal hemorrhage. Tuberculosis and histoplasmosis cause adrenal calcifications and may be associated with Addison's disease. CT findings of adrenal calcifications include:

- Coarse, punctate calcification in one or both glands without a mass being evident is char-acteristic of remote adrenal hemorrhage (Fig. 16-10).
- Adrenal tumors in children that calcify are neuroblastoma and ganglioneuroma.
- Adrenal tumors in adults that calcify include adrenal carcinoma, pheochromocytoma, ganglioneuroma, and metastases.
- Wolman's disease is a rare autosomal reces-sive condition associated with enlarged, cal-cified adrenal glands, hepatomegaly, and splenomegaly.

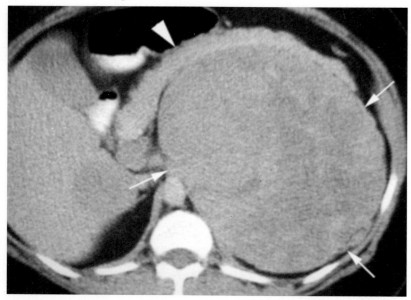

FIGURE 16-8 **Adrenal carcinoma.** A huge solid heterogeneous mass *(arrows)* replaces the left adrenal gland. The pancreas *(arrowhead)* is anteriorly displaced by the mass confirming that the origin of the tumor is in the retroperitoneum.

☐ HYPERFUNCTIONING ADRENAL LESIONS

Adrenal Hyperplasia

Adrenal hyperplasia is usually associated with adrenal endocrine hyperfunction. CT findings include:

- The adrenal glands most commonly are uniformly enlarged but maintain their normal adrenal shape (Fig. 16-11). Thickness of the limbs of the gland exceeds 10 mm.
- A multinodular pattern of adrenal hyperplasia may also occur. The appearance may be indistinguishable from multiple small adrenal metastases.
- Biochemical hyperplasia may be associated with a normal size and imaging appearance of the adrenal glands.

Cushing's Syndrome

Cushing's syndrome is produced by excess secretion of glucocorticoids. About 70% of patients have bilateral adrenal hyperplasia, 20%

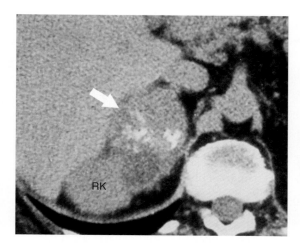

FIGURE 16-9 **Adrenal carcinoma calcification.** Unenhanced CT shows a solid mass *(arrow)* with coarse calcifications arising from the right adrenal gland. The tumor invaded the upper pole of the right kidney (RK).

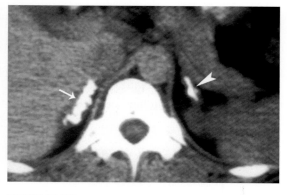

FIGURE 16-10 **Adrenal calcifications.** The right adrenal gland *(arrow)* is completely and densely calcified. The left adrenal gland *(arrowhead)* is similarly calcified.

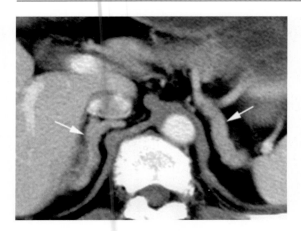

FIGURE 16-11 **Adrenal hyperplasia.** Both adrenal glands *(arrows)* show diffuse thickening of their limbs.

have a benign hyperfunctioning adrenal adenoma, and 10% have adrenocortical carcinoma. CT findings in Cushing's syndrome include:

- Adenomas are round or oval and are usually less than 2 cm in diameter.
- Hyperfunctioning adenomas are indistinguishable from nonhyperfunctioning adenomas.

Conn's Syndrome

Primary hyperaldosteronism is caused by a benign hyperfunctioning adenoma (80%) or by bilateral adrenal hyperplasia (20%). Adrenal carcinoma rarely is a cause of hyperaldosteronism.

Adrenogenital Syndrome

Excess secretion of androgens may cause a congenital or acquired condition. Congenital adrenogenital syndrome results from congenital enzyme deficiency and is associated with bilateral adrenal hyperplasia. Acquired adrenogenital syndrome is usually caused by a hyperfunctioning benign adrenal adenoma (80%), but 20% are associated with adrenal cortical carcinoma.

Pheochromocytoma

Pheochromocytoma is a catecholamine-secreting tumor that arises from chromaffin cells of the sympathetic nervous system. Most (90%) are benign, unilateral, and arise in the adrenal medulla. About 10% are extra-adrenal, with the most common location being the organ of

Zückerkandl near the origin of the inferior mesenteric artery. About 10% are bilateral, and 10% are associated with multiple endocrine neoplasia syndromes or tuberous sclerosis. CT findings of pheochromocytoma include:

- CT most often shows a round homogeneous mass with attenuation without contrast about equal to normal liver.
- Cystic change, central necrosis, and calcifications may be present (Fig. 16-12).
- Contrast enhancement with the old ionic contrast agents has been reported to precipitate hypertensive crisis in some patients. Nonionic contrast appears be safe to administer.
- Tumors are highly vascular and enhance avidly.
- Metaiodobenzylguanidine or indium–111 pentetreotide scintigraphy may be used to locate extra-adrenal pheochromocytoma not identified by CT.

☐ PROBLEMATIC ADRENAL MASSES

Benign, nonhyperfunctioning, adrenal adenomas are common incidental findings on cross-sectional imaging examinations. Up to 5% of CT scans obtained for other reasons demonstrate an adrenal mass. Even in patients with known malignancy, benign adrenal masses are more common than metastases to the adrenal glands. However, accurate tumor staging requires definitive diagnosis of adrenal lesions. A variety of imaging strategies have been reported.

Imaging differentiation of benign adenomas from metastases is based on the increased fat content found within most functioning adrenocortical adenomas. Cholesterol is a precursor of adrenocortical hormones, and cholesterol, fatty acids, and neutral fats are stored within functioning adrenal cells. CT and chemical shift magnetic resonance (MR) imaging are based on detection of increased fat content within benign tumors.

Notably, the lipid in benign adenomas is intracytoplasmic within adrenal cortical cells, whereas the lipid in myelolipomas is macroscopic and within fat cells. Thus, myelolipomas measure fat density on CT, whereas adenomas measure low density but usually not as low as subcutaneous fat.

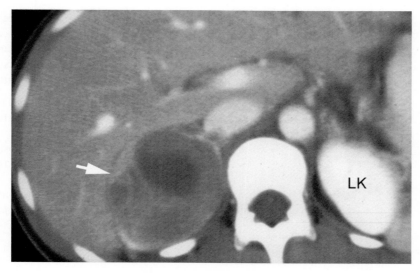

FIGURE 16-12 **Pheochromocytoma.** An unsuspected pheochromocytoma is seen as a heterogeneous mass *(arrow)* arising from the right adrenal. Necrosis and cystic change are present. Nonionic contrast media was administered by intravenous bolus without adverse effect. Hypertensive crisis has been precipitated by intravenous injection of ionic contrast agents in patients with pheochromocytoma. The left kidney (LK) enhances avidly.

General Features of Benign Adrenal Adenomas

Patients with benign, nonhyperfunctioning adenomas have no symptoms related to adrenal function and have normal adrenal hormone levels. Adenomas are found in 9% of cases at autopsy. CT findings include:

- Adrenal adenomas are sharply defined, homogeneous, round masses usually smaller than 3 cm (Fig. 16-13). On noncontrast CT scans, adenomas are hypodense compared with normal liver.
- Contrast enhancement tends to be moderate in intensity and relatively uniform throughout the tumor. Washout of contrast is significantly more rapid with benign adenomas than with metastases. This important feature is used to characterize benign adenomas that are low in fat content (lipid-poor adenomas).
- Because of the variability in contrast administration and timing of the CT imaging, adenomas cannot be definitively characterized as benign on a single postcontrast scan.
- A small adrenal mass with the characteristics described that remains stable in size and appearance on follow-up examination for 6 months or more is likely to be benign.

General Features of Metastases to the Adrenals

Metastases to the adrenal glands are found in 27% of patients with epithelial malignancies at autopsy studies. The most common primary tumors are lung and breast adenocarcinoma and melanoma. CT findings include:

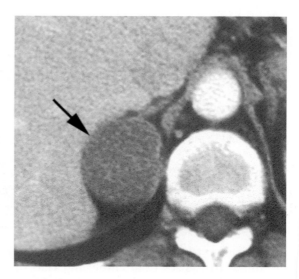

FIGURE 16-13 **Benign adrenal adenoma.** Even though this CT scan is performed after intravenous contrast administration, the uniform low density of this lipid-rich benign adrenal adenoma *(arrow)* is easily appreciated.

- Larger metastases (>3 cm) tend to be more heterogeneous and lobulated in contour with less well-defined margins. Hemorrhage and calcification are common. Enhancement tends to be heterogeneous (Fig. 16-14). These large, heterogeneous, irregular lesions should not be confused with benign adrenal adenomas. Most adrenal masses larger than 5 cm are malignant (metastasis or adrenal carcinoma).
- Cystic changes may be present. Cystic metastases have thick, irregular walls that enhance with contrast.
- Smaller metastases (<3 cm) tend to be homogeneous, round, and relatively well defined. These lesions may be indistinguishable from benign adenomas. Size is not a useful criterion for distinguishing benign adenomas from metastases (Fig. 16-15).

Features That Characterize Benign Adenomas and Adrenal Metastases

Boland and Korobkin provide excellent summaries of a large number of studies that have analyzed CT attenuation criteria to differentiate benign from malignant lesions. CT differentiation is based on high lipid content, rapid contrast washout that characterizes benign adrenal adenomas, or both.

- *Unenhanced CT attenuation.* On unenhanced CT, a mean attenuation value *less than 10 H* is indicative of a benign adenoma (specificity 98%, sensitivity 71%). This criterion defines lipid-rich, benign adrenal adenomas (Fig. 16-16). Approximately 70% of benign adenomas are lipid-rich and can be characterized by unenhanced CT attenuation. The remaining 30% of benign adenomas are lipid-poor and will not be characterized as benign by this criterion. Using less than 20 H as a threshold attenuation value yields a specificity of 84% with a sensitivity of 88%. A threshold value of less than 2 H yields specificity of 100% with sensitivity of 47%.
- To use threshold values of CT attenuation, the region-of-interest cursor must be properly placed within the central one half to two thirds of the mass. Any regions of calcification or necrosis should be excluded from the cursor measurement. Lesions with large areas of necrosis or cystic change cannot be characterized by calculations of contrast washout.
- *Enhanced CT attenuation.* Attenuation values of benign adenomas and metastases on routine contrast-enhanced CT scans show too much overlap to be clinically useful in differentiation. Unfortunately, many adrenal masses are discovered on

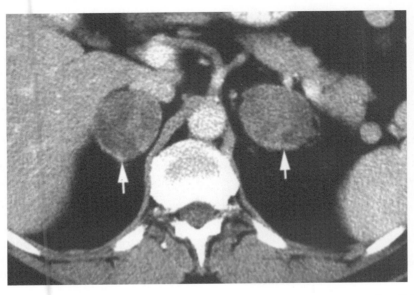

FIGURE 16-14 **Bilateral adrenal metastases.** Adrenal metastases *(arrows)* from lung carcinoma are relatively well defined but heterogeneous in density. Compare with the uniform low density of the benign adenoma in Figure 16-13.

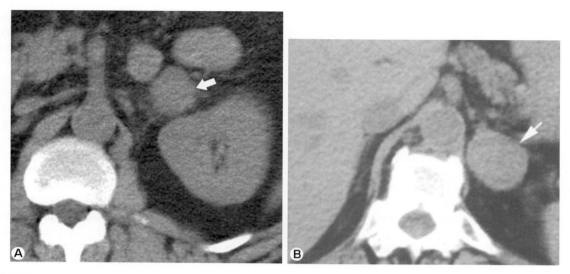

FIGURE 16-15 **Problematic adrenal lesions.** *A,* This well-defined adrenal nodule *(arrow)* was a benign adenoma. *B,* This well-defined adrenal nodule *(arrow)* was a metastasis from lung carcinoma.

postcontrast CT scans. These patients usually require reimaging to accurately characterize their lesions.

- *Percentage enhancement washout.* Although absolute attenuation values after contrast have not been proved to be diagnostic, benign adenomas show a characteristic brisk washout of the contrast agent that can be used to characterize the lesions as benign. Metastases show a characteristically

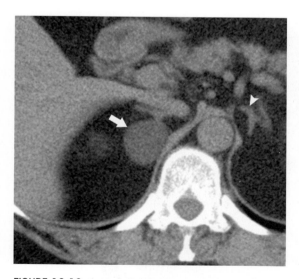

FIGURE 16-16 **Benign adenoma: lipid-rich.** Well-defined, 2.5-cm mass *(arrow)* arising from the right adrenal gland measures −2 H in CT attenuation. These CT characteristics define a benign, lipid-rich, adrenal adenoma. A portion of the normal left adrenal gland is evident *(arrowhead).*

slow washout of contrast agent. Korobkin provides an explanation of the terms used in several studies. *Enhancement* is defined as enhanced attenuation minus nonenhanced attenuation. *Enhancement washout* is calculated by comparing immediate postcontrast scans with delayed postcontrast scans (usually obtained at 10–15 minutes after injection). Enhancement washout is defined as initial enhanced attenuation minus delayed enhanced attenuation. *Percentage enhancement washout* is defined as enhancement washout divided by enhancement multiplied by 100%. This calculation requires attenuation measurement on a noncontrast CT. *Relative percentage enhancement washout* is defined as enhancement washout divided by immediate enhanced attenuation and multiplied by 100%. This calculation requires attenuation measurements on only immediate and delayed postcontrast CT images. *Relative percentage washout greater than 40% to 50%* is highly indicative of benign adenoma. Korobkin used a threshold washout of greater than 40%, whereas Peña used a threshold washout of greater than 50%. Both studies reported specificity and sensitivity of 100% comparing immediate postcontrast scans with 10- to 15-minute delay postcontrast scans. Attenuation of the adrenal mass is measured on the immediate (dynamic) postcontrast images and on the delayed postcontrast images. Enhancement washout analysis appears to be highly reliable in assessment of both lipid-rich and lipid-poor benign adrenal adenomas.

Example: CT of an adrenal lesion performed according to the protocol outlined in the next section yielded the following data (Fig. 16-17):

Precontrast attenuation: +26 H

Immediate (1-minute) postcontrast attenuation: +94 H

Delayed (15-minute) postcontrast attenuation: +30 H

Enhancement = immediate − precontrast = 94 − 26 = 68 H

Enhancement washout = immediate − delayed = 94 − 30 = 64 H

Percentage enhancement washout = (enhancement washout/enhancement) × 100% = 64/68 × 100% = 94%

Relative percentage enhancement washout = (enhancement washout/immediate attenuation) × 100% = 64/94 × 100% = 68%

This study is diagnostic of a benign, lipid-poor, adrenal adenoma.

- Adrenal carcinomas have not yet been adequately studied to determine if the criteria outlined above can be applied to

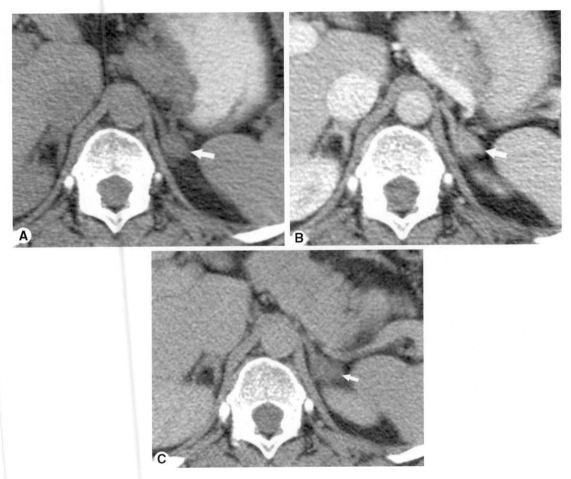

FIGURE 16-17 **Lipid-poor adenoma.** *A,* Small left adrenal mass *(arrows)* measures +26 H on unenhanced CT. This attenuation is not compatible with a lipid-rich adenoma. A decision was made to proceed with intravenous contrast after the adrenal protocol outlined at the end of this chapter. *B,* The immediate postcontrast scan demonstrates that the mass avidly enhances to +94 H. *C,* The 15-minute delay postcontrast scan shows rapid washout of contrast agent with attenuation of the mass now measuring +30 H. Relative percentage enhancement washout is 68%, which is considered diagnostic of a lipid-poor adenoma.

differentiate adrenal adenomas from small adrenal carcinomas. Most carcinomas will be accurately diagnosed by their large size, extensive necrosis, and hemorrhage usually present, or by the common presence of metastases at presentation.

- Attenuation values less than 10 H and washout of contrast more than 60% recently have been reported with small pheochromocytomas.
- *Chemical shift MR* may be used to accurately characterize lipid-rich adenomas. Fat and water protons process at different frequencies. Gradient-echo image sequences can be performed so that fat and water proton signals can be separated within an imaged voxel. At 1.5 Tesla, fat and water protons are out of phase at echo time of 2.3 milliseconds and in-phase at echo time of 4.6 milliseconds. Fat-containing adenomas show a distinct decrease in signal intensity on out-of-phase images (water and fat signal cancel out each other) compared with in-phase images (additive signal of water and fat) (Figs. 16–18 and 16–19). Subjective assessment of signal loss is equally accurate to quantitative measurements of signal loss. Although MR is equally accurate to noncontrast CT for characterization of lipid-rich adenomas, it offers no advantage over CT. Only the lipid-rich adenomas that can be definitively characterized by noncontrast CT can be characterized by in-phase/out-of-phase MR. Limited attempts to assess gadolinium washout on MR have not been successful.
- Lesions that are not adequately characterized by CT or MR may require image-guided percutaneous biopsy. This procedure has been shown to be safe and effective. CT is routinely used to guide the biopsy procedure.

CT Protocol for Characterization of Adrenal Masses

A variety of protocols can be used effectively. Spiral single-slice and multislice CT allows for thin collimation to decrease volume average artifact in the small glands. CT protocols include the following:

- Adrenal CT is routinely performed with spiral technique and collimation of 3 to 5 mm with matching table speed. Multislice CT allows prospective or retrospective slice reconstruction at 1-mm thickness. Oral contrast is given to opacify and distend bowel to avoid confusion with adrenal lesions.
- Nonenhanced CT is obtained through both adrenal glands. If CT attenuation of the adrenal mass is less than 10 H, a diagnosis of lipid-rich adrenal adenoma is made, and no further evaluation is needed.
- If on noncontrast CT the attenuation of the adrenal mass is greater than 10 H, then a contrast-enhanced CT is performed. A 150 mL bolus of nonionic 60% contrast is given intravenously by power injector. Immediate postcontrast images are obtained approximately 1 minute after the onset of contrast injection. Delayed images of the adrenal glands are obtained at 15 minutes after contrast injection. Attenuation of the adrenal mass is measured on the immediate postcontrast scan and is compared with the delayed postcontrast scan.
- If enhancement washout is more than 50% and if attenuation is less than 35 H at 15 minutes, then a diagnosis of lipid-poor benign adrenal adenoma is made.
- If enhancement washout is less than 50% or if 15-minute delay mass attenuation is greater than 35 H, then the mass remains indeterminate, and adrenal biopsy may be indicated.

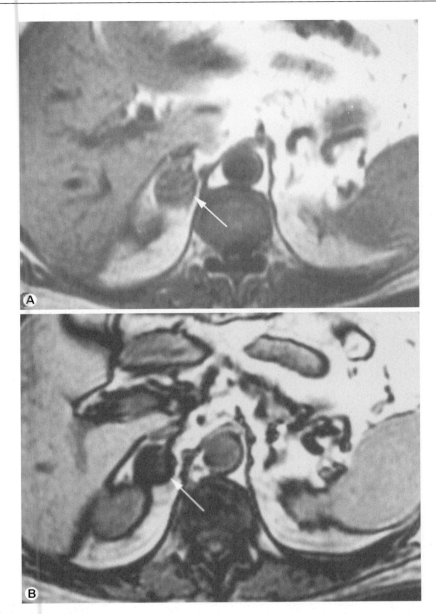

FIGURE 16-18 **Magnetic resonance (MR) benign adrenal adenoma.** *A,* In-phase MR image shows an adrenal mass *(arrow)* that is near muscle in signal intensity. *B,* Out-of-phase MR image shows a marked decrease in signal intensity of the mass *(arrow),* indicating high fat content.

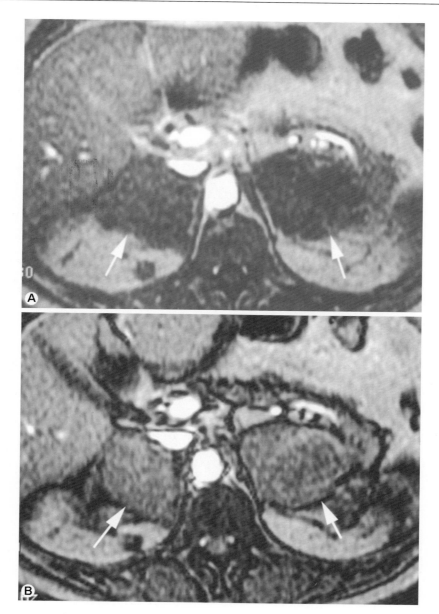

FIGURE 16-19 **Magnetic resonance (MR) adrenal metastases.** *A,* In-phase MR image shows bilateral ill-defined adrenal masses *(arrows)* of relatively low signal intensity. *B,* Out-of-phase MR image shows an increase rather than a decrease in signal intensity. This patient has metastatic sarcoma.

SUGGESTED READING

BLAKE MA, KRISHNAMOORTHY SK, BOLAND GW, et al: Low-density pheochromocytoma on CT: A mimicker of adrenal adenoma. AJR Am J Roentgenol 181:1663–1668, 2003.

BOLAND GWL, LEE MJ, GAZELLE GS, et al: Characterization of adrenal masses using unenhanced CT: An analysis of the CT literature. AJR Am J Roentgenol 171:201–204, 1998.

BRANT WE: Adrenal glands and kidneys. In Brant WE, Helms CA (eds): Fundamentals of Diagnostic Radiology 2nd ed. Baltimore, Lippincott Williams & Wilkins, 1999, pp 769–775.

BURKS DW, MIRVIS SE, SHANMUGANATHAN K: Acute adrenal injury after blunt abdominal trauma: CT findings. AJR Am J Roentgenol 158:503–507, 1992.

CAOILI EM, KOROBKIN M, FRANCIS IR, et al: Delayed enhancement CT of lipid-poor adrenal adenomas. AJR Am J Roentgenol 175:1411–1415, 2000.

CIRILLO RL, BENNETT WF, VITELLAS KM, et al: Pathology of the adrenal gland: Imaging features. AJR Am J Roentgenol 170:429–435, 1998.

CYRAN KM, KENNEY PJ, MEMEL DS, YACOUB I: Adrenal myelolipoma. AJR Am J Roentgenol 166:395–400, 1996.

DOPPMAN JL, CHROUSOS GP, PAPINCOLAOU DA, et al: Adrenocorticotropin-independent macronodular adrenal hyperplasia: An uncommon cause of primary adrenal hypercortisolism. Radiology 216:797–802, 2000.

DUNNICK NR, KOROBKIN M, FRANCIS I: Adrenal radiology: Distinguishing benign from malignant adrenal masses. AJR Am J Roentgenol 167:861–867, 1996.

FUJIYOSHI F, NAKAJO M, FUKUKURO Y, TSUCHIMOCHI S: Characterization of adrenal tumors by chemical shift fast low-angle shot MR imaging: Comparison of four methods of quantitative evaluation. AJR Am J Roentgenol 180:1649–1657, 2003.

FULCHER AS, NARLA LD, HINGSBERGEN EA: Pediatric case of the day (Wolman disease). Radiographics 18:533–535, 1998.

KAWASHIMA A, SANDLER CM, ERNST RD, et al: Imaging of nontraumatic hemorrhage of the adrenal gland. Radiographics 19:949–963, 1999.

KAWASHIMA A, SANDLER CM, FISHMAN EK, et al: Spectrum of CT findings in nonmalignant disease of the adrenal gland. Radiographics 18:393–412, 1998.

KENNEY PJ, STANLEY RJ: Calcified adrenal masses. Urol Radiol 9:9–15, 1987.

KENNEY PJ, WAGNER BJ, RAO P, HEFFESS CS: Myelolipoma: CT and pathologic features. Radiology 208:87–95, 1998.

KLOOS RT, GROSS MD, FRANCIS IR, et al: Incidentally discovered adrenal masses. Endocr Rev 16:460–484, 1996.

KOROBKIN M: CT characterization of adrenal masses: The time has come. Radiology 217:629–632, 2000.

KOROBKIN M, BRODEUR FJ, FRANCIS IR, et al: CT time-attenuation washout curves of adrenal adenomas and nonadenomas. AJR Am J Roentgenol 170:747–752, 1997.

KOROBKIN M, GIORDANO TJ, BRODEUR FJ, et al: Adrenal adenomas: Relationship between histologic lipid and CT and MR findings. Radiology 200:743–747, 1996.

KREBS TL, WAGNER BJ: MR imaging of the adrenal gland: Radiologic-pathologic correlation. Radiographics 18:1425–1440, 1998.

MAYO-SMITH WW, LEE MJ, MCNICHOLAS MMJ, et al: Characterization of adrenal masses (< 5 cm) by use of chemical shift MR imaging: Observer performance versus quantitative measures. AJR Am J Roentgenol 165:91–95, 1995.

MITCHELL DG, CROVELLO M, MATTEUCCI T, et al: Benign adrenocortical masses: Diagnosis with chemical shift MR imaging. Radiology 185:345–351, 1992.

MITCHELL DG, NASCIMENTO AB, ALAM F, et al: In vivo observations, and high-resolution in vitro chemical shift MR imaging-histologic correlation. Acad Radiol 9:430–436, 2002.

MUKHERJEE JJ, PEPPERCORN PD, REZNEK RH, et al: Pheochromocytoma: Effect of nonionic contrast medium in CT on circulating catecholamine levels. Radiology 202:227–231, 1997.

NEWHOUSE JH, HEFFESS CS, WAGNER BJ, et al: Large degenerated adrenal adenomas: Radiologic-pathologic correlation. Radiology 210:385–391, 1999.

OTAL P, ESCOURROU G, MAZEROLLES C, et al: Imaging features of uncommon adrenal masses with histopathologic correlation. Radiographics 19:569–581, 1999.

OUTWATER EK, SIEGELMAN ES, HUANG AB, BIRNBAUM BA: Adrenal masses: Correlation between CT attenuation value and chemical shift ratio at MR imaging with in-phase and opposed-phase sequences. Radiology 200:749–752, 1996.

OUTWATER EK, SIEGELMAN ES, RADECKI PD, et al: Distinction between benign and malignant adrenal masses: Value of T1-weighted chemical-shift MR imaging. AJR Am J Roentgenol 165:579–583, 1995.

PEÑA CS, BOLAND GWL, HAHN PF, et al: Characterization of indeterminate (lipid-poor) adrenal masses: Use of washout characteristics at contrast-enhanced CT. Radiology 217:798–802, 2000.

Rao P, Kenney PJ, Wagner BJ, Davidson AJ: Imaging and pathologic features of myelolipoma. Radiographics 17:1373–1385, 1997.

Rozenblit A, Morehouse HT, Amis ES Jr: Cystic adrenal lesions: CT features. Radiology 201:541–548, 1996.

Sivit CJ, Ingram JD, Taylor GA, et al: Posttraumatic adrenal hemorrhage in children: CT findings in 34 patients. AJR Am J Roentgenol 158:1299–1302, 1992.

Szolar DH, Kammerhuber FH: Adrenal adenomas and nonadenomas: Assessment of washout at delayed contrast-enhanced CT. Radiology 207:369–375, 1998.

van Gils APG, Falke THM, van Erkel AR, et al: MR imaging and MIBG scintigraphy of pheochromocytomas and extraadrenal functioning paragangliomas. Radiographics 11:37–57, 1991.

17

Gastrointestinal Tract

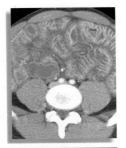

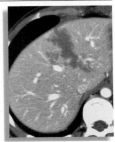

William E. Brant, M.D.

☐ BASIC PRINCIPLES

CT complements endoscopy and barium examination of the gastrointestinal tract by better demonstration of intramural and extraintestinal components of gastrointestinal disease, including disease in the mesentery, peritoneal cavity, lymph nodes, and liver. CT is used for the following reasons: (1) to diagnose the presence of gastrointestinal disease; (2) to evaluate its nature and extent; and (3) to demonstrate complications such as abscess, phlegmon, fistula, and perforation. CT is excellent for determining the extent of gastrointestinal disease but is seldom specific for its nature.

The gastrointestinal tract is shown on every CT scan of the abdomen. The intestinal lumen should be distended and opacified for routine abdominal CT by administration of 700 to 800 mL of 2% to 3% iodinated, or barium, contrast agent at least 1 hour before scanning. CT examination dedicated to evaluation of the gastrointestinal tract requires cleansing of the colon (by barium enema preparation), fasting for at least 4 hours (to keep the stomach empty), and oral contrast medium administration. Studies should be optimized by oral administration of gas-producing crystals, colon insufflation with air,

and changing the patient's position to maximize gastrointestinal distention in the area of a suspected pathologic process. Water is an excellent contrast agent for the lumen of the stomach and upper intestinal tract. Intravenous contrast medium is used to assess enhancement of known lesions, demonstrate blood vessels, and evaluate the solid organs of the abdomen. Thin-section (≤5 mm) scans improve lesion definition. Short scan times (≤1 second) improve image quality by limiting motion artifact. Collapsed bowel loops without intraluminal contrast medium enhancement may mimic adenopathy and mass lesions. However, when scans are obtained during the arterial phase of bolus contrast medium enhancement, identification of enhanced bowel wall confirms the nature of nondistended bowel.

A CT hallmark of intestinal disease is thickening of the bowel wall. When fully distended, the bowel wall is 1 to 2 mm in thickness. When collapsed, the bowel wall should not exceed 3 to 4 mm, except in the stomach near the esophageal junction where the normal stomach wall may be 2 cm in thickness when collapsed. The CT appearance of wall thickening is helpful in differentiating benign from malignant wall thickening (Table 17-1). Benign, pathologic

TABLE 17-1

Benign Versus Malignant Bowel Wall Thickening

Benign	Malignant
Homogeneous attenuation	Heterogeneous attenuation
Symmetric	Asymmetric
Circumferential	Eccentric
Thickening < 1 cm	Thickening > 1–2 cm
Segmental or diffuse involvement	Focal mass
"Double-halo sign"	Abrupt transition
Dark inner ring	Lobulated contour
Bright outer ring	Spiculated contour
"Target sign"	Narrowed bowel lumen
Bright inner ring	Enlarged lymph nodes
Dark middle ring	Liver metastases
Bright outer ring	

wall thickening usually does not exceed 1 cm and is homogeneous in attenuation, circumferential, symmetric, and segmental in distribution. The "double halo" and "target" appearance of the intestine in cross section is caused by inflammation, edema, and hyperemia and is best demonstrated on contrast-enhanced scans. Neoplastic wall thickening is thicker (1–2 cm), asymmetric, nodular, lobulated, or spiculated in contour and tends to narrow the intestinal lumen. Benign wall thickening is caused by inflammatory bowel disease, intestinal ischemia, and intramural hemorrhage. Neoplastic wall thickening is produced by adenocarcinoma, lymphoma, and leiomyosarcoma.

☐ ESOPHAGUS

Anatomy

The esophagus is a muscular tube that extends from the cricopharyngeus muscle at the level of the cricoid cartilage to the stomach. The major portion of its length is within the middle mediastinum. The cervical portion extends from the level of the C6 vertebral body to the thoracic inlet. A short abdominal segment extends below the diaphragm to the gastroesophageal junction. The esophagus is lined by squamous epithelium to the gastric junction where the mucosa abruptly changes to columnar epithelium. The lack of serosal covering allows early invasion by esophageal tumors into periesophageal tissues. The musculature of the esophageal wall is striated

in the upper third, striated and smooth muscle in the middle third, and solely smooth muscle in the distal third.

On CT, the esophagus appears as an oval of soft-tissue density often containing air or contrast material within its lumen (Fig. 17-1). When distended, the wall of the esophagus should not exceed 3 mm in thickness. In the neck and upper thorax, the esophagus courses between the trachea and the spine. In the lower thorax, the esophagus courses to the right of the descending aorta between the left atrium and the spine. The esophagus enters the abdomen through the esophageal hiatus and courses to the left to join the stomach. The edges of the diaphragmatic crura forming the esophageal hiatus are seen often as prominent, teardrop-shaped structures partially surrounding the esophagus.

Technical Considerations

The esophagus is studied using contiguous 5-mm or thinner slices from the level of the larynx to the stomach. When esophageal tumors are evaluated, scanning is continued through the liver to look for metastases. Oral contrast agent is given to distend the stomach and the gastroesophageal junction. Intravenous contrast medium is useful to evaluate mediastinal vessels and to detect varices. Attempts to fully distend the esophagus during CT scanning are not consistently successful. Oral administration of dilute barium paste may aid in coating the esophageal mucosa.

Esophageal Carcinoma

Because of the lack of serosal covering, carcinoma spreads beyond the esophagus early in its course, resulting in a poor prognosis. Ninety percent of tumors are squamous cell carcinoma, with the remaining 10% being adenocarcinoma arising in Barrett's esophagus in the distal esophagus. It must be recognized that the CT findings in esophageal carcinoma may be duplicated by benign disease. Diagnosis depends on biopsy. CT is performed to assess the extent of disease and to identify those patients for whom the disease cannot be resected. The CT findings in esophageal carcinoma include:

- Irregular thickening of the wall of the esophagus more than 3 mm (Fig. 17-2)

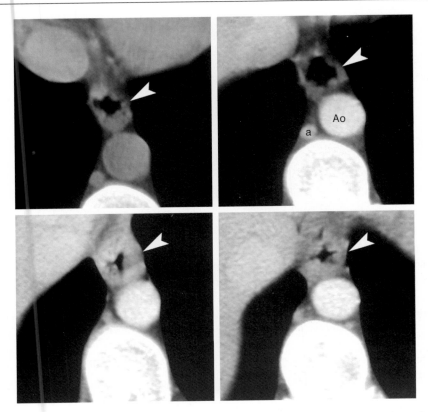

FIGURE 17-1 **Normal esophagus.** Multiple sequential slices demonstrate the normal appearance of the esophagus *(arrowheads)* on CT. The descending thoracic aorta (Ao) and azygos vein (a) are also seen.

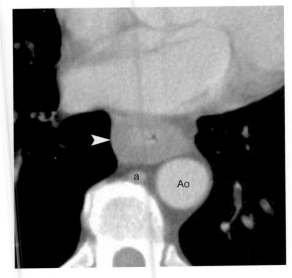

FIGURE 17-2 **Carcinoma: esophagus.** Squamous cell carcinoma of the esophagus causes circumferential thickening *(arrowhead)* of the wall of the esophagus with narrowing of the lumen. a, azygos vein; Ao, thoracic aorta.

- Intraluminal polypoid mass
- Eccentric narrowing of the lumen
- Dilatation of the esophagus above the area of narrowing
- Invasion of periesophageal tissues: fat, aorta, trachea
- Metastases to lymph nodes, liver, and other organs
- Tumor invasion of the trachea or bronchi is suggested by tumor that displaces or indents the posterior airway wall (90% accurate)
- Tumor invasion of the aorta is suggested by an arc of contact between the tumor and aorta of greater than 90 degrees; an arc less than 45 degrees indicates no invasion, and an arc between 45 and 90 degrees is indeterminate; these findings are about 80% accurate
- Esophageal carcinoma spreads to paraesophageal, other mediastinal, gastrohepatic ligament, and left gastric nodal chains (Fig. 17-3); microscopic disease in normal-sized nodes, and lymph node enlargement caused by benign conditions, limits the CT

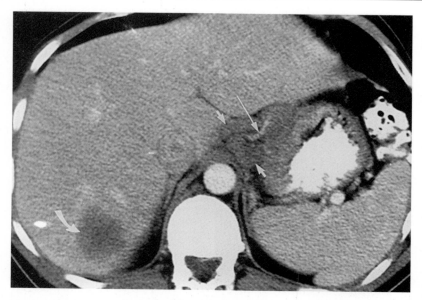

FIGURE 17-3 **Carcinoma of the gastroesophageal junction.** Carcinoma arising near the gastroesophageal junction has spread to the liver *(curved arrow)* and to lymph nodes *(short arrows)* surrounding the celiac axis *(long arrow).*

accuracy of nodal involvement by esophageal carcinoma to 39% to 85%.

- Tumor recurrence after esophagectomy is well demonstrated by CT; tumors may recur anywhere within the mediastinum, in distant lymph nodes in the neck or abdomen, and in liver, lung, pleural space, adrenal glands, or peritoneal cavity.

Esophageal Leiomyoma

Leiomyoma is the most common benign tumor of the esophagus. Smooth muscle tumors of the esophagus are true leiomyomas and are not classified as gastrointestinal stromal tumors. Most are asymptomatic until becoming very large and causing dysphagia. Endoscopy demonstrates a submucosal mass, usually easily differentiated from carcinoma. CT findings of esophageal leiomyoma include:

- On CT, it appears as a smooth, well-defined, 2- to 8-cm mass of uniform soft-tissue density. The esophageal wall is eccentrically thickened, and the lumen is deformed. A large, well-defined mass is much more likely to be a leiomyoma than a carcinoma.
- Leiomyomas are multiple in 3% to 4% of patients.
- Leiomyosarcomas tend to grow intraluminally, are usually large (>5 cm), have heterogeneous attenuation, and may ulcerate.

Esophageal Varices

Esophageal varices are most often caused by portal hypertension but may occur with superior vena cava obstruction. The major complication is hemorrhage. CT findings of esophageal varices include:

- Varices are clearly recognized on postcontrast scans as well-defined, enhancing nodular and tubular densities adjacent to the esophagus and within its wall (Fig. 17-4).
- Varices cause scalloped thickening of the esophageal wall that may be indistinguishable from tumor or inflammation without the use of contrast medium enhancement.
- Signs of cirrhosis, portal hypertension, and other portosystemic collateral vessels may also be present.

Esophagitis

Causes of esophagitis include gastroesophageal reflux, radiation, and infection. Infectious esophagitis is most commonly seen in immunosuppressed patients. Causative organisms include *Candida*, herpes simplex, cytomegalovirus, and tuberculosis. CT findings of esophagitis include:

- The major CT finding is a relatively long segment of circumferential wall thickening (>5 mm).

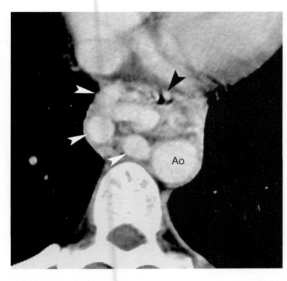

FIGURE 17-4 **Esophageal varices.** Numerous large enhancing varices *(white arrowheads)* resulting from cirrhosis and portal hypertension surround and indent the distal esophagus *(black arrowhead)*. Ao, thoracic aorta.

- Presence of a target sign helps to differentiate esophagitis from other causes of wall thickening.
- Strictures are seen as areas of luminal narrowing with dilatation of the esophagus above the lesion.
- Severe esophagitis may lead to deep ulcers, perforation, mediastinitis, and abscess.

Esophageal Perforation

Esophageal perforation may be traumatic, may be iatrogenic after instrumentation, or may result from neoplasm or inflammation. Boerhaave syndrome is spontaneous rupture of the esophagus associated with violent vomiting. Because it may be fatal, prompt recognition of esophageal perforation is essential. Underlying esophageal disease is often present. CT findings include:

- Periesophageal fluid or contrast and extra-luminal mediastinal air are the most specific findings (Fig. 17-5).
- The wall of the esophagus is usually thickened.
- Pleural effusions are common.

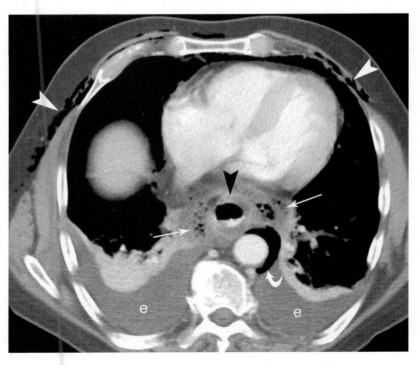

FIGURE 17-5 **Perforation of the esophagus.** Perforation of the distal esophagus during a stenting procedure for esophageal stricture is evidenced by extensive air in the mediastinum *(straight arrows)*, around the aorta *(curved arrow)*, and in the subcutaneous tissues of the chest *(white arrowheads)*. The esophagus *(black arrowhead)* has a thickened wall. Bilateral pleural effusions (e) are evident.

☐ **STOMACH**

Anatomy

The posteriorly located gastric fundus is seen on CT sections through the dome of the diaphragm. The esophagus joins the stomach a short distance below the fundus. A prominent pseudotumor, caused by thickening of the gastric wall due to incomplete distention, is often seen near the gastroesophageal junction. Additional distention with more air or contrast agent will eliminate this pseudotumor. The body of the stomach sweeps toward the right. The antrum crosses the midline of the abdomen between the left lobe of the liver and the pancreas to join the duodenal bulb in the region of the gallbladder.

The normal gastric wall should not exceed 5 mm in thickness when the stomach is well distended. Rugal folds are commonly visualized even with good distention. Like the esophagus, benign and malignant conditions produce similar CT findings. CT is performed to document the extent of extraluminal disease.

Technical Considerations

The stomach must be filled with positive contrast medium or distended with air or water for optimal assessment by CT. Oral contrast agent or water (200–300 mL) is routinely given to fill the stomach just before the patient lies down on the CT couch. Alternatively, distention of the stomach with air may be achieved by giving gas-producing crystals (4–6 g of citrocarbonate granules with 16–30 mL water) instead of the opaque contrast agent. The patient can be repositioned, in prone or decubitus positions, to optimize distention of the different portions of the stomach with air or contrast agent. Scanning is performed using contiguous slices of 5 mm or thinner.

Hiatus Hernia and Gastric Volvulus

Hiatus hernia is a protrusion of any portion of the stomach into the thorax. A major reason to recognize a hiatus hernia is to avoid mistaking it for a tumor. CT findings include:

- On CT, a sliding hiatus hernia (95% of hiatus hernias) is identified by recognition of gastric folds appearing above the esophageal hiatus (Fig. 17-6). The herniated stomach

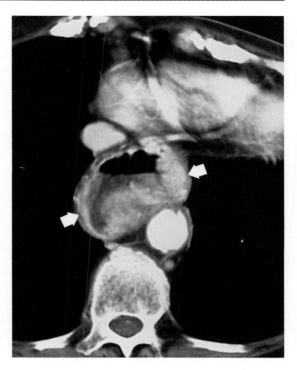

FIGURE 17-6 **Hiatus hernia.** A portion of the stomach extends through the esophageal hiatus to form a hiatal hernia *(arrows)*. Gastric folds are evident. Fluid retained within the herniated stomach forms an air–fluid level.

may create an air- or contrast-filled mass contiguous with the esophagus above and the remainder of the stomach below.

- The edges of the esophageal hiatus are often widely separated, exceeding 15 mm in width.
- With a paraesophageal hernia the gastric cardia and gastroesophageal junction are below the esophageal hiatus and the fundus of stomach is above the hiatus adjacent to the distal esophagus. A variant of paraesophageal hernia is coexistence of a sliding hiatal hernia with the paraesophageal intrathoracic fundus.
- In organoaxial rotation, the stomach rotates around its long axis resulting in the convex greater curvature of the stomach being positioned in the chest anteriorly, superiorly, and to the right of the lesser curvature.
- In the much less common mesenteroaxial rotation, the stomach turns upside down. The antrum and pylorus are superior and in the chest, whereas the fundus is near the diaphragm.

- The term *gastric volvulus* refers to abnormal gastric rotation associated with strangulation and obstruction. Emergency surgical repair is needed.

Thickened Gastric Wall

Thickening of the gastric wall, either focal or diffuse, is an important but nonspecific sign of gastric disease. With good technique, which includes aggressive distention of the stomach with air or contrast agent, wall thickening greater than 5 mm can be considered abnormal. Causes include carcinoma, lymphoma, gastric inflammation (peptic or Crohn's disease), perigastric inflammation (pancreatitis), and radiation. CT may show gastric ulcers as collections of contrast agent within a thickened wall. Penetrating ulcers appear as a sinus tract, marked by contrast agent or air, extending to adjacent structures.

Gastritis

Gastritis is a common disease with numerous causes including alcohol; aspirin; nonsteroidal antiinflammatory drugs; and viral, fungal, or *Helicobacter pylori* infection. CT findings of gastritis include:

- Thickened gastric folds are the best CT sign of gastritis.
- Wall thickening is often focal and most common in the antrum.

- The mucosa may enhance brightly during arterial phase because of hyperemia, causing a three-layer wall appearance that differentiates this benign condition from malignant wall thickening.
- Emphysematous gastritis is a rare life-threatening condition characterized by air within the thickened gastric wall. It is caused by invasion of the gastric wall by gas-producing *Escherichia coli*.

Gastric Carcinoma

Adenocarcinoma is the cause of 95% of gastric malignancy. CT is used to stage disease and identify patients whose disease is not surgically resectable. CT findings for gastric carcinoma include:

- The primary tumor appears as focal, nodular, or irregular thickening of the gastric wall (Fig. 17-7) or as a polypoid, soft-tissue density, intraluminal mass.
- Diffuse wall thickening with narrowing of the lumen is indicative of scirrhous carcinoma (linitis plastica).
- Extension of tumor into the perigastric fat is nearly always present when wall thickness exceeds 2 cm (Fig. 17-8). The serosal surface is blurred and strands and nodules of tumor are seen in the adjacent fat.
- Perigastric lymph nodes are considered to be involved when the short axis diameter is greater than 6 mm. Round shape and

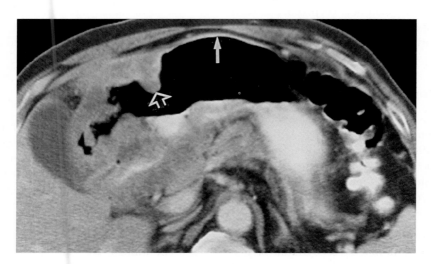

FIGURE 17-7 Gastric carcinoma. Nodular thickening of the wall of the gastric antrum *(open arrow)* is striking in comparison to the normal wall of the gastric body *(closed arrow)*.

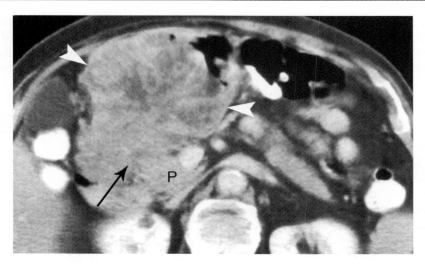

FIGURE 17-8 **Large gastric carcinoma.** Adenocarcinoma of the distal stomach produces a large heterogeneous mass *(arrowheads)* containing low-attenuation areas of necrosis and hemorrhage. The tumor has extended through the stomach wall, obliterated the fat plane between the stomach and the pancreas, and invaded *(arrow)* the pancreas (P).

heterogeneous or marked enhancement are additional signs of nodal involvement. Nodes near the celiac axis and in the gastro-hepatic ligaments are most likely to be involved.

- Hematogenous metastases go first to the liver, then to lungs, adrenal glands, kidneys, bones, and brain.
- Peritoneal carcinomatosis may occur.
- Local recurrence of gastric carcinoma appears as focal wall thickening at the anastomosis or in the remaining stomach. Nodal recurrence is most common along the course of the hepatic artery or in the para-aortic region. Peritoneal recurrence is seen in the cul-de-sac, on peritoneal surfaces, or on the surface of bowel.

Gastric Lymphoma

The stomach is the most common site of involvement for primary gastrointestinal lymphoma. Most cases (90% to 95%) are non–Hodgkin's lymphoma of B-cell origin. Mucosa-associated lymphoid tissue lymphoma is an indolent form of lymphoma with a significantly better prognosis. CT findings include:

- Gastric lymphoma may cause a polypoid mass, diffuse wall infiltration with feature-less walls, or markedly thickened walls with nodular, thickened folds.

- CT features that favor lymphoma rather than carcinoma include more dramatic thickening of the stomach wall (>3 cm), involvement of more than one region of the gastrointestinal tract, transpyloric spread of tumor (occurs in 30% of patients with gastric lymphoma), and more wide-spread adenopathy above and below the level of the renal hilum (Fig. 17-9). Luminal narrowing is typical of carcinoma but rare with lymphoma.
- Low-grade, mucosa-associated lymphoid tissue lymphomas are superficial spreading lesions that are seen as mucosal nodularity, shallow ulcers, and minimal fold thickening.
- High-grade lymphomas tend to be seen as bulky mass lesions or marked fold and wall thickening.

Gastrointestinal Stromal Tumors

The belief that gastrointestinal mesenchymal tumors arise from a common precursor cell (the Cajal cell) has led to the term *gastrointestinal stromal tumor* (GIST). Most GISTs arise in the muscularis propria throughout the gastrointestinal tract with 60% to 70% of these tumors arising in the stomach and 20% to 30% arising in the small bowel. Lesions are rare in the colon and rectum. Other primary sites of origin include the omentum, mesentery, and retroperitoneum. Gastric tumors previously identified as

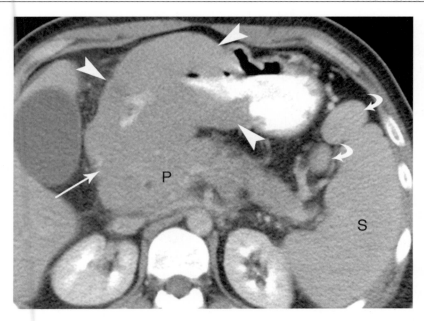

FIGURE 17-9 **Gastric lymphoma.** Non–Hodgkin's lymphoma causes a large mass that massively thickens the wall of the distal stomach *(arrowheads).* Compare with Figure 17-8. Note the homogeneous attenuation of lymphoma compared with the large adenocarcinoma. Lymphoma also obliterates the fat plane *(arrow)* between the stomach and the pancreas (P). The spleen (S) and two splenules *(curved arrows)* were enlarged.

leiomyomas, leiomyosarcomas, and leiomyoblastomas are currently primarily classified as GISTs. Approximately 10% to 30% of GISTs are malignant. GISTs are differentiated from true leiomyomas and leiomyosarcomas by the presence of KIT (CD117) protein, a tyrosine kinase growth factor receptor that is tested for by immunohistochemical stain. Only in the esophagus are leiomyomas more common than GISTs. In other portions of the gastrointestinal tract, GISTs are the most common mesenchymal tumor. Most tumors present with gastrointestinal bleeding resulting from mucosal ulceration. GISTs are rarely seen in patients younger than 40 years old. CT findings of GIST include:

- Tumors arise from the bowel wall and grow away from the gut lumen to project into the abdominal cavity. Size varies from millimeters to 30 cm. Small lesions that are homogeneous in attenuation are usually benign (Fig. 17-10).
- Ulceration of the luminal surface is seen in 50% of lesions.
- Cystic degeneration, hemorrhage, and necrosis are common especially in large lesions (Fig. 17-11). The tumor cavity may communicate with the gut lumen and con-

tain air or oral contrast. Calcification in the tumor is rare.
- Contrast enhancement is seen in viable tumor, most commonly in the periphery of the mass.
- Risk for malignancy is increased in tumors that arise outside of the stomach or are larger than 5 cm. Metastases are most common in the liver and the peritoneal cavity.

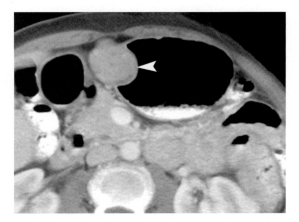

FIGURE 17-10 **Benign gastric stromal tumor.** A wall mass *(arrowhead)* of uniform attenuation and enhancement projects both into the gastric lumen and into the abdominal cavity.

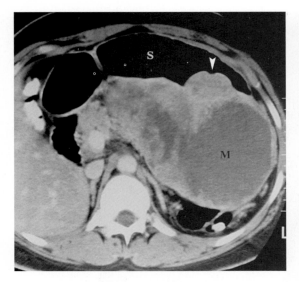

FIGURE 17-11 **Malignant gastric stromal tumor.** A huge heterogeneous mass (M) arises from the posterior wall of the stomach (S). Large low-density areas within the mass correspond to hemorrhage and necrosis. An ulcer crater *(arrowhead)* is identified within a nodular tumor projection into the gastric lumen.

Gastric Varices

Gastric varices occur as a result of portal hypertension or splenic vein thrombosis. CT findings include:

- Varices appear as well-marginated clusters of rounded and tubular densities in, or adjacent to, the wall of the stomach, most commonly in the fundal region. Bright enhancement with intravenous contrast clinches the diagnosis (Fig. 17-12).
- CT signs of liver disease and other portosystemic collateral vessels are often present.
- Gastric varices without esophageal varices is a hallmark finding associated with splenic vein thrombosis.

☐ **SMALL BOWEL**

Anatomy

The duodenum extends from the pylorus to the ligament of Treitz forming the familiar C-loop. The duodenum becomes retroperitoneal at the right free edge of the hepatoduodenal ligament, closely related to the neck of the gallbladder. The descending duodenum passes to the right of the pancreatic head to just below the uncinate process where the duodenum turns to the

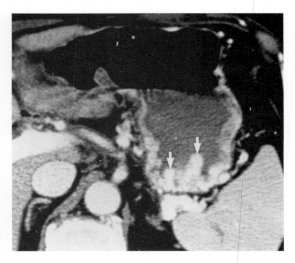

FIGURE 17-12 **Gastric varices.** Bolus intravenous contrast medium administration causes bright enhancement of varices *(arrows)* in the wall of the gastric fundus in this patient with alcoholism and portal hypertension.

left. The horizontal portion crosses anterior to the inferior vena cava and aorta and posterior to the superior mesenteric vein and artery. The fourth portion ascends just left of the aorta to the ligament of Treitz where it becomes the intraperitoneal jejunum.

The jejunum occupies the left upper abdomen, whereas the ileum lies in the right lower abdomen and pelvis. Jejunal loops are feathery with distinct folds. Ileal loops are featureless with thin walls. Opacification of the lumen with oral contrast media is essential to adequately evaluate the bowel. Unopacified small bowel may mimic adenopathy and abdominal masses. The small bowel mesentery contains many vessels that are easily visualized when outlined by fat. The normal luminal diameter of the small bowel does not exceed 2.5 cm. The normal wall thickness is less than 3 mm.

Technical Considerations

Opacification of the small bowel with oral contrast agent is mandatory for high-quality abdominal CT. It is nearly impossible to administer too much oral contrast. A 1% to 3% concentration of oral contrast agent is optimal for CT. This concentration is obtained by adding 3 mL 60% oral contrast solution to 100 mL water. We give 400-mL doses of this mixture 12 hours, 2 hours, 30 minutes, and immediately before CT scanning. To study the small bowel, we obtain sequential

5-mm or thinner slices through the abdomen and pelvis. When the duodenum is the organ of primary interest, administration of 0.1 mg glucagon intravenously is helpful in stopping peristalsis and in distending the bowel. An intravenous contrast agent is optional for the small bowel itself but is helpful for assessment of the remainder of the abdomen.

Small Bowel Edema and Wall Thickening

Like the other portions of the gastrointestinal tract, edema and wall thickening are nonspecific signs seen in a wide variety of disease states. Wall thickening greater than 15 mm, or associated with mesenteric mass, suggests neoplasm. Wall thickening less than 15 mm (Fig. 17-13), with normal or increased density mesenteric fat, suggests inflammatory disease or noninflammatory edema (ischemia, trauma, hypoalbuminemia, lymphatic obstruction, or radiation).

Small Bowel Diverticula

Small bowel diverticula may cause unusual collections of fluid, air, contrast material, or soft-tissue density in the fat and tissues adjacent to the bowel. These must not be mistaken for abscesses, pancreatic pseudocysts, or tumors. Rescanning the patient will often demonstrate a significant change in the appearance of diverticula. Typically, diverticula appear as mucosal sacs without folds and containing air or contrast located adjacent to a loop of bowel (Fig. 17-14).

Small Bowel Tumors

Both benign and malignant small bowel neoplasms are uncommon. CT demonstrates about 73% of small bowel tumors, which appear as soft tissue mass or wall thickening. CT is useful in demonstrating extraluminal tumor growth, involvement of adjacent structures, adenopathy, and complications such as fistulas or necrosis. CT findings include:

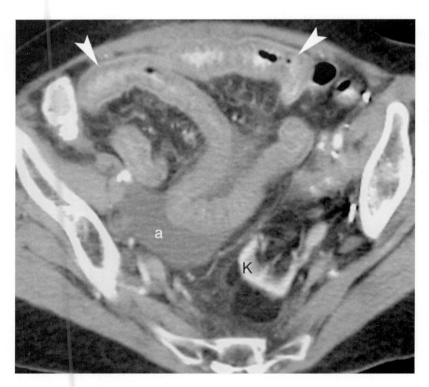

FIGURE 17-13 **Wall thickening caused by radiation enteritis.** Small bowel loops in the pelvis demonstrate diffuse circumferential wall thickening *(arrowhead)* associated with radiation enteritis. A pelvic kidney (K) shows diffuse atrophy also caused by radiation therapy. Ascites (a) is present.

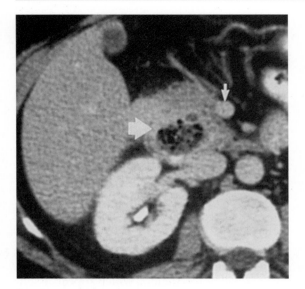

FIGURE 17-14 **Duodenal diverticulum.** A diverticulum, arising from the second portion of the duodenum, is seen as a mass *(large arrow)* containing air and fluid that displaces the superior mesenteric vein *(small arrow)*.

- *Lymphomas* appear as single or multiple, often large (9 cm) soft-tissue masses or as focal or diffuse nodular wall thickening (Fig. 17-15). Ulceration is common. The ileum is the most common location. Mesenteric or retroperitoneal adenopathy is seen in half of cases.
- *Hematogenous metastases* to the small bowel are common. The most common primaries are malignant melanoma, breast, lung, and renal cell carcinoma. Lesions from melanoma are small and round and may cause intussusception. Metastases may be single or multiple, flat or polypoid, submucosal or ulcerative producing a "target" appearance.
- *Carcinoid* tumors occur most commonly in the appendix (50%) and mesenteric small bowel (20%). They are the second most common small bowel malignancy. All tumors have the potential to metastasize and are considered malignant, although some may have an indolent course. The primary tumor tends to be small and difficult to detect on CT. They appear as a brightly enhancing wall mass. Aggressive tumors tend to be larger than 2 cm and have necrosis and ulceration. Tumor invasion of the bowel wall induces a dramatic fibrosing reaction in the mesentery that is the hallmark of CT diagnosis. Linear strands of fibrosis radiate into the mesenteric fat from the soft-tissue mass or focal wall thickening of the primary tumor (Fig. 17-16). Liver metastases are always present in patients with carcinoid syndrome. Metastases are hypervascular and are best seen on arterial phase images.
- *Adenocarcinoma* of the small bowel is a rare lesion that is most common in the duodenum (50%). Tumors appear as a constricting annular mass with abrupt irregular margins, a distinct polypoid nodule, or as an ulcerative mass. Only a short segment of bowel is involved. Partial or complete obstruction may be present (Fig. 17-17).

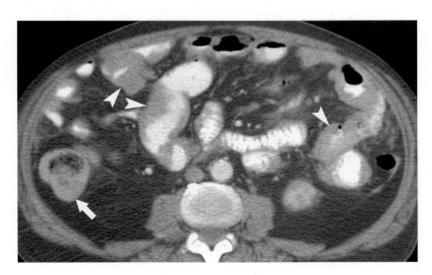

FIGURE 17-15 **Small bowel lymphoma.** Small bowel loops in the central abdomen demonstrate variable wall thickening *(arrowheads)*. The cecum *(arrow)* also shows wall thickening indicative of lymphoma.

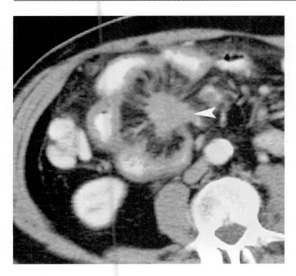

FIGURE 17-16 **Carcinoid tumor.** A carcinoid tumor arising in the ileum causes a mass *(arrowhead)* in the small bowel mesentery. Characteristic thick fibrotic strands radiate from the mass to the adjacent bowel, which shows wall thickening.

- *Leiomyosarcomas* tend to be large (11 cm) and exophytic with prominent central necrosis.

Crohn's Disease

Crohn's disease is characterized by inflammation of the bowel mucosa, bowel wall, and mesentery with marked submucosal edema. These features are nicely reflected in the CT appearance:

- The small bowel, especially the terminal ileum, is affected in 80% of patients, and the colon is affected in 50%.

- Circumferential thickening of the bowel wall is a hallmark of disease (Fig. 17-18). Thickening is most often 1 to 2 cm but can be up to 3 cm. Wall thickening may be homogeneous or have a stratified "target" or "double halo" appearance caused by bands of edema.
- Acutely inflamed bowel demonstrates marked wall enhancement after intravenous contrast administration. The degree of enhancement correlates with the intensity of inflammation.
- The "comb sign" produced by hyperemic thickening of the vasa recta is a sign of active disease. The swollen blood vessels produce a comblike appearance extending from the thickened bowel wall into the mesenteric fat.
- Wall thickening results in strictures narrowing of the bowel lumen in advanced disease.
- "Skip areas" of normal bowel intervened between diseased segments are characteristic of Crohn's disease.
- Diffuse haziness and increased density of the mesenteric fat is evidence of mesenteric inflammation.
- Fistulas and sinus tracts between bowel loops (Fig. 17-19) or to the bladder, adjacent muscle, or the skin surface are characteristic of Crohn's disease.
- Extramural abscesses appear as fluid collections in the mesentery. Mesenteric lymph nodes may be enlarged.
- Mesenteric abscesses containing fluid, air, or contrast material are present.

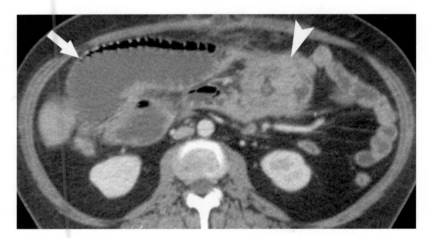

FIGURE 17-17 **Adenocarcinoma of the jejunum.** An irregular solid mass *(arrowhead)* that caused obstruction of the proximal small bowel *(arrow)* proved to be an adenocarcinoma arising in the jejunum.

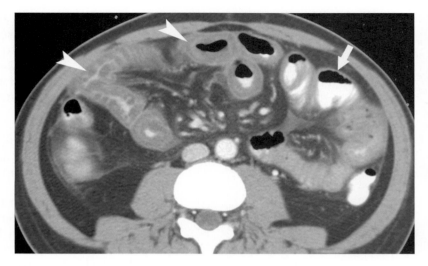

FIGURE 17-18 Crohn's disease: wall thickening. Many loops of small bowel show circumferential wall thickening *(arrowheads)*, whereas others *(arrow)* are unaffected representing skip lesions.

CT is excellent in documenting the extraluminal manifestations of the disease.

Small Bowel Obstruction

CT is reported to be 90% to 95% sensitive for detecting small bowel obstruction (SBO) and 47% to 73% sensitive in identifying its cause. CT findings include:

- If the bowel is significantly distended on a plain radiograph, administration of oral contrast is not needed. Intravenous contrast is recommended because it provides enhancement of the bowel wall and better visualization of pathologic processes.
- *Complete mechanical* SBO appears as dilatation of proximal small bowel (>2.5 cm) with a distinct transition zone to col-

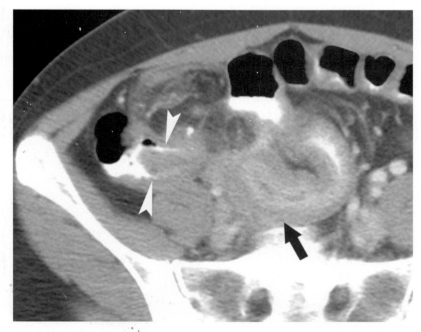

FIGURE 17-19 Crohn's disease: fistulas. Ileum *(arrow)* in the right lower quadrant demonstrates marked wall thickening and matting of bowel loops caused by inflammation of the mesentery. A double-tract bowel lumen *(arrowhead)* is seen indicating formation of ileoileal fistula.

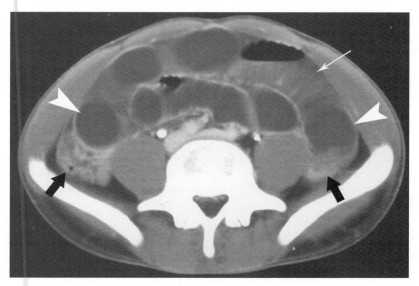

FIGURE 17-20 **Small bowel obstruction.** CT demonstrates diffuse dilatation of small bowel *(arrowheads)*. Most loops contain fluid. Small bowel is identified by its central location and the valvulae conniventes *(white arrow)*. The colon *(black arrows)* is collapsed. Adhesions were the cause of this obstruction.

lapsed distal bowel (Fig. 17-20). No oral contrast passes the transition zone. The colon is collapsed and contains minimal fluid or gas.

- *Paralytic ileus* appears as dilatation of both proximal and distal small bowel without a transition zone. The colon is distended with fluid and gas and may contain oral contrast. However, a totally collapsed descending colon is common in nonobstructive ileus and should not be mistaken for evidence of a transition zone.
- *Partial mechanical SBO* appearance falls between complete SBO and ileus. The proximal bowel is less dilated, and the transition zone is less distinct. The bowel distal to the obstruction is not completely collapsed. The colon is normal or slightly dilated and contains moderate amounts of fluid and gas. The "small bowel feces" is uncommon but highly indicative of partial SBO. Intestinal transit is slowed, resulting in increased water absorption that causes small bowel content to resemble feces.
- *CT enteroclysis* is useful in the evaluation of equivocal cases. A tube is placed in the fourth portion of the duodenum and 1 to 1.5 L dilute contrast agent is infused into the small bowel to maximize bowel visualization.
- Adhesions cause 50% to 75% of SBOs but are not directly visualized by CT. Abrupt transition from dilated to nondilated bowel with-

out other findings suggests adhesions as the cause. Beaklike narrowing at the transition zone is characteristic of adhesions but is uncommon.

- Tumor, abscess, intussusception, inflammation, and hernia causing obstruction are identified by characteristic signs.
- *Closed loop obstruction* has a greater morbidity and mortality rate than simple obstruction. Closed loop obstruction refers to a loop of bowel occluded at two adjacent points along its course, usually caused by adhesions or internal hernia. The obstructed loop may twist, resulting in volvulus. The "beak" or "whirl" sign may be seen at the obstruction and volvulus. Dilated bowel loops with stretched and prominent mesenteric vessels converging on a site of obstruction suggest closed loop obstruction. *Strangulation* refers to closed loop obstruction with intestinal ischemia. Strangulation is suggested by associated mild circumferential thickening of the bowel wall with the low-density concentric rings indicative of wall edema ("target" and "halo" signs). Poor or absent enhancement of the bowel wall is indicative of ischemia.
- *Intussusception* is an uncommon cause of SBO in adults. Causes include lipoma and other benign submucosal tumors, carcinoma, metastatic disease, and lymphoma. CT

demonstrates characteristic findings (Fig. 17-21). The distal receiving segment (intussuscipiens) is markedly dilated and has a thickened wall. Its lumen contains an eccentric, soft-tissue mass (intussusceptum) with an adjacent crescent of fat density that represents the invaginated mesentery. The mass causing the intussusception can often be identified at the leading end of the intussusceptum.

☐ MESENTERY

Sclerosing Mesenteritis

Sclerosing mesenteritis refers to an inflammatory disorder of unknown cause affecting the mesentery. It usually involves the small bowel mesentery but may also affect the mesocolon. The lesion is a mixture of chronic inflammation (mesenteric panniculitis), fat necrosis (mesenteric lipodystrophy), and fibrosis (retractile mesenteritis). Patients may present with abdominal pain. CT findings include:

- Inflammation causes fat within the mesentery to show hazy increased attenuation and small lymph nodes. This appearance has been termed *misty mesentery*. Misty mesentery may result from hemorrhage or edema from any cause or from lymphoma.

- Continuing inflammation may coalesce into a soft-tissue mass that envelops the mesenteric vessels. Preservation of fat around enveloped vessels (the "fat ring sign") is characteristic.

Cystic Mesenteric Masses

Cystic lesions primary to the mesentery are more common than primary mesenteric neoplasms. CT findings include:

- Mesenteric and omental cysts are cystic lymphangiomas. They are generally unilocular, thin walled, and contain serous fluid. Internal hemorrhage may occur.
- Cystic mesothelioma is a rare benign tumor that presents as a unilocular or multilocular mesenteric mass.
- Cystic teratomas contain fat and calcifications.

Mesenteric Neoplasms

A wide variety of lesions may produce solid masses within the mesentery:

- *Lymphoma* is the most common malignancy seen in the mesentery. Lymphoma of the small bowel demonstrates focal nodular or circumferential wall thickening. Mesenteric

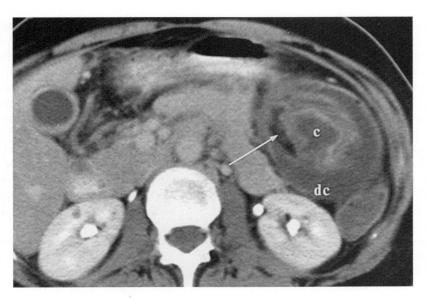

FIGURE 17-21 **Intussusception.** An adenoma arising in the cecum served as a lead mass for a colocolonic intussusception. This image demonstrates a portion of the cecum (c) inside the lumen of the descending colon (dc). Note the intraluminal crescent of fat density *(arrow)*, which represents the cecal mesentery.

involvement may consist of enlarged individual mesenteric nodes or large confluent masses (Fig. 17-22). Lymphomatous masses characteristically "sandwich" mesenteric vessels between thin layers of spared mesenteric fat (the "sandwich" sign).

- *Metastases* to the mesentery are far more common than primary tumors arising in the mesentery. Metastatic spread to the mesentery may occur by direct extension (carcinoid), lymphatic flow (bowel malignancies), hematogenous spread to bowel wall (melanoma and breast cancer), and peritoneal seeding (ovarian and colon cancers).
- *Mesenteric fibromatosis (desmoid tumor)* arises most commonly in the mesentery of the small bowel. With Gardner's syndrome, tumors are also found in the abdominal wall. The lesion consists of bland fibroblastic cells suspended in collagenous stroma. This produces a well-defined, homogeneous, solid mass without hemorrhage, necrosis, or cystic change (Fig. 17-23).
- *GISTs* that arise in the mesentery or omentum tend to be large (>10 cm) and demonstrate prominent hemorrhage, necrosis, and cystic change.
- *Sarcomas* that arise in the mesentery or omentum are indistinguishable from GISTs. Tissue types include leiomyosarcoma, fibro-

sarcoma, malignant fibrous histiocytoma, and liposarcoma.

☐ APPENDIX

Anatomy

The normal appendix can be seen on CT as a thin-walled tubular structure surrounded by mesenteric fat. It may be collapsed or filled with air, fluid, or contrast material. The normal appendix does not exceed 6 mm in diameter and has a sharp outer contour defined by homogeneous low-density fat (Fig. 17-24). The origin of the appendix is between the ileocecal valve and the cecal apex, always on the same side of the cecum as the valve. Approximately one third of appendixes course inferomedially from the cecum, whereas two thirds are retrocecal.

Appendicitis

Acute appendicitis is the most common cause of acute abdominal pain affecting 6% of the population. CT has a 95% to 98% sensitivity in its diagnosis:

- CT findings diagnostic of acute appendicitis are a distended appendix (>6 mm in diameter), thickened walls that enhance, and

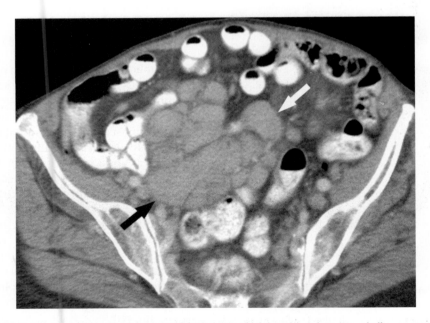

FIGURE 17-22 **Mesenteric lymphoma.** Multiple bloated lymphomatous lymph nodes coalesce into a bulky mesenteric mass *(arrows).*

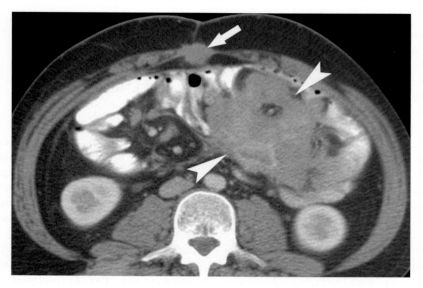

FIGURE 17-23 **Mesenteric fibromatosis.** In a patient with Gardner's syndrome after total colectomy, mesenteric fibromatosis (desmoid tumor) causes a homogeneous soft-tissue mass *(arrowheads).* A desmoid tumor is also seen in the anterior abdominal wall *(arrow).*

periappendiceal inflammatory changes with stranding in the fat (Fig. 17-25).

- Detection of an appendicolith appearing as a ringlike or homogeneous calcification within, or adjacent to, a phlegmon or abscess is diagnostic of appendicitis. Appen-

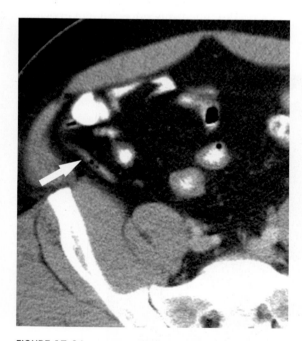

FIGURE 17-24 **Normal appendix.** The wormlike normal appendix *(arrow)* extends from the cecum. The periappendiceal fat provides sharp definition of the wall with no inflammatory infiltration.

dicoliths may be seen in 28% of adult patients with acute appendicitis. Examining CT images with bone windows aids in the detection of appendicoliths.

- Appendicitis confined to the distal tip is more difficult to diagnose. The proximal appendix may be collapsed or filled with air or contrast material. The inflamed distal appendix is distended (average, 13 mm) with thickened enhancing wall and periappendiceal fat stranding. A transition zone between normal thin appendiceal wall and thickened wall with narrowed lumen is seen.

- Complications associated with perforated appendicitis include phlegmon, seen as a periappendiceal soft-tissue mass (>20 H), and abscess, seen as a fluid collection (<20 H). Phlegmons and abscesses smaller than 3 cm generally resolve on antibiotic treatment, whereas abscesses larger than 3 cm usually require surgical or catheter drainage.

- Additional complications that may be demonstrated by CT include SBO, hepatic abscess, and mesenteric vein thrombosis.

- Differential diagnosis of right lower quadrant inflammatory change, without visualization of an abnormal appendix or appendicolith, includes Crohn's disease, cecal diverticulitis, perforated cecal carcinoma, mesenteric adenitis, and pelvic inflammatory disease.

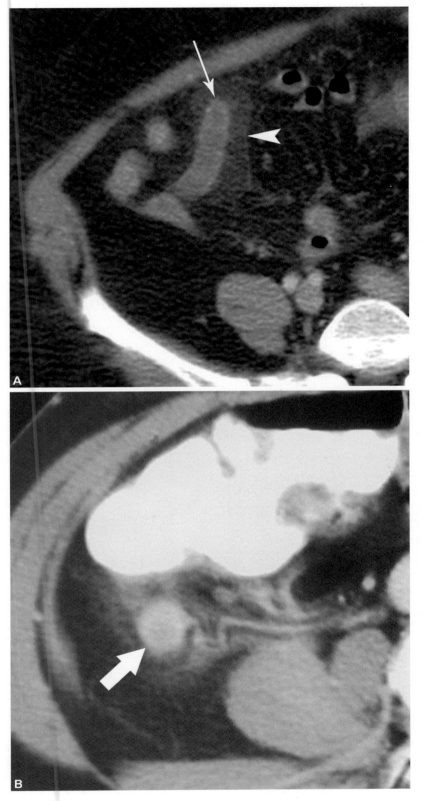

FIGURE 17-25 **Acute appendicitis.** Four different examples of acute appendicitis are provided. *A,* The swollen appendix, measuring 9 mm in diameter, is identified by its bulbous tip *(arrow).* The periappendiceal fat is infiltrated by edema *(arrowhead). B,* The inflamed appendix *(arrow)* is shown in cross section. The wall of the appendix enhances markedly, and extensive inflammation is present in the surrounding fat.

Continued

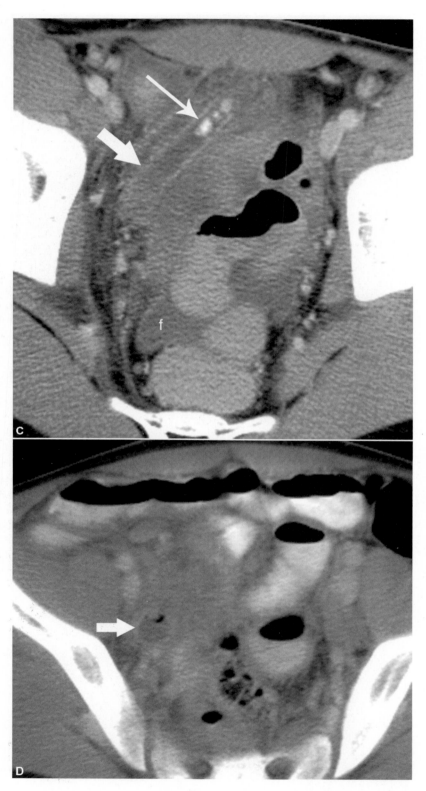

FIGURE 17-25 Cont'd *C, A* row of high-attenuation appendicoliths *(long arrow)* are seen occluding the proximal appendix *(short arrow)*, which is dilated with an enhancing will. Fluid (f) in the cul-de-sac is indicative of perforation, which was confirmed at surgery. *D,* The appendix *(arrow)* is difficult to identify because of the surrounding fluid and inflammation. Examination of serial images is needed to identify its origin from the cecum and its bulbous tip.

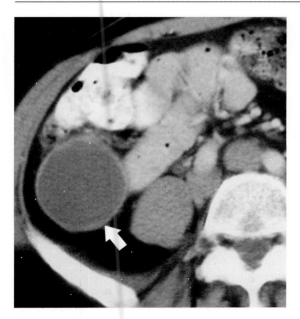

FIGURE 17-26 **Mucocele of the appendix.** The appendix *(arrow)* is markedly dilated and filled with fluid. At surgery, the appendix was filled with mucin and a small obstructing benign mucinous cystadenoma was discovered.

Mucocele of the Appendix

Mucocele refers to a distended appendix filled with mucus. Mucinous neoplasms are the most common cause of mucocele. On CT, a mucocele appears as a well-encapsulated, cystic mass with thin walls that may be calcified (Fig. 17-26). Size is variable up to 15 cm. Mucoceles smaller than 2 cm diameter are likely to caused by a simple retention cyst near the appendix origin; those larger than 2 cm are usually caused by a mucinous neoplasm. Curvilinear calcification is seen in the wall in 50% of patients.

☐ COLON AND RECTUM

Anatomy

The colon is easily identified by its location and its haustral markings when it is distended by air or contrast agent. Mottled fecal material also serves as a marker of the colon and rectum. The scout view of the abdominal CT should be inspected to determine the general outline and course of the colon. The cecum generally occupies the iliac fossa, although, because of its variably long mesentery, it may be found almost anywhere in the abdomen. Its identity is confirmed by recognizing the ileocecal valve or appendix. The ascending colon occupies a posterior and lateral position in the right flank. The hepatic flexure makes one or more sharp bends near the undersurface of the liver and gallbladder. The transverse colon sweeps across the abdomen on a long and mobile mesentery. Because of its anterior position, the transverse colon is usually filled with air when patients are supine on the CT couch. The splenic flexure makes one or more tight bends near the spleen. The descending colon extends caudad down the left flank. Remember that the ascending and descending portions of the colon are retroperitoneal. The peritoneum sweeps over their anterior surfaces and extends laterally to form the paracolic gutters that distend with fluid when ascites is present. The sigmoid colon begins in the left iliac fossa and extends a variable distance craniad before it dives toward the rectum. The sigmoid becomes the rectum at the level of the third sacral segment. The rectum distends to form the rectal ampulla, and then abruptly narrows to form the anal canal. Fat around the colon is normally uniformly of low density. Soft-tissue stranding densities in the pericolic fat are indicative of inflammatory changes or neoplastic invasion.

The peritoneum covering the anterior surface of the rectum extends to the level of the vagina forming the rectovaginal pouch of Douglas. In male individuals, the peritoneum extends to the seminal vesicles, 2.5 cm above the prostate, forming the rectovesical pouch. Three anatomic compartments are important to recognize when staging rectal carcinoma: (1) the peritoneal cavity above the peritoneal reflections, (2) the extraperitoneal compartment between the peritoneum and the levator ani muscle that forms the pelvic diaphragm, and (3) the perineum identified by the triangular ischiorectal fossa inferior and lateral to the levator ani. The lower two thirds of the rectum are extraperitoneal. On CT, the thickness of the wall of the normal colon does not exceed 3 mm.

Technical Considerations

For routine scanning, the rectum and colon usually can be adequately opacified by giving contrast agents orally. Scanning is then carried out through the entire abdomen and pelvis. Demonstration of subtle findings is improved by narrow collimation (3–5 mm) through a defined area of abnormality. Intravenous contrast medium enhancement is optional but usually is helpful.

Virtual Colonoscopy

CT colonography is becoming a viable alternative to invasive colonoscopy to screen for colorectal cancer. The procedure begins with diligent bowel preparation identical to that used for invasive colonoscopy. A rectal tube is inserted and the colon is insufflated with carbon dioxide or room air. Multidetector CT of the entire extent of the colon with the patient in supine position is obtained in a single breath hold using 1.25- to 2.5-mm collimation and a reconstruction interval of 1 mm. The scan is repeated with the patient in prone position. Commercially available software programs that provide endoluminal display and "fly-through" capabilities provide three-dimensional volume rendering imaging processing. Image viewing and interpretation is usually performed using both standard two-dimensional axial CT reconstructions and the three-dimensional volume-rendered images on a computer workstation. Most colon cancers are thought to develop from an adenomatous polyp. Polyp detection exceeds 90% for lesions 6 mm and larger. The role of virtual colonoscopy in screening for colorectal cancer is still being debated. CT findings include:

- Polyps are seen as well-defined oval or round intraluminal projections usually seen best in profile (Fig. 17-27).
- Polyps smaller than 5 mm are nearly all hyperplastic and are considered by most to be clinically insignificant (99% hyperplastic, 1% adenomatous). Polyps in the 6- to 9-mm range may contain dysplasia or rarely cancer (<1%); however, 50% of lesions in this size range are adenomas. Polyps in the range of 10 to 15 mm have an 80% risk for being an adenoma and a 1% to 5% risk for being a cancer. Polyps larger than 2 cm have a 40% risk for being cancerous.
- Cancers appear as larger intraluminal masses with nodular contours and irregular mucosal surfaces.
- Narrowing of the lumen suggests constricting annular carcinomas
- Flat adenoma and annular constricting lesions are the major sources of interpretation error.

- Incidental extracolonic findings are present in up to 11% of patients. These include adrenal masses, renal cysts, gallstones and kidney stones, and unsuspected renal cancers.

Colorectal Carcinoma

Colon cancer is the second leading cause of cancer death in the United States. Seventy percent of colon cancers occur in the rectosigmoid region. The remainder are scattered fairly evenly throughout the rest of the colon. Colon cancer spreads by: (1) direct extension with penetration of the colon wall, (2) lymphatic drainage to regional nodes, (3) hematogenous routes through portal veins to the liver, and (4) intraperitoneal seeding. CT has become routine for the preoperative staging (Table 17-2) and surgical planning. However, the accuracy of CT staging ranges from 17% for early lesions (Dukes stage B) to 81% for advanced lesions (Dukes stage D). Inaccuracies arise from nonspecific CT signs of tumor spread through the bowel wall and a high incidence of tumor-involved lymph nodes being smaller than 10 mm. CT findings of colorectal carcinoma include:

- The primary tumor may be a colon polyp. These are nearly always larger than 1 cm.
- Most cancers appear as a soft-tissue mass that narrows the lumen of the colon (Fig. 17-28). Central low attenuation represents hemorrhage or necrosis. Air within the tumor indicates ulceration.
- Flat lesions appear as focal, lobulated thickening of the bowel wall (>3 mm).
- "Apple core" lesions demonstrate irregular bulky circumferential wall thickening with marked and irregular narrowing of the bowel lumen (Fig. 17-29).
- Linear soft-tissue densities extending from the colonic mass into pericolic fat suggest, but are not diagnostic of, extension of tumor through the bowel wall.
- Loss of fat planes between the tumor and adjacent structures suggest local invasion.
- Regional lymph nodes larger than 1 cm are considered positive for metastatic disease. However, some nodes smaller than 1 cm may contain tumor and some nodes larger than 1 cm may not contain tumor, limiting the value of CT.

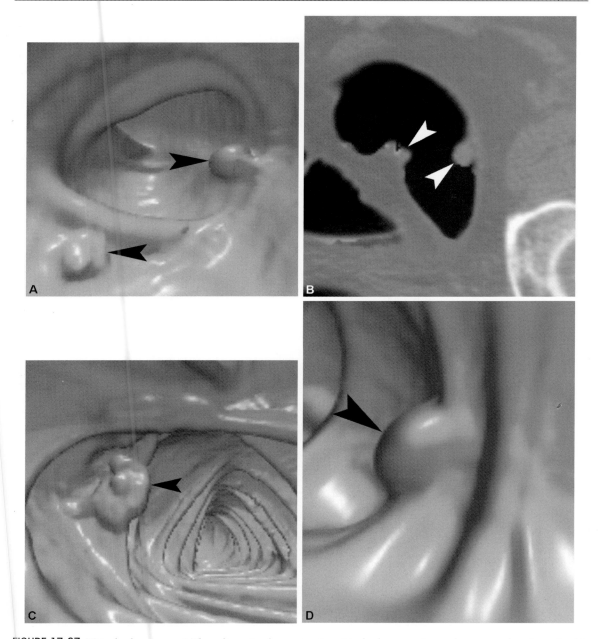

FIGURE 17-27 **Virtual colonoscopy.** *A*, Three-dimensional reconstruction virtual colonoscopy image shows two polyps *(arrowheads)* projecting into the colon lumen. Several colonic folds are visible. *B*, Source CT image shows the same two polyps *(arrowheads)* as in *A*. *C*, A villous polyp *(arrowhead)* with a lobulated contour is demonstrated. *D*, A well-defined polyp *(arrowhead)* projects off a fold.

- Distant metastases are seen in the liver (75%), lung (5% to 50%), adrenal gland (14%), and elsewhere.
- Complications of colon malignancy include bowel obstruction, perforation, and fistula formation (Fig. 17-30).
- Calcifications in the primary tumor and metastases occur with mucinous adenocarcinoma.

- Edema may cause thickening of the wall of the colon proximal to the tumor. Obstructing colon cancers may cause ischemic colitis proximal to the tumor.

Colorectal Cancer Recurrence

CT is more valuable in the detection of colorectal cancer recurrence than it is for initial staging.

TABLE 17-2

Staging of Colorectal Cancer

Modified Dukes Classification	TNM Classification		
	T	N	M
A—Penetration into but not through the bowel wall	T1—Tumor invades submucosa	N0	M0
	T2—Tumor invades muscularis propria		
B—Penetration through the bowel wall	T3—Tumor invades through the muscularis propria into subserosa or into nonperitonealized pericolic or perirectal tissues	N0	M0
	T4—Tumor perforates the visceral peritoneum or invades adjacent organs or structures		
C—Lymph node involvement regardless of extent of bowel wall penetration	Any T	N1—Metastases in from one to three regional lymph nodes	M0
		N2—Metastases in more than four regional lymph nodes	
D—Distant metastases present	Any T	Any N	M1—Distant metastases

M = distant metastases; N = lymph nodes; T = primary tumor.
Modified from Iyer RB, Silverman PM, DuBrow RA, Charnsangave C: Imaging in the diagnosis, staging, and follow-up of colorectal cancer. AJR Am J Roentgenol 179:3–13, 2002.

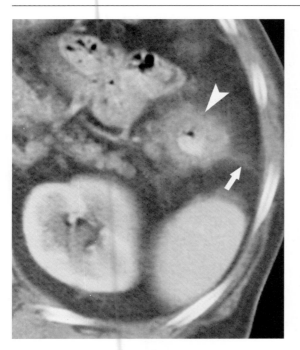

FIGURE 17-28 Colon carcinoma: wall thickening.
A carcinoma of the descending colon causes thickening of the colon wall *(arrowhead)* and narrowing of the lumen. Stranding densities *(arrow)* extending into the pericolonic fat suggest tumor extension through the bowel wall.

One third of patients who have undergone a colorectal cancer resection will experience development of recurrent disease; most (70% to 80%) will experience recurrence within 2 years. About half of the colon cancer recurrences occur at the site of the original tumor, whereas the remainder recur at distant sites, especially in the liver. Multiple sites of tumor recurrence are more common than a solitary site of recurrence. CT findings of recurrence include:

- Recurrences appear as irregular masses, often with a low-density necrotic center and an enhancing periphery.
- Presacral soft-tissue densities, seen in patients with abdominoperineal resection, may be recurrent tumor or fibrosis. Percutaneous biopsy is generally required for confirmation.

Colon Lymphoma

Colon lymphoma is less common than gastric or small bowel lymphoma but has a striking and fairly characteristic CT appearance; for example:

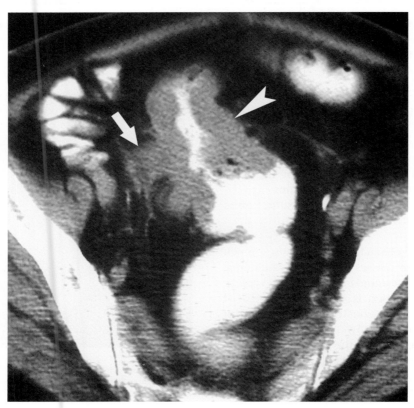

FIGURE 17-29 Rectal carcinoma: apple core lesion. The rectum demonstrates marked wall thickening *(arrowhead)* with severe and irregular narrowing of the lumen. Spread of tumor into perirectal fat is evident *(arrow)*.

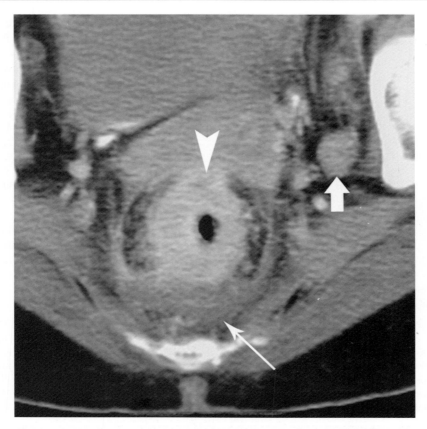

FIGURE 17-30 **Rectal carcinoma: perforation.** The rectal wall *(arrowhead)* is markedly and circumferentially thickened with an ill-defined outer margin. The presacral area of low density *(long arrow)* suggests focal perforation. An enlarged metastatic internal iliac lymph node *(short arrow)* is evident.

- Marked thickening of the bowel wall, often exceeding 4 cm
- Homogeneous soft-tissue mass without calcification or necrosis (Fig. 17-31)
- Minimal to no enhancement of the mass with intravenous contrast medium
- Regional and diffuse adenopathy, often massive.

Lymphoma characteristically causes much larger soft-tissue masses than does carcinoma. The absence of desmoplastic reaction is typical; and the colon lumen is commonly dilated or normal, rather than constricted, at the site of tumor involvement. Bowel obstruction is uncommon. Patients with the acquired immunodeficiency syndrome have a much greater incidence of colon involvement with lymphoma than the general population.

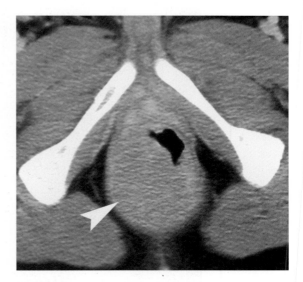

FIGURE 17-31 **Lymphoma rectum.** In a patient with AIDS, non–Hodgkin's lymphoma causes a bulky rectal mass *(arrowhead)* that distorts the rectal lumen.

Lipoma

CT can be used to make a specific and noninvasive diagnosis of gastrointestinal lipoma by demonstrating homogeneous fat density (−80 to −120 H) within a sharply defined tumor. Most lipomas are 2 to 3 cm, are round or ovoid, and are clinically silent. Some may bleed or are a cause of intussusception. Lipomas occur most commonly in the colon (65% to 75%) and small bowel (20% to 25%) and uncommonly in the stomach (5%), esophagus, and pharynx.

Acute Diverticulitis

Diverticulosis describes small saclike outpouchings of mucosa and submucosa through the muscular layers of the wall of the colon. Diverticula are most common in the sigmoid colon but may occur throughout the colon. The incidence of diverticulosis increases with age affecting more than 80% of the population older than 85 years. Obstruction of the neck of a diverticulum by feces, undigested food particles, or inflamma-

tion results in acute diverticulitis. Microperforation of the diverticulum causes pericolic inflammation. The inflammatory process commonly spreads to adjacent diverticula to affect a short or long segment of colon. CT findings of acute diverticulitis include:

- Diverticula are easily visualized on CT as small, rounded collections of air, feces, or contrast material outside the lumen of the colon. Size ranges from 1 mm to 2 cm. Thickening of the muscular wall of the colon is common.
- Acute diverticulitis demonstrates on CT a colon segment with wall thickening hyperemic contrast enhancement and inflammatory changes that extend into the pericolic fat (Fig. 17-32). Identification of diverticula in the involved segment confirms the diagnosis of acute diverticulitis.
- Because most diverticula occur along the mesenteric surface of the colon, perforation caused by diverticulitis is confined initially to between the leaves of the mesocolon.

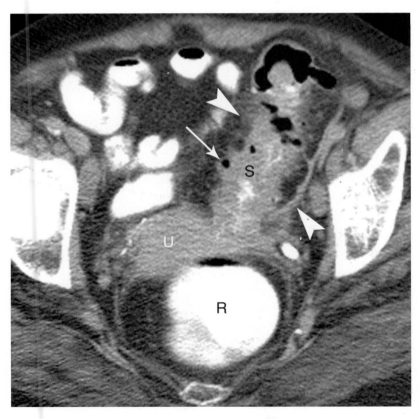

FIGURE 17-32 **Acute diverticulitis: uncomplicated.** The sigmoid colon (S) demonstrates wall thickening in luminal narrowing. Pericolonic inflammation is manifest by fascial thickening and stranding in the pericolic fat *(arrowheads)*. Several diverticula *(long arrow)* are evident in the inflamed portion of the colon. R, rectum; U, uterus.

The inflammatory mass that forms is both extraluminal and extraperitoneal. CT is better suited to documentation of this extraluminal disease than is barium enema.

- Sinus tracts and fistulas may extend to adjacent organs or the skin and are represented by linear fluid or air collections. Air in the bladder suggests the possibility of colovesical fistula.
- Abscess formation may be extensive (Fig. 17-33). Obstruction of the colon or urinary tract may result from the inflammatory process.
- Diverticulitis of the right colon may be confused with acute appendicitis or Crohn's disease.
- The CT appearance of diverticulitis overlaps that of colon cancer. Fluid in the sigmoid mesentery with engorgement of mesenteric vessels favors diverticulitis. Enlarged lymph nodes in the mesentery and presence of an intraluminal mass favors cancer. Equivocal cases require biopsy.

Colitis

Patients with colitis commonly present with vague abdominal symptoms. CT is often the first imaging study that is obtained. Thickening of the colon wall is the CT hallmark of colitis. Wall thickness more than 3 mm when the colon is distended is abnormally thickened. Bowel with mural thickening commonly demonstrates homogeneous mural enhancement or a "target" or "halo" appearance. The target or halo appearance is highly indicative of an inflammatory or infectious process rather than a neoplasm. CT findings of colitis include:

- *Ulcerative colitis* (UC) is characterized by inflammation and diffuse ulceration of the colon mucosa. The disease starts in the rectum and extends proximally to involve part or all of the colon. The CT hallmarks of UC are wall thickening with lumen narrowing (Fig. 17-34). The inflammatory pseudopolyps that result from extensive mucosal ulceration are sometimes seen on CT.

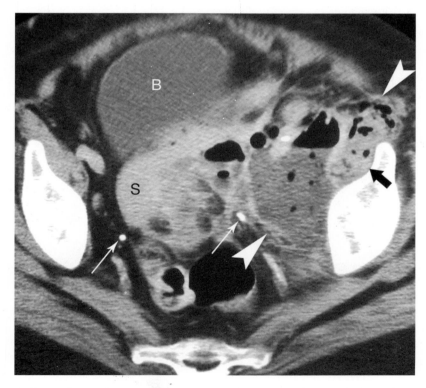

FIGURE 17-33 **Acute diverticulitis: perforation and abscess.** Diverticulitis arising in the sigmoid colon (S) has ruptured and caused a large pelvic abscess *(arrowheads)* containing air and fluid. The left iliopsoas muscle *(black arrow)* is involved by the abscess. Note the proximity of the ureters *(white arrows)* to the inflammatory process. They can easily become involved and obstructed. B, bladder.

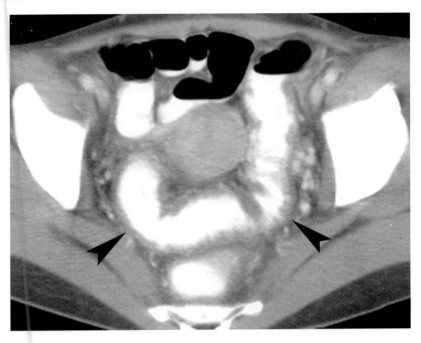

<u>FIGURE 17-34</u> **Ulcerative colitis.** The findings of ulcerative colitis on CT often are not dramatic. This scan demonstrates wall thickening *(arrowheads)* and pericolic inflammatory changes involving the sigmoid colon and rectum. These findings are indicative of colitis but are not specific for cause.

Mural thickening is usually in the range of 7 to 8 mm and commonly demonstrates the target or halo appearance. Narrowing of the rectal lumen with thickening of the rectal wall and widening of the presacral space are characteristic. Edematous stranding and mildly enlarged lymph nodes may be seen in the pericolic fat and mesocolon.

- *Crohn's colitis* is characterized by transmural inflammation that usually affects the terminal ileum and proximal colon, and then extends distally. Bowel wall thickening in Crohn's colitis is typically 10 to 20 mm compared with the 7 to 8 mm for UC. With Crohn's disease, the outer wall is irregular, whereas with UC the outer wall is smooth. Acute active disease shows layering of the colon wall (target and halo signs), whereas chronic disease with fibrosis show homogeneous enhancement of the colon wall. Fibrous and fat proliferation in the mesentery ("creeping fat") separates bowel loops with extensive fat-containing fibrous strands. Lymph nodes up to 1 cm are seen in the mesentery. Fistulas and sinus tracts are additional characteristics of Crohn's disease (Fig. 17-35). These may lead to intraabdominal abscesses, which occur in 15% to

20% of patients. Phlegmons are poorly defined inflammatory masses that occur in the mesentery or omentum.

- *Pseudomembranous colitis* results from overgrowth of *Clostridium difficile* in the colon as a complication of antibiotic therapy. A cytotoxic enterotoxin produced by the bacillus ulcerates the mucosa and creates pseudomembranes of mucin, fibrin, inflammatory cells, and sloughed mucosal cells. A pancolitis or segmental colitis with irregular wall thickening (up to 30 mm) and shaggy endoluminal contour is characteristic. Submucosal edema is marked resulting in the "accordion pattern" of disease that is characteristic of pseudomembranous colitis on CT (Fig. 17-36).
- *Typhlitis* or neutropenic colitis refers to a potentially fatal infection of the cecum and ascending colon in patients who are neutropenic and severely immunocompromised. It is classically seen in patients with leukemia who are undergoing chemotherapy. CT demonstrates marked wall thickening (10–30 mm), low-density edema with the cecal wall, and pericecal fluid and inflammation (Fig. 17-37). Colon wall ischemia leads to pneumatosis, necrosis, and perforation.

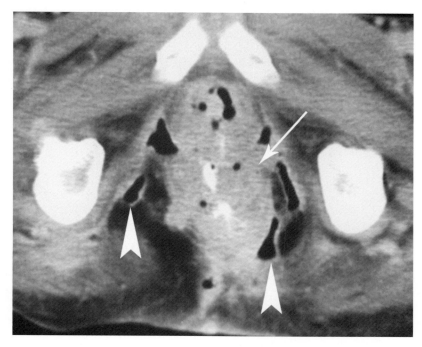

FIGURE 17-35 **Crohn's colitis: perianal fistulas.** CT shows marked irregular thickening of the wall of the rectum *(arrow)*, infiltration of the perirectal fat, and perianal fistulas extending into the ischiorectal fossa *(arrowheads)*. The presence of fistulas is typical of Crohn's colitis.

- *Ischemic colitis* occurs most commonly in the setting of low cardiac output in a patient with extensive but nonocclusive vascular disease. Most patients are older than 70 years. CT features are mild to moderate circumferential thickening of the colon wall in a segment of colon corresponding to an anatomic vascular distribution. Watershed areas at the splenic flexure and rectosigmoid are most commonly affected. Submucosal

edema produces the target or halo sign on postcontrast scans. Stranding and inflammation are seen in the pericolic fat. Hemorrhage and pneumatosis may occur in the bowel wall.
- *Radiation colitis* occurs only within the area treated by radiation. CT in the acute phase demonstrates mild wall thickening and pericolic stranding confined to the radiation port. Chronic radiation injury is seen 6

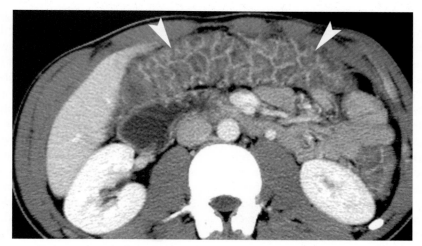

FIGURE 17-36 **Pseudomembranous colitis.** The transverse colon *(arrowheads)* demonstrates the "accordion pattern" of irregular wall thickening characteristic of *Clostridium difficile* colitis.

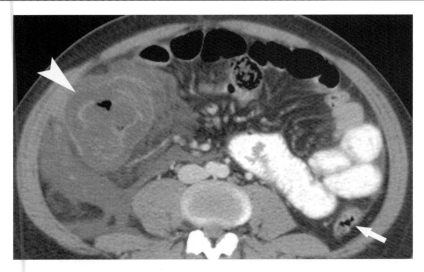

FIGURE 17-37 **Typhilitis.** The ascending colon *(arrowhead)* and cecum demonstrate dramatic wall thickening, poor enhancement, and pericolic fluid collections and edema. The descending colon *(arrow)* is unaffected. This patient was neutropenic from chemotherapy.

to 24 months after treatment and appears as mural thickening with prominent stranding in expanded pericolic fat. These findings are seen most often in the rectum and sigmoid in patients who have undergone pelvic radiation.

- *Infectious colitis* may be caused by bacteria (Shigella, Salmonella, Campylobacter, *Yersinia, Staphylococcus*), fungi (histoplasmosis, mucormycosis, actinomycosis), viruses (herpes, cytomegalovirus), parasites (amebiasis), or tuberculosis. Differentiation is based on clinical findings because CT findings are nonspecific. Wall thickening with homogeneous enhancement or wall edema affects all or portions of the colon. Inflammatory change is seen in pericolic fat. Air–fluid levels are seen in the colon because of increased volumes of fluid mixed with feces.
- *Enterohemorrhagic colitis* is caused by specific strain of E. coli most commonly acquired from undercooked ground beef. Patients present with cramps and watery diarrhea that progresses to bloody diarrhea. CT demonstrates wall thickening to 20 mm of segments of the colon with submucosal edema (target sign) and stranding of the pericolic fat.
- *Toxic megacolon* is a potentially fatal complication of many types of colitis. The CT hallmarks are dilatation of the colon (>5 cm) with thinning of the colon wall, pneumatosis, and perforation.

Pneumatosis Intestinalis and Ischemic Bowel

Pneumatosis intestinalis is the term applied to all cases of intramural intestinal gas. This is an imaging sign, not a diagnosis. At least 58 causative factors ranging from life threatening to insignificant have been reported. The major causes can be grouped into four categories. *Bowel necrosis* is the most important because it is life threatening. Bowel necrosis may occur with any cause of bowel ischemia, volvulus, necrotizing enterocolitis, typhilitis, or sepsis. *Mucosal disruption* related to peptic ulcers, endoscopy, enteric tubes, trauma, child abuse, UC, or Crohn's disease may cause pneumatosis. *Increased mucosal permeability* is associated with immunosuppression in AIDS, organ transplantation, chemotherapy, steroid therapy, or graft versus host disease. In *pulmonary conditions*, such as chronic obstructive pulmonary disease, asthma, cystic fibrosis, chest trauma, or mechanical ventilation, air from disrupted alveoli may dissect along the bronchopulmonary interstitium to the mediastinum and retroperitoneum to along the visceral vessels to the bowel wall. The key is to differentiate patients with pneumatosis indicative of significant disease from those in whom pneumatosis is an incidental finding. The clinical condition of the patient is key. Patients who are asymptomatic can be observed safely. Those who are critically ill with evidence of bowel ischemia require urgent surgery. Patients with bowel ischemia usually have predisposing con-

SUGGESTED READING

ABBARA S, KALAN MMH, LEWICKI AM: Intrathoracic stomach revisited. AJR Am J Roentgenol 181: 403–414, 2003.

APPLEGATE KE, SIVIT CJ, MYERS MT, PSCHESANG B: Using helical CT to diagnose acute appendicitis in children: Spectrum of CT findings. AJR Am J Roentgenol 176:501–505, 2001.

BA-SSALAMAH A, PROKOP M, UFFMAN M, et al: Dedicated multidetector CT of the stomach: Spectrum of diseases. Radiographics 23:625–644, 2003.

BERKOVICH GY, LEVINE MS, MILLER WT Jr: CT findings in patients with esophagitis. AJR Am J Roentgenol 175:1431–1434, 2000.

BETTS MT, HUO EJ, MILLER FH: Gastrointestinal and genitourinary smooth-muscle tumors. AJR Am J Roentgenol 181:1349–1354, 2003.

BIRNBAUM BA, WILSON SR: Appendicitis at the millennium. Radiology 215:337–348, 2000.

BUCKLEY JA, FISHMAN EK: CT evaluation of small bowel neoplasms: Spectrum of disease. Radiographics 18:379–392, 1998.

BUETOW PC, BUCK JL, CARR NJ, PANTONGRAG-BROWN L: Colorectal adenocarcinoma: Radiologic-pathologic correlation. Radiographics 15: 127–146, 1995.

CHOU CK: CT manifestations of bowel ischemia. AJR Am J Roentgenol 178:87–91, 2002.

FERRUCCI JT: Colon cancer screening with virtual colonoscopy: Promise, polyps, politics. AJR Am J Roentgenol 177:975–988, 2001.

FERRUCCI JT: Virtual colonoscopy for colon cancer screening: Further reflections on polyps and politics. AJR Am J Roentgenol 181:795–797, 2003.

FURUKAWA A, SAOTOME T, YAMASAKI M, et al: Cross-sectional imaging in Crohn disease. Radiographics 24:689–702, 2004.

FURUKAWA A, YAMASAKI M, FURUICHI K, et al: Helical CT in the diagnosis of small bowel obstruction. Radiographics 21:341–355, 2001.

GIMENEZ A, FRANQUET T, ERASMUS JJ, et al: Thoracic complications of esophageal disorders. Radiographics 22:S247–S258, 2002.

GORE RM, BALTHAZAR EJ, GHAHREMANI GG, MILLER FH: CT features of ulcerative colitis and Crohn's disease. AJR Am J Roentgenol 167:3–15, 1996.

HENG Y, SCHUFFER MD, HAGGITT RC, ROHRMANN CA Jr: Pneumatosis intestinalis: A review. Am J Gastroenterol 90:1747–1757, 1995.

HORTON KM, ABRAMS RA, FISHMAN EK: Spiral CT of colon cancer: Imaging features and role in management. Radiographics 20:419–430, 2000.

HORTON KM, CORL FM, FISHMAN EK: CT evaluation of the colon: Inflammatory disease. Radiographics 20:399–418, 2000.

HORTON KM, FISHMAN EK: Current role of CT in imaging of the stomach. Radiographics 23:75–87, 2003.

HORTON KM, KAMEL I, HOFMANN L, FISHMAN EK: Carcinoid tumors of the small bowel: A multitechnique imaging approach. AJR Am J Roentgenol 182:559–567, 2004.

HORTON KM, LAWLER LP, FISHMAN EK: CT findings in sclerosing mesenteritis (panniculitis): Spectrum of disease. Radiographics 23:1561–1567, 2003.

IYER RB, SILVERMAN PM, DUBROW RA, CHARNSANGAVE C: Imaging in the diagnosis, staging, and follow-up of colorectal cancer. AJR Am J Roentgenol 179:3–13, 2002.

IYER RB, SILVERMAN PM, TAMM EP, et al: Diagnosis, staging, and follow-up of esophageal cancer. AJR Am J Roentgenol 181:785–793, 2003.

JAYARAMAN MV, MAYO-SMITH WW, MOVSON JS, et al: CT of the duodenum: An overlooked segment gets its due. Radiographics 21:S147–S160, 2001.

KAWAMOTO S, HORTON KM, FISHMAN EK: Pseudomembranous colitis: Spectrum of imaging findings with clinical and pathologic correlation. Radiographics 19:887–897, 1999.

KIM H-C, LEE JM, KIM SH, et al: Primary gastrointestinal stromal tumors in the omentum and mesentery: CT findings and pathologic correlations. AJR Am J Roentgenol 182:1463–1467, 2004.

LEVY AD, REMOTTI HE, THOMPSON WM, et al: Gastrointestinal stromal tumors: Radiologic features with pathologic correlation. Radiographics 23: 283–304, 2003.

MACARI M, BINI EJ, JACOBS SL, et al: Filling defects at CT colonography: Pseudo- and diminutive lesions (the good), polyps (the bad), flat lesions, masses, and carcinomas (the ugly). Radiographics 23: 1073–1091, 2003.

MILLER FH, MA JJ, SCHOLZ FJ: Imaging features of enterohemorrhagic *Escherichia coli* colitis. AJR Am J Roentgenol 177:619–623, 2001.

NOH HM, FISHMAN EK, FORASTIERE AA, et al: CT of the esophagus: Spectrum of disease with emphasis on esophageal carcinoma. Radiographics 15:1113–1134, 1995.

PEAR BL: Pneumatosis intestinalis: A review. Radiology 207:13–19, 1998.

PICKHARDT PJ, CHOI JR, HWANG I, et al: Computed tomographic colonoscopy to screen for colorectal neoplasia in asymptomatic adults. N Engl J Med 349:2191–2200, 2003.

PICKHARDT PJ, LEVY AD, ROHRMANN CA Jr, KENDE AI: Primary neoplasms of the appendix: Radiologic spectrum of disease with pathologic correlation. Radiographics 23:645–662, 2003.

RAO PM: Technical and interpretative pitfalls of appendiceal CT imaging. AJR Am J Roentgenol 171:419–425, 1998.

RHA SE, HA HK, LEE S-H, et al: CT and MR imaging findings of bowel ischemia from various primary causes. Radiographics 20:29–42, 2000.

SHETH S, HORTON KM, GARLAND MR, FISHMAN EK: Mesenteric neoplasms: CT appearances of primary and secondary tumors and differential diagnosis. Radiographics 23:457–473, 2003.

WIESNER W, KHURANA B, JI H, ROS PR: CT of acute bowel ischemia. Radiology 226:635–650, 2003.

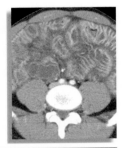

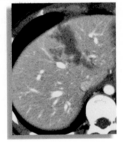

18

Pelvis

William E. Brant, M.D.

☐ ANATOMY

The true (lesser) pelvis is divided from the false (greater) pelvis by an oblique plane extending across the pelvic brim from the sacral promontory to the symphysis pubis. The true pelvis contains the rectum, bladder, pelvic ureters, and prostate and seminal vesicles in the male, or vagina, uterus, and ovaries in the female individual. The false pelvis is open anteriorly and is bounded laterally by the iliac fossae. It contains small bowel loops and portions of the ascending, descending, and sigmoid colon.

Muscle groups form prominent anatomic landmarks on CT. The psoas muscles extend from the lumbar vertebra through the greater pelvis to join with the iliacus muscles arising from the iliac fossa. The iliopsoas muscles exit the pelvis anteriorly to insert on the lesser trochanters of the femurs. The obturator internus muscles line the interior surface of the lateral walls of the true pelvis. Involvement of these muscles by pelvic tumors precludes surgical resection of the tumor. The piriformis muscles arise from the anterior sacrum and exit the pelvis through the greater sciatic foramen to insert on the greater trochanter of the femur. The piriformis forms a portion of the lateral wall of the true pelvis. The pelvic diaphragm, which is composed of the levator ani anteriorly and the coccygeus posteriorly, stretches across the pelvis to separate the pelvic cavity from the perineum. The pelvic diaphragm is penetrated by the rectum, urethra, and vagina.

The pelvis is divided into three major anatomic compartments (Figs. 18-1 and 18-2). These are important to understand because anatomic compartments allow determination of the origin and spread of disease. The *peritoneal cavity* extends to the level of the vagina forming the pouch of Douglas in female individuals, or to the level of the seminal vesicles forming the rectovesical pouch in male individuals. The *extraperitoneal space* of the pelvis is continuous with the retroperitoneal space of the abdomen. Pathologic processes from the pelvis may spread preferentially into the retroperitoneal compartments of the abdomen. The retropubic space (of Retzius) is continuous with the posterior pararenal space and the extraperitoneal fat of the abdominal wall. Fascial planes also allow communication with the scrotum and labia. The presacral space between sacrum and rectum normally contains only fat. Any soft-tissue density in this space is abnormal and must be explained. The *perineum* lies below the pelvic diaphragm. On CT, the most obvious portion of the perineum is the ischiorectal fossa. This fossa

355

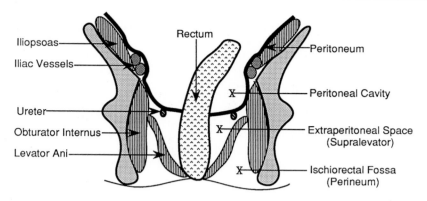

FIGURE 18-1 **Anatomic compartments of the pelvis.** Diagram of a posterior coronal section at the level of the rectum demonstrates the major anatomic compartments of the pelvis.

is seen as a triangular area of fat density extending between the obturator internus laterally, the gluteus maximus posteriorly, and the anus and urogenital region medially.

The arteries and veins define the location of the major lymphatic node chains in the pelvis

(Fig. 18-3). The aorta and vena cava divide to form the common iliac vessels at the level of the top of the iliac crest. The common iliac vessels divide at the pelvic brim, marked on CT by the transition between the convex sacral promontory and the concave sacral cavity. The internal

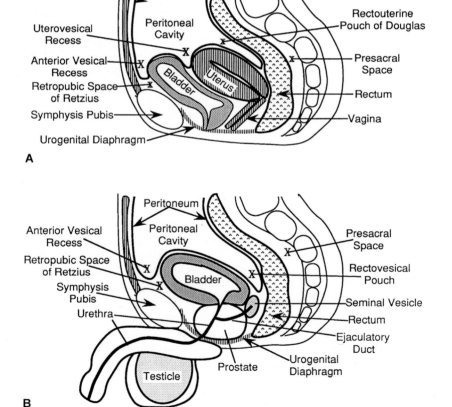

FIGURE 18-2 **Anatomic compartments of the pelvis.** Diagrams of midline sagittal planes through a female *(A)* and a male *(B)* pelvis demonstrate the pelvic compartments and peritoneal recesses and their relations to pelvic organs.

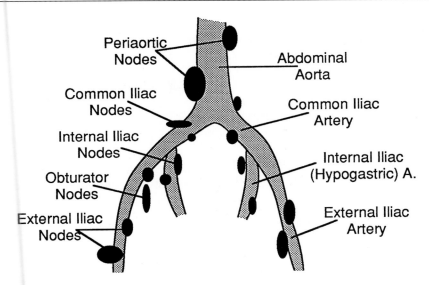

FIGURE 18-3 Pelvic lymph node chains. Diagram of the aortic bifurcation and the iliac arteries illustrates the classification and naming of pelvic lymph nodes.

iliac (hypogastric) vessels course posteriorly across the sciatic foramen dividing rapidly into smaller branches. The external iliac vessels course anteriorly adjacent to the iliopsoas to exit the pelvis at the inguinal ligament. Pelvic lymph nodes are classified with their accompanying vessels and are correspondingly named the common iliac, internal iliac, and external iliac nodal chains. The obturator nodes are satellites of the external iliac chain and course along the midportion of the obturator internus. Inguinal nodes in the subcutaneous tissue near the common femoral vessels drain the perineum but not the true pelvis. Pelvic lymph nodes are considered pathologically enlarged when they exceed 10 mm in short axis.

The bladder is best appreciated on CT when filled with urine or contrast agent. The normal bladder wall does not exceed 5 mm in thickness when the bladder is distended. The dome of the bladder is covered by peritoneum, whereas its base and anterior surface are extraperitoneal. The ureters course anterior to the psoas, cross over the common iliac vessels at the pelvic brim, pass on either side of the cervix, and insert into the bladder trigone. In male individuals, the ureters insert into the bladder just above the prostate at the level of the seminal vesicle.

The vagina is seen in cross section as a flattened ellipse of soft tissue between the bladder and rectum. An inserted tampon will outline the cavity of the vagina with air density and is useful in marking the vagina for pelvic CT. The

level of the cervix is recognized by the transition from the elliptical shape of the vagina to the rounded shape of the cervix. Contrast-filled ureters are frequently identified in close proximity to the cervix. The uterus is seen as a homogeneous, smooth-outlined oval of soft-tissue density. The myometrium is highly vascular, causing the uterus to enhance more than most pelvic organs. Assessment of the uterus on CT is made difficult by variation in position and flexion of the uterus and the amount of bladder filling. The broad ligament is a sheetlike fold of peritoneum that drapes over the uterus and extends laterally to the pelvic sidewalls. Between the leaves of the broad ligament is the *parametrium,* which is loose connective tissue and fat through which pass the fallopian tubes, uterine and ovarian blood vessels and lymphatics, the pelvic ureters, and the round ligament. Determination of tumor extension into the parametrium is an important part of gynecologic tumor staging. The fallopian tube forms the superior free edge of the broad ligament, best seen when outlined by ascites. The cardinal ligaments extend laterally from the cervix to the obturator internus muscles, forming the base of the broad ligament. The cardinal ligaments appear on CT as triangular densities extending laterally from the cervix. The round ligaments extend from the uterine fundus through the internal inguinal ring to terminate in the labia majora. Uterosacral ligaments extend in an arc from the cervix to the anterior sacrum. Uterine arteries branch from the hypogastric trunk and course in the parametrium just superior to the cardinal ligaments. Enhanced parametrial blood vessels are commonly prominent on bolus-enhanced CT scans. Normal ovaries are sometimes difficult to identify on CT. Because they are mobile, they may be anywhere in the pelvis, but they are most commonly seen adjacent to the uterine fundus. They appear as oval soft-tissue densities, approximately $2 \times 3 \times 4$ cm. The presence of cystic follicles allows positive identification of the ovaries.

The normal prostate gland is seen at the base of the bladder as a homogeneous, rounded, soft-tissue organ up to 4 cm in maximal diameter. Prostate zonal anatomy is not demonstrated by CT. A well-defined plane of fat separates the prostate from the obturator internus. This fat plane may be invaded by carcinoma. Denonvilliers' fascia provides a particularly tough barrier between the prostate and rectum, usually preventing spread of disease from one organ to the other. The paired seminal vesicles produce a characteristic "bow tie"–shaped, soft-tissue structure in the groove between the bladder base and the prostate. Normal testes are easily identified in the scrotum as homogeneous oval structures 3 to 4 cm in diameter. The spermatic cord can be recognized in the inguinal canal as a thin-walled oval structure of fat density containing small dots representing the vas deferens and spermatic vessels.

TECHNICAL CONSIDERATIONS

The ideal technique for CT imaging of the pelvis requires optimal bowel opacification. We give 500 mL dilute contrast agent orally the evening preceding the examination and repeat the dose 45 to 60 minutes before the examination. The colon and rectum can be distended by placing a tube in the rectum and insufflating with 20 puffs of air, or to the limit of patient comfort. All patients are asked to avoid urination for 30 to 40 minutes before the examination to allow bladder filling. Intravenous contrast medium is routinely given by mechanical injector at 2 to 3 mL/second for a total dose of 150 mL of 60% contrast agent. Scanning through the pelvis is performed with contiguous 3- to 5-mm-thick slices. We routinely scan the abdomen as well in patients with known or suspected pelvic malignancy. To optimize contrast medium enhancement of pelvic organs, we scan the pelvis first, then the abdomen.

BLADDER

Bladder Carcinoma

Bladder cancer may be superficial and confined to the mucosa. However, with invasion of the bladder wall musculature, risk for spread to regional and distant nodes increases. As the number and size of nodal metastases increases, so does the risk for hematogenous spread to bone and lung. CT is useful for the staging of advanced disease but is not accurate in defining early-stage disease. The key elements of staging are depth of tumor invasion into the bladder wall and the involvement of adjacent and distant sites by tumor. TMN staging has become the staging method most often used. Most (95%) malignant bladder tumors are transitional cell carcinomas that carry a risk for multiple synchronous tumors in the ipsilateral ureter and renal collecting system. Squamous cell carcinomas (5%) are usually associated with chronic inflammation. CT findings are as follows:

- The primary tumor appears as a focal thickening of the bladder wall or as a soft-tissue mass projecting into the bladder lumen (Fig. 18-4). Early postcontrast scans may demonstrate a weakly enhancing mural nodule on a background of low-attenuation urine. Delayed scans show a soft-tissue filling defect on a background of high-attenuation, contrast-opacified urine. Masses may be plaquelike, polypoid, or papillary.
- Calcifications are seen in 5% of transitional cell carcinomas.
- Perivesical spread is seen as soft-tissue density in the perivesical fat (Fig. 18-5). Extension to the pelvic sidewall precludes complete surgical resection.
- Pelvic lymph nodes larger than 10 mm in short axis are considered positive for metastatic disease. Smaller nodes are unlikely to be involved.
- Hematogenous metastases are most common in liver, lungs, bones, and adrenal glands.
- Rare bladder tumors to be considered in the differential diagnosis include pheochromocytoma, leiomyoma, lymphoma, sarcoma, and metastases.

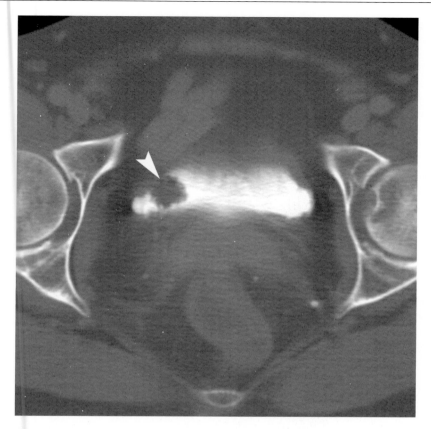

FIGURE 18-4 **Transitional cell carcinoma of the bladder: polypoid.** Bone windows provide the best visualization of a polypoid frondlike mass *(arrowhead)* projecting into the bladder lumen and seen as a filling defect within the intraluminal contrast material.

☐ UTERUS

Leiomyoma

Leiomyomas (fibroids) are found in up to 40% of women older than 30 years. As frequent findings, their CT features should be recognized; for example:

- Leiomyomas appear as homogeneous or heterogeneous masses that may be hypodense, isodense, or hyperdense relative to enhanced myometrium (Fig. 18-6). Diffuse enlargement of the uterus and lobulation of its contour are common.
- Coarse dystrophic mottled calcifications within the mass are common and characteristic.
- Cystic degeneration produces interior low density and may convert the mass into a large cavity.
- Pedunculated leiomyomas may appear as adnexal rather than uterine masses.

- Leiomyomas cannot be accurately differentiated from rare leiomyosarcomas by CT appearance alone. Rapid growth of a uterine mass in a postmenopausal woman suggests malignancy. Leiomyosarcomas appear as large masses with prominent, irregular, low-attenuation areas of necrosis and hemorrhage.

Carcinoma of the Cervix

Although CT has been used to stage cervical carcinoma, MR is preferable in most instances. CT is useful to stage advanced disease and to detect recurrence. Cervical malignancies are squamous cell carcinomas (85%) and adenocarcinomas (15%) that spread primarily by direct extension to adjacent organs and tissues. Lymphatic spread to regional nodes is common. Hematogenous spread to lung, bone, and brain is uncommon and occurs late in the course of disease. The accuracy of CT staging is in the

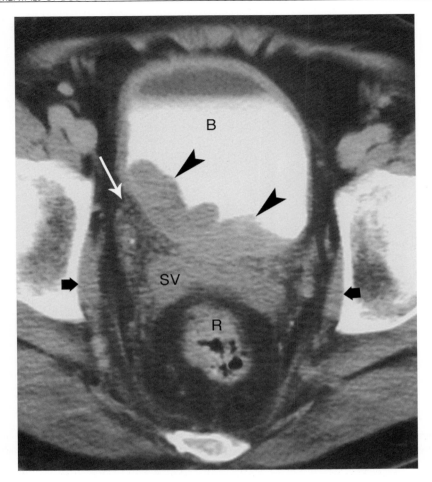

FIGURE 18-5 **Transitional cell carcinoma of the bladder: wall thickening.** Spreading tumor *(arrowheads)* thickens the bladder wall and projects into the bladder lumen (B) near the trigone. Tiny nodules and strandlike densities *(white arrow)* infiltrate the normal clear fat triangle between the bladder and the seminal vesicles (SV). In this case, the tumor did penetrate the bladder wall and infiltrate the perivesical fat. However, this finding is not a reliable indication of tumor spread. The obturator internus muscles *(black arrows)* are clearly not involved, indicating that this tumor is potentially resectable. Clear fat separates these muscles from the perivesical tumor nodules. R, rectum.

range of 58% to 88% compared with 70% to 100% reported for MR (Table 18-1). CT findings include:

- The normal cervix enhances variably on early postcontrast scans but is uniformly enhanced on scans obtained with a delay of several minutes. The primary tumor may be low attenuation or isoattenuating compared with normal cervix (Fig. 18-7). Low attenuation is caused by reduced vascularity, necrosis, or ulceration. The primary tumor may enlarge the cervix (>3.5 cm in diameter).
- Fluid collections in the uterine cavity, representing serous fluid, blood, or pus, are com-

mon because of tumor obstruction of the cervix.
- Spread of tumor by direct extension (Figs. 18-8 and 18-9) is seen as thick, irregular tissue strands or masses fanning out from the cervix into the parametrium often encasing the ureters, extending into the vagina, or to the pelvic sidewalls (obturator internus muscle). Normal broad, round, cardinal, and uterosacral ligaments should not be mistaken for tumor extension. Encasement of the ureter is a specific sign of parametrial invasion.
- Extension to the pelvic sidewall is indicated when tumor nodules are seen within 3 mm

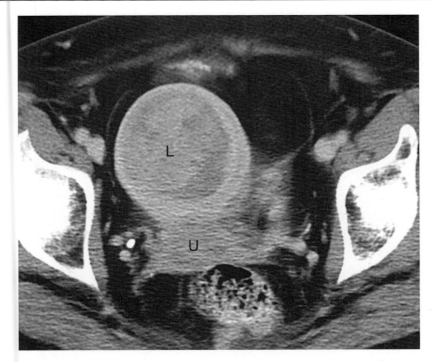

FIGURE 18-6 **Leiomyoma uterus.** A large leiomyoma (L) extends anteriorly from the uterus (U).

of the obturator internus or piriformis muscles. Tumor invasion is seen as an enhancing mass within enlarged muscles.

- Invasion of the bladder or rectum is indicated by loss of the perivesical or perirectal fat plane, nodular thickening of the wall of the bladder or rectum, or mass within the bladder or rectum. Air within the bladder suggests fistula formation.

- Enlarged lymph nodes (>10 mm in short axis) are strong evidence of metastatic involvement, but cervical carcinoma will commonly involve nodes without enlarging them. These small but involved nodes cannot be differentiated from benign nodes by CT.

- Recurrences appear as soft-tissue masses anywhere in the pelvis but most commonly

TABLE 18-1

Staging of Cervical Carcinoma (International Federation of Obstetrics and Gynecology 1995)

Stage	Description
0	Carcinoma in situ
I-A	Tumor confined to cervix; invasive cancer identified only microscopically
I-B	Clinically evident lesions confined to cervix
II	Tumor extends beyond cervix but not to pelvic sidewall or lower third of vagina
II-A	No parametrial invasion
II-B	Invades parametrium
III	Tumor extends to pelvic side wall, involves the lower third of vagina, or causes hydronephrosis or a nonfunctioning kidney
III-A	Invades lower third of vagina but does not extend to pelvic sidewall
III-B	Extends to pelvic side wall, or causes hydronephrosis or nonfunctioning kidney
IV-A	Tumor involves bladder or rectal mucosa
IV-B	Tumor spreads to distant organs

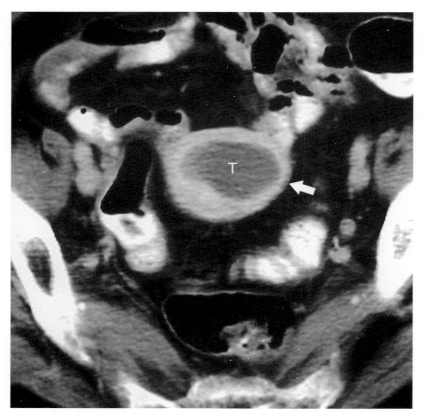

FIGURE 18-7 **Cervical carcinoma, stage IB.** Postcontrast CT demonstrates a squamous cell carcinoma of the cervix as a low-attenuation tumor (T) confined within the enhancing cervix. The cervical tissue is asymmetrically thinned on the left *(arrow)*, but the paracervical tissues are not invaded.

at the top of the vaginal vault in patients who have undergone hysterectomy. Enlarged nodes are also suggestive of recurrence. Percutaneous biopsy is usually needed to confirm the diagnosis.

Endometrial Malignancy

Carcinoma of the endometrium is the most common invasive gynecologic malignancy. Peak incidence occurs at 55 to 65 years of age. Most tumors (90%) are endometrioid adenocarcinomas. Clear cell and papillary serous subtypes are more aggressive. Müllerian mixed tumor is a sarcoma of the endometrium. The tumor spreads first by invasion of the myometrium, then by lymphatic channels to regional nodes, or by direct extension through the uterine wall to parametrial tissues. When the uterine serosa is penetrated, diffuse peritoneal spread may occur. Hematogenous spread to lung, bone, liver, and brain is much more common with endometrial than cervical cancer. Because the tumor is isodense with uterine tissue on unenhanced CT, all studies should be performed with intravenous contrast enhancement. CT staging is reported to be 58% to 88% accurate compared with 83% to 92% accuracy for MR. Surgical staging is the method of choice (Table 18-2). Imaging staging is useful in patients with advanced disease or patients who are difficult to examine. CT findings include:

- The primary tumor appears as a hypodense mass within the endometrial cavity (Fig. 18-10). The uterine cavity is frequently fluid filled because of tumor obstruction. The uterus may be greatly enlarged. The tumor typically enhances less than the surrounding myometrium.
- Depth of myometrium invasion is assessed on postcontrast images. The invading tumor is hypodense to enhanced myometrium. CT is only 58% to 61% accurate in evaluating depth of myometrial invasion.

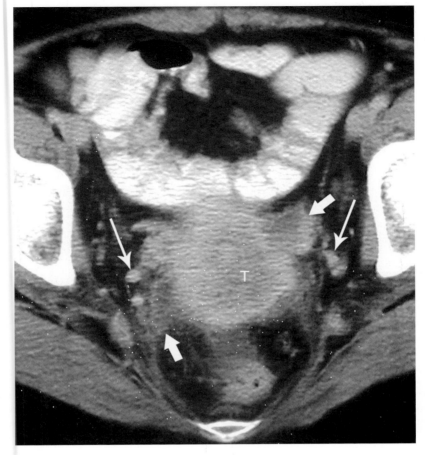

FIGURE 18-8 **Cervical carcinoma, stage IIB.** In this patient, the cervical tumor (T) is slightly lower in attenuation than the enhancing cervix. However, extension of tumor into the parametrium *(short arrows)* is apparent. Soft-tissue density approaches the ureters *(long arrows)* but does not involve them.

- Cervical invasion is indicated by heterogeneous enlargement of the cervix.
- Irregular uterine margins and strands and nodules of soft tissue extending into adjacent fat are evidence of parametrial invasion.
- Enlarged pelvic lymph nodes (>1 cm) indicate tumor involvement. However, as with other pelvic tumors, CT will miss microscopic nodal metastases that do not enlarge the nodes. CT can be used to guide percutaneous biopsy of suspicious lymph nodes.
- Müllerian mixed tumor is suggested by massive enlargement of the uterus, large areas of necrosis and hemorrhage within the tumor, and rapid growth of metastases.
- Tumor recurrences appear as pelvic soft-tissue masses or nodal enlargement. Most recurrences occur within 2 years.

☐ OVARY

Ovarian Cancer

Ovarian malignancy encompasses a wide range of histologic tumor types, but most share a common pattern of spread and similar range of CT appearances. Two thirds of ovarian cancers are cystic, 25% are bilateral, and 85% are endocrinologically nonfunctional. The primary route of tumor spread is diffusion throughout the peritoneal cavity, present in 70% of cases at the time of diagnosis. Direct extension to pelvic organs, lymphatic spread to nodes, and hematogenous spread to lung, liver, and bone also occur. Most patients will go directly to surgery for initial staging, hysterectomy, salpingo-oophorectomy, omentectomy, and tumor debulking without preoperative imaging. CT is, however, the imaging method of choice for documenting residual

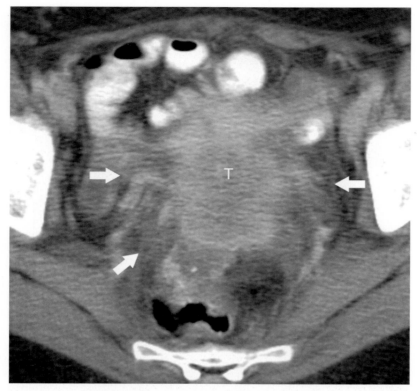

FIGURE 18-9 Cervical carcinoma, stage IIIB. Ill-defined tumor mass (T) of squamous cell carcinoma of the cervix shows extensive nodular stranding *(arrows)* of the parametrium, indicating tumor invasion. The left ureter was obstructed at this level indicating a stage IIIB lesion.

tumor response to therapy and for detection of postoperative recurrence. Magnetic resonance remains inferior to CT, primarily because of difficulty in differentiating intraperitoneal tumor from bowel. Staging accuracy of CT is 70% to 90% (Table 18-3). CT findings of ovarian malignancy include:

- The primary tumor is usually cystic with thick, irregular walls; internal septations; and prominent soft-tissue components (Fig. 18-11). Uniformly solid tumors and mixed cystic/solid tumors also occur. Calcifications may be evident in both the primary tumor and metastases.

TABLE 18-2

Staging of Endometrial Carcinoma (International Federation of Obstetrics and Gynecology 1988)

Stage	Description
0	Carcinoma in situ
I-A	Tumor growth limited to endometrium
I-B	Tumor invades <50% thickness of myometrium
I-C	Tumor invades ≥50% thickness of myometrium
II-A	Tumor invades endocervical glands
II-B	Tumor invades cervical stroma
III-A	Tumor involves adnexa or peritoneal fluid cytology is positive
III-B	Tumor invades the vagina
III-C	Tumor involves pelvic or para-aortic nodes
IV-A	Tumor involves bladder or rectal mucosa, extends beyond true pelvis, or both
IV-B	Distant metastases (outside of pelvis)

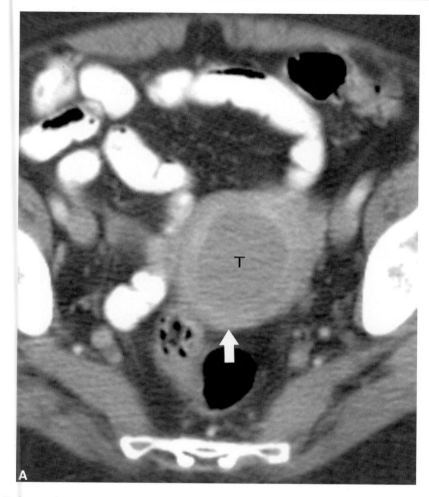

FIGURE 18-10 **Endometrial carcinoma, stage IB.** *A,* Low-density tumor mass (T) of endometrial carcinoma fills the uterine cavity. A few millimeters of posterior myometrium *(arrow)* were invaded by this neoplasm. *Continued*

- Tumor extension to adjacent pelvic organs is suggested by distortion or irregular interface between tumor and myometrium, obliteration of tissue planes between tumor and bladder or colon, less than 3-mm separation between tumor and intrapelvic muscles, and displacement or encasement of pelvic blood vessels.
- Direct tumor extension commonly involves the uterus, colon, small bowel, and bladder.
- Peritoneal implants are seen as often subtle, thickening, soft-tissue nodules or enhancement of peritoneal surfaces (see Figs. 9-4 to 9-6). Key areas to carefully examine include the undersurfaces of the diaphragm, the paracolic gutters, the cul-de-sac, and the surface of bowel. The presence of ascites makes peritoneal implants more evident on CT. "Omental cake" refers to irregular, often marked thickening of the greater omentum separating bowel from the anterior abdominal wall. The greater omentum, normally fat density, is soft-tissue density when involved by tumor. CT will commonly miss even extensive peritoneal seeding when the tumor nodules are small (<5 mm).
- Bowel involvement is evidenced by thickening of the bowel wall, matting together of bowel loops, and evidence of bowel obstruction.
- The presence of ascites usually indicates peritoneal spread even if peritoneal tumor nodules are not visualized.
- Lymphatic metastases usually follow gonadal lymphatics, skipping pelvic nodes, to involve nodes at the renal hilum.

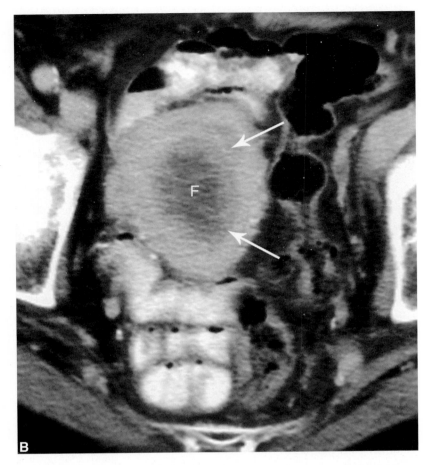

FIGURE 18-10 Cont'd *B*, In another patient, bloody fluid (F) is seen within the uterine cavity. Endometrial tumor *(arrows)* is intermediate in density between the dark fluid and the enhancing myometrium. This tumor also invades less than 50% thickness of the myometrium.

TABLE 18-3

Staging of Ovarian Carcinoma (International Federation of Obstetrics and Gynecology)

Stage	Description
I	Tumor limited to ovaries
I-A	Limited to one ovary, no malignant ascites
I-B	Limited to both ovaries, no malignant ascites
I-C	Stage I-A or I-B with malignant ascites
II	Tumor involves one or both ovaries with pelvic extension
II-A	Tumor involves uterus or fallopian tubes, no malignant ascites
II-B	Tumor extends to other pelvic tissues, no malignant ascites
II-C	Stage II-A or II-B with malignant ascites
III	Tumor involves one or both ovaries with peritoneal implants outside of the pelvis, retroperitoneal lymph node metastases, or both
III-A	Microscopic peritoneal implants outside of pelvis
III-B	Macroscopic peritoneal implants outside of pelvis 2 cm or less
III-C	Peritoneal implants outside of pelvis more than 2 cm or regional lymph node metastases
IV	Distant metastases including liver parenchyma

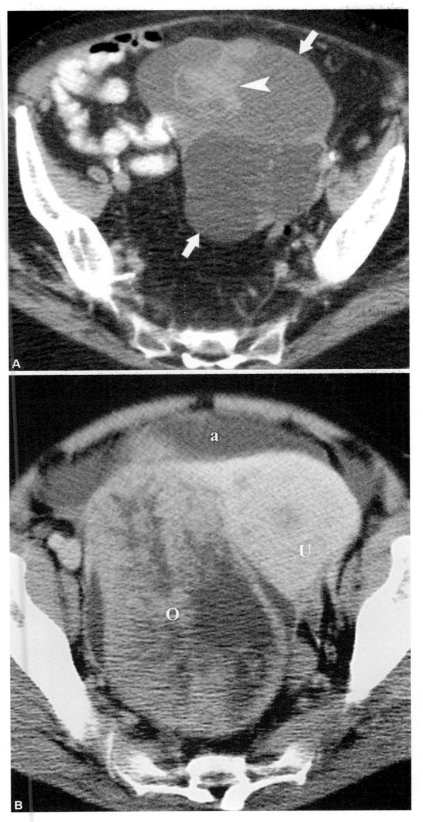

FIGURE 18-11 **Ovarian carcinoma.** *A*, A large, predominantly cystic mass *(arrows)* occupies the central pelvis. The mass contains septa of irregular thickness and a prominent lobulated solid component *(arrowhead)*, which are typical findings of ovarian carcinoma. *B*, A large mass (O) with predominant solid components arises from the right ovary and displaces the uterus (U) anteriorly and leftward. Ascites (a) is present, strongly indicating intraperitoneal spread of tumor.

Benign Adnexal Masses

Although ultrasonography is the primary imaging modality for female pelvic masses, adnexal masses may be discovered incidentally on CT. CT may also be used to further characterize difficult examinations. A few conditions to consider are:

- *Normal ovaries.* Normal ovaries are seen as oval soft tissue masses approximately $4 \times 3 \times 2$ cm in size. Follicles are best seen on postcontrast scans (Fig. 18-12). Visualization of follicles provides definitive identification of the ovary. Normal follicles are thin-walled, low-attenuation cysts smaller than 3 cm in size. Ovaries can be difficult to identify and may be confused with bowel, blood vessels, and lymph nodes.
- *Functional ovarian cyst.* Benign ovarian cysts, including follicular and corpus luteum cysts, are common incidental findings. On CT, they are well defined, are thin walled (<3 mm), have homogeneous internal density near water, and are less than 3 cm in size (Fig. 18-13). Atypical cysts can be re-examined with ultrasound to determine if they resolve after one or two menstrual cycles.
- *Benign cystic teratoma.* The presence of fat-density fluid, teeth, bone, hair, or fat–fluid levels allows definitive CT diagnosis in most cases (Fig. 18-14). Dermoid plugs are

conglomerations of tissue and hair seen as soft-tissue nodules inside the cysts.
- *Ovarian cystadenoma.* Benign ovarian tumors tend to have regular thin walls, fine septations, no solid components, and no associated ascites (Fig. 18-15). Definitive differentiation of benign from malignant cystic ovarian tumors is not possible with CT.
- *Endometriomas* arise from deposits of endometrial glands and stroma on peritoneal surfaces. Most (80%) arise on the ovary. The wall is initially thin but may thicken and become irregular with time. Internal contents are high in attenuation reflecting blood. Coexisting endometrial deposits on adjacent tissues may cause scarring and retraction simulating malignant disease.

Pelvic Inflammatory Disease

Pelvic inflammatory disease (PID) refers to infection and inflammation of the endometrium, fallopian tubes, and ovaries. Infection is caused by *Neisseria gonorrhoeae* or *Chlamydia trachomatis* or is polymicrobial. CT is commonly the initial imaging study. CT findings include:

- Early findings include thickening of the fallopian tubes and enlargement (edema) and abnormal enhancement of the ovaries.
- More advanced pelvic inflammatory disease presents with dilated fallopian tubes filled

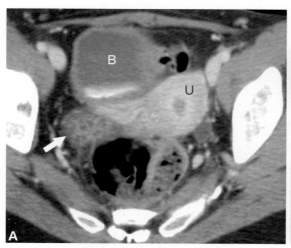
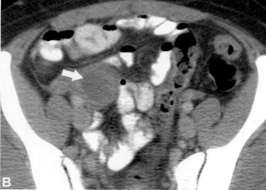

FIGURE 18-12 **Normal ovary.** *A,* A normal right ovary *(arrow)* containing numerous follicles is seen adjacent to the uterus (U) and posterior to the bladder (B). Administration of intravenous contrast has enhanced the walls of the follicles making them more visible than on noncontrast scans. *B,* In another patient, aged 34 years, a thin-walled, 2.5-cm cyst *(arrow)* is seen on the right ovary. This is a normal physiologic structure. No further evaluation or follow-up is necessary.

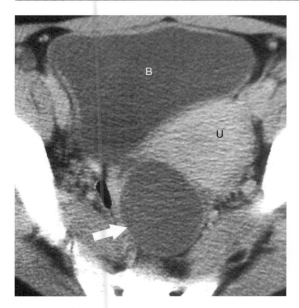

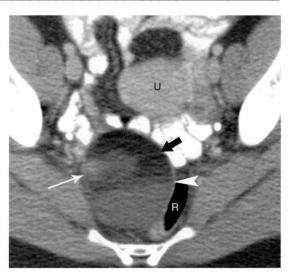

FIGURE 18-13 **Functional ovarian cyst.** CT shows a thin-walled, uniformly low-attenuation, 4.5-cm cyst *(arrow)* in the right adnexal adjacent to the uterus (U) and posterior to the bladder (B). These characteristics are most indicative of a functional ovarian cyst. Follow-up with ultrasound 10 weeks later confirmed complete resolution.

FIGURE 18-14 **Benign cystic teratoma.** A mass posterior to the uterus (U) and impinging on the rectum (R) is definitively characterized by CT to be a benign cystic teratoma. Fat-density fluid *(black arrow)* representing sebum is characteristic. Compare the density of the fluid to intrapelvic and subcutaneous fat. Suspended hair within the sebum produces a fluid level *(arrowhead),* and a dermoid plug *(white arrow)* produces a soft-tissue nodule.

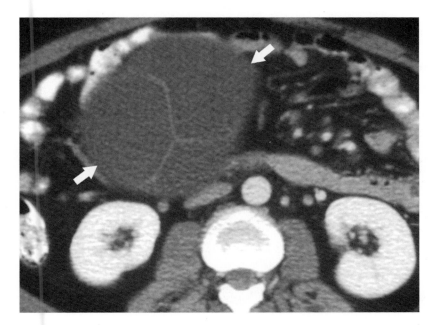

FIGURE 18-15 **Benign mucinous ovarian cystadenoma.** A large cystic mass *(arrows)* containing homogeneous low-attenuation fluid extends out of the pelvis. The outer walls are so thin as to be not discernible. Thin septa (<3 mm) are evident within the mass. Surgical removal and pathologic examination is needed to confirm a benign diagnosis.

with high-attenuation fluid (pyosalpinx) and complex fluid collections with septa, debris, fluid-fluid levels or gas in the adnexa. This inflammatory mass is called a tubo-ovarian abscess (Fig. 18-16).

- The inflammatory process may incorporate adjacent small or large bowel, obstruct the ureters, and inflame and thicken the bladder wall.

Adnexal Torsion

The ovary, fallopian tube, or both structures twist on the vascular pedicle causing vascular compromise. Torsion may be partial only impairing venous drainage, complete occluding arterial supply, or intermittent. Unrelieved torsion may result in hemorrhagic infarction of the ovary. Because patients present with often severe pain, CT may provide the initial images. CT findings of adnexal torsion include:

- Most cases of torsion involve an adnexal mass, most commonly a benign cystic teratoma, hydrosalpinx, or functional cyst. The wall of the mass thickens, and its contents may become hemorrhagic with torsion.
- Major findings are thickening of the wall of the fallopian tube, smooth thickening of the wall of the mass, ascites, and deviation of the uterus to the affected side.
- The twisted vascular pedicle may be visualized.

☐ PROSTATE

Benign Prostatic Hypertrophy

Benign prostatic hypertrophy results in nodular enlargement of the prostate with constriction of the urethra and obstruction to bladder emptying. It is indistinguishable from prostate

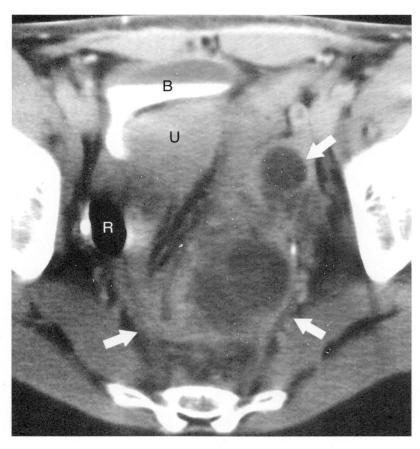

FIGURE 18-16 **Tubo-ovarian abscess.** A poorly marginated cystic and solid inflammatory mass *(arrows)* displaces the rectum (R), uterus (U), and bladder (B) anteriorly and rightward. The left ovary and dilated left fallopian tube are incorporated within the mass but are not definitively identified.

carcinoma on CT. CT findings of benign prostatic hypertrophy include:

- The prostate is enlarged and commonly has a lobulated contour (Fig. 18-17). Nodules may cause high- and low-density regions within the prostate with variable enhancement.
- Cystic degeneration and coarse calcifications are common.
- The bladder base is elevated and the prostate projects upward into the bladder lumen.
- Bladder wall thickening and trabeculation result from bladder outlet obstruction. Diverticula may project through the bladder wall.

Prostate Cancer

Prostate cancer is the second most common malignancy in male individuals. Prostate carcinoma spreads by direct extension to periprostatic tissues and the seminal vesicles. Lymphatic spread is similar to bladder cancer with early involvement of internal iliac and obturator nodes and later involvement of para-aortic nodes. Hematogenous spread to the axial skeleton via vertebral veins is particularly characteristic. CT does not demonstrate intraprostatic architecture and is poor at demonstrating intraprostatic tumor. CT staging of prostate cancer is neither sensitive nor specific enough to be clinically useful. CT findings include:

- Enlargement of the prostate is common and may be caused by benign prostatic hypertrophy, tumor growth, or both. Nodules or stranding densities in the periprostatic fat are signs of tumor extension outside the prostate gland.
- Asymmetric size of the seminal vesicles and infiltration of fat between the bladder base, prostate, and seminal vesicles are evidence of tumor involvement. Bladder involvement is difficult to detect accurately. Rectal invasion is rare.

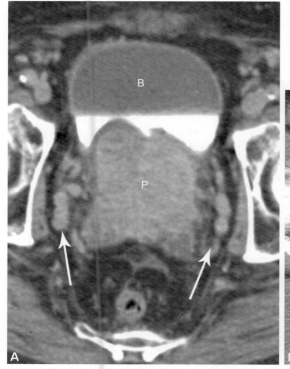
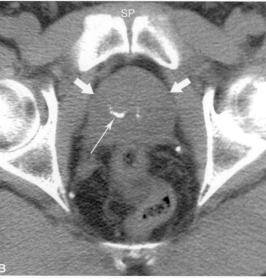

FIGURE 18-17 **Benign prostatic hypertrophy.** *A,* Delayed postcontrast CT shows a large heterogeneous prostate (P) bulging into the base of the bladder (B). The wall of the bladder shows mild hypertrophy reflecting outflow obstruction caused by prostatic enlargement. Prominent periprostatic vessels *(arrows)* are evident. This is a common and benign finding confirmed by documenting contrast enhancement of the venous structures. *B,* A noncontrast CT in another patient shows the characteristic course and linear calcifications *(thin arrow)* associated with benign prostatic hypertrophy and chronic prostatitis. The prostate *(fat arrows)* is mildly enlarged. The symphysis pubis (SP) is the anatomic landmark for the normal location of the prostate.

- Nodes larger than 10 mm are usually involved with metastatic tumor.

☐ TESTES

Testicular Cancer

Testicular germ cell tumors can be separated into seminomas and nonseminomas. Seminomas (40% to 50%) are treated with orchiectomy and radiation and generally do not require retroperitoneal node dissection. Nonseminomas are radioresistant, are treated with orchiectomy and chemotherapy, and generally do require retroperitoneal node dissection for staging. Lymphatic spread of tumor is most common, with nodal involvement following an orderly ascending pattern. Initial spread is along gonadal lymphatics following testicular veins to renal hilar nodes. Alternatively, lymphatic metastases may follow the external iliac chain to the para-aortic nodes. Internal iliac and inguinal nodes are generally not involved. Lymphatic spread to the mediastinum and hematogenous spread to the lungs rarely occurs without para-aortic disease, except for choriocarcinoma, which spreads hematogenously early. CT is 73% to 97% accurate for initial tumor staging and for

detection of recurrences. CT findings of testicular cancer include:

- Pelvic and retroperitoneal adenopathy is most pronounced on the side of involvement. Nodal enlargement near the ipsilateral renal hilum is particularly characteristic. Inguinal nodes are involved only when the scrotum is invaded by tumor. Bulky nodal mets may have low attenuation internally as a result of tumor necrosis.
- Absence of the spermatic cord identifies the side of orchiectomy.

Undescended Testes

Undescended testes may be located anywhere along the course of testicular descent from the lower pole of the kidney to the superficial inguinal ring. Undescended testes are at high risk for development of malignancy (48-fold risk) and for torsion (10-fold risk). CT is reported 95% sensitive for detection of ectopic testes. CT findings include:

- The undescended testis appears as an oval soft-tissue density up to 4 cm (Fig. 18-18).

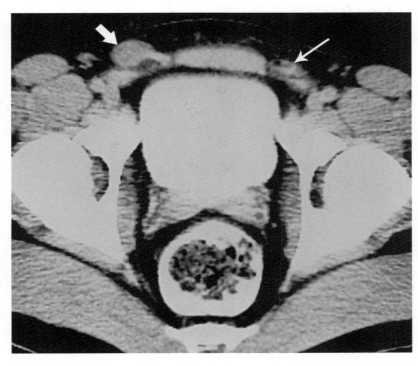

FIGURE 18-18 **Undescended testis.** An undescended testis *(fat arrow)* is seen in the right inguinal canal near the internal inguinal ring. A normal spermatic cord *(skinny arrow)* in the inguinal canal is seen on the left.

Undescended testes are usually atrophic. CT detection of intra-abdominal testes requires optimal bowel opacification and intravenous contrast medium enhancement to opacify normal structures.

- Testes in the inguinal canal can be easily identified on CT as long as you know where to look. The inguinal canal runs an oblique, medially directed course through the flat muscles of the abdominal wall between the deep and superficial inguinal rings. The deep (internal) inguinal ring is located midway between the anterosuperior iliac spine and the symphysis pubis. The superficial (external) inguinal ring is located just above the pubic crest.

SUGGESTED READING

CASILLAS J, JOSEPH RC, GUERRA JJ Jr: CT appearance of uterine leiomyomas. Radiographics 10:999–1007, 1990.

FOSHAGER MC, WALSH JW: CT anatomy of the female pelvis: A second look. Radiographics 14:51–66, 1994.

JEONG YY, KANG HK, CHUNG TW, et al: Uterine cervical carcinoma after therapy: CT and MR imaging findings. Radiographics 23:969–981, 2003.

JEONG YY, OUTWATER EK, KANG HK: Radiographics 20:1445–1470, 2000.

KUNDRA V, SILVERMAN PM: Imaging in the diagnosis, staging, and follow-up of cancer of the urinary bladder. AJR Am J Roentgenol 180:1045–1054, 2003.

PANNU HK, BRISTOW RE, MONTZ FJ, FISHMAN EK: Multidetector CT of peritoneal carcinomatosis from ovarian cancer. Radiographics 23:687–701, 2003.

PANNU HK, CORL FM, FISHMAN EK: CT evaluation of cervical cancer: Spectrum of disease. Radiographics 21:1155–1168, 2001.

RHA SE, BYUN JY, JUNG SE, et al: CT and MR imaging features of adnexal torsion. Radiographics 22:283–294, 2002.

RHA SE, BYUN JY, JUNG SE, et al: CT and MRI of uterine sarcomas and their mimickers. AJR Am J Roentgenol 181:1369–1374, 2003.

SAM JW, JACOBS JE, BIRNBAUM BA: Spectrum of CT findings in acute pyogenic pelvic inflammatory disease. Radiographics 22:1327–1334, 2002.

WOODWARD PJ, HOSSEINZADEH K, SAENGER JS: Radiologic staging of ovarian carcinoma with pathologic correlation. Radiographics 24:225–246, 2004.

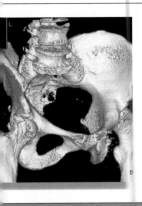

PART THREE

MUSCULOSKELETAL SYSTEM

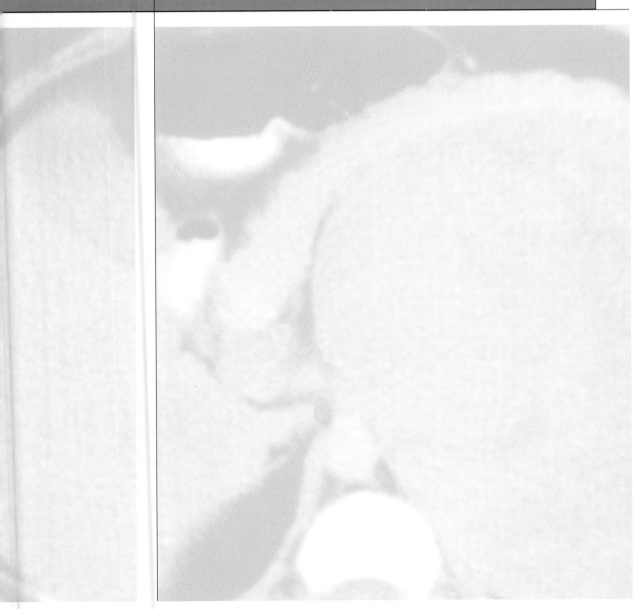

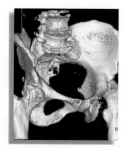

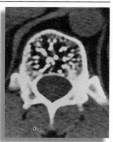

19

CT in Musculoskeletal Trauma

Nancy M. Major, M.D.

The use of CT in the musculoskeletal system has been markedly affected by the introduction of magnetic resonance imaging (MRI). Even though MRI has become the diagnostic modality of choice for many entities that were formerly imaged with CT, there continue to be areas where CT is superior and will remain appropriate. The advent of helical CT scanning has impacted the musculoskeletal applications, primarily in the setting of trauma, and availability of rapid, thin sections for re-formations and 3-D reconstructions. This chapter examines the use of CT in the musculoskeletal system for evaluation of trauma.

☐ TRAUMA

CT has proved to be extremely important in trauma, both in the axial (central) and the appendicular (peripheral) skeleton. MRI has been the modality of choice for evaluation of occult fractures, but CT has completely replaced conventional tomography in evaluating trauma to the skeleton.

Plain films are still used as the screening examination for spine trauma. However, CT should be performed to evaluate the extent of bony abnormality in spinal trauma. CT is often performed in conjunction with MRI, which can evaluate associated cord or nerve root injury in patients experiencing neurologic deficits. A CT (or MRI) examination is necessary regardless of the plain film findings when neurologic deficits are present. If no neurologic deficits are present, plain films are usually sufficient. However, if the plain films are nondiagnostic or raise questions that cannot be answered by the clinical examination, CT should be performed.

Spiral CT enables rapid acquisition of multiple thin-section images over a large area. The slice thickness will vary depending on the anatomic location in the spine, the number of vertebral body levels to be examined, and the need for re-formations. In general, thin slices (1.5 mm) will allow for more acceptable re-formations but are not recommended over large areas of the spine unless spiral CT is available, because of the enormous number of slices necessary to evaluate the area in question.

Re-formations, including three-dimensional (3-D) reconstructions, can be made rapidly with the currently available computer systems. In most instances of trauma, re-formations in at least one plane are recommended. 3-D reconstructions rarely aid in helping make the diagnosis, but many surgeons appreciate the overview and the different perspective that a 3-D image

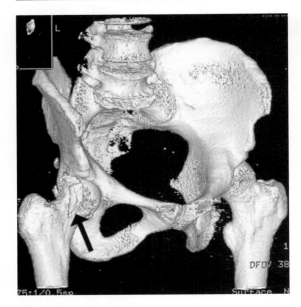

FIGURE 19-1 Three-dimensional (3-D) image of superior acetabular fracture. *Arrow* identifies the fracture. The diagnosis was readily made on the conventional radiograph, but the 3-D image was useful for the clinician in preoperative planning.

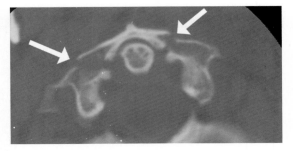

FIGURE 19-2 Jefferson fracture. Axial image through C1 vertebral body shows two obvious fractures of the bony ring *(arrows)* not clearly demonstrated on conventional radiography. Spinal fractures identified with conventional radiography should be further evaluated with CT.

allows. Two types of 3-D reconstructions exist: surface rendering and volume rendering. Surface rendering fails to show any detail deep to the surface of the bony structures and is believed by most not to produce as smooth or as true a depiction as volume rendering. Different investigators seem to prefer one type of rendering over the other for a variety of reasons having much to do with personal preference, as well as with which technique their computer software will allow. In general, volume rendering technique seems to be the more reliable method of 3-D reconstructions.

In general, 3-D reconstructions are performed when the surgeon requests it, usually for surgical planning. This is often done for fractures of the acetabulum, scapula, calcaneus, and complicated fractures of the pelvis (Fig. 19-1).

☐ SPINE

Cervical

A typical example of a cervical spine fracture that is more completely evaluated with CT is a Jefferson fracture, that is, a burst fracture of the C1 ring (Fig. 19-2). Any vertebral body fractures with bony fragments in the central canal should be examined with CT (Fig. 19-3).

Minor trauma can occasionally result in a fracture if there is an underlying bony abnormality present within the vertebral body such as metastatic disease (Fig. 19-4). CT can demonstrate the extent of bony involvement, as well as show the soft-tissue mass. These findings can also be seen with MRI.

Lumbar

Compression deformities of the lumbar spine are seen regularly on routine evaluation. When this observation is made in the setting of trauma, an acute fracture is difficult to exclude as a cause of this finding particularly if patients have pain

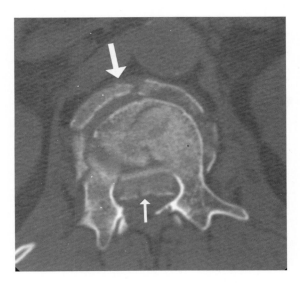

FIGURE 19-3 L1 burst fracture. Axial image through L1 vertebral body shows fractures through the vertebral body with extension into the posterior elements. A displaced fragment is noted extending into the central canal *(small arrow)*. Anteriorly, the outer margin of L1 is noted *(large arrow)*.

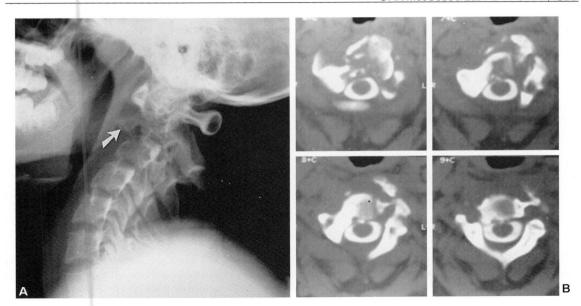

FIGURE 19-4 **Eosinophilic granuloma with a fracture.** *A,* Lateral C-spine film in a 12-year-old with neck pain shows disruption of the C2 vertebral body with a large fragment in the retropharyngeal space *(arrow).* *B,* Axial images from a CT myelogram show a comminuted fracture of C2 with effacement of the cerebrospinal fluid and mild mass effect on the cord.

referable to this area. If the pedicles appear wide on the conventional anteroposterior radiograph, that suggests the posterior elements are involved and the fracture is unstable. If there is no interpedicular widening, the patient is often treated with brace or corset immobilization when symptomatic. If neurologic symptoms are present, an MRI can be performed. In the lumbar spine, a common post-traumatic entity that is clearly shown with CT is spondylolysis (pars defect). Although many claim it is necessary to use sagittal re-formations to identify pars defects, the defect can be easily seen by examining the midvertebral body axial slice. Structures present at this level include the basivertebral plexus, which is always in the posterior aspect at the midvertebral body level, and the pedicles. On this slice, the lamina should be a continuous bony ring—any defect is a pars break (Fig. 19-5). A pars defect can be overlooked particularly if the defect is smooth along its margins resembling facet joints. For this reason, any break in the bony ring that occurs on the slice that has the basivertebral plexus is a spondylolysis until proved otherwise. Another way to determine if a pars defect is present is to recognize there should not be contiguous facet joints on all axial images through the vertebral body. If facet joints are noted on each image, a pars defect is likely.

An uncommon but potentially serious sequela of spondylolysis is a fibrocartilaginous mass that can develop at the pars defect or fracture site to such a degree that it encroaches on the thecal sac or nerve roots (Fig. 19-6). This

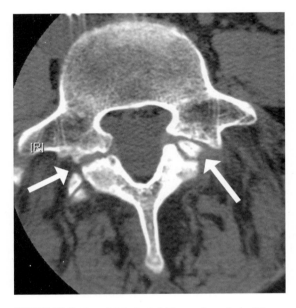

FIGURE 19-5 **Spondylolysis.** Axial image through the L5 vertebral body shows linear disruption of the lamina *(arrows)* bilaterally. On the mid-body image through the vertebral body, a complete bone ring should be present. Right facet joint is noted adjacent to the pars break.

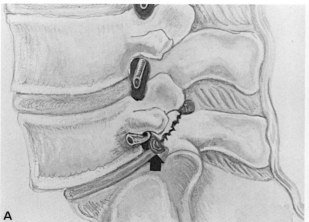
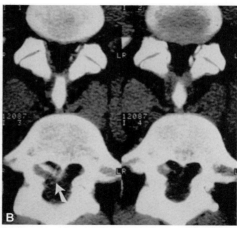

FIGURE 19-6 Fibrocartilaginous mass at spondylolysis. *A,* Drawing showing how a fibrocartilaginous mass *(arrow)* at pars break can impinge on a nerve root in the neuroforamen. *B,* Axial CT image through L5 in a patient with spondylolysis, and spondylolisthesis shows a soft-tissue mass in the central canal *(arrow)* that has encroached on the right lateral recess and the thecal sac. This can be readily identified on magnetic resonance imaging performed for the evaluation of disc disease.

mass is a potential source of symptoms and should be searched for in patients who have a pars defect. If not recognized, a surgical fusion across that level would result in missing what could be the main cause of the patient's symptoms. This fibrocartilaginous mass has been likened to excess callus that can occur across a long bone fracture that has been inadequately immobilized.

In conclusion, evaluation of a fracture of the spine identified on plain films requires CT with re-formations. CT is also recommended in the setting of inadequate plain films, neurologic deficits, or both.

☐ PELVIS/HIP

A fracture that can be mistaken for metastatic disease is an insufficiency fracture of the sacrum. This is found primarily in two types of patients: patients with osteoporosis and patients who have had prior radiation to the pelvis. Patients with these insufficiency fractures present with low back or sacral pain and may have a normal plain film or a plain film that shows patchy sclerosis of one or both sacral alae (Fig. 19-7). A radionuclide bone scan is characteristic and should be pathognomonic because of its geographic appearance throughout half (unilateral fracture) or all of the sacrum (bilateral fracture) (see Fig. 19-7*B*). The fracture line generally parallels the sacroiliac joint. Stress fractures of

the sacrum can occur as a result of athletics and have been reported in long-distance runners. These individuals generally have normal bone density and are often misdiagnosed as having disk disease. CT can show the fracture line paralleling the sacroiliac joint or increased sclerosis representing callus formation.

CT of the hip is routinely done in most centers when loose bodies are considered or when the position of fracture fragments needs to be determined precisely (Fig. 19-8). In instances where metal might be present in the joint (bullets, shrapnel, or fixation pins or screws from surgery), CT can still be used, with useful information almost always obtained despite metallic streak artifacts (Fig. 19-9). Re-formations often diminish the metallic streak artifact, making interpretation less difficult. It is important in patients who have sustained hip dislocations to have CT performed after the reduction to assess for fracture fragments or loose bodies in the joint space. The presence of these findings, if not recognized and treated, will lead to irregular articulation and accelerated wear of the cartilage in the joint.

☐ EXTREMITIES

Fractures of the scapula, with or without glenohumeral dislocation, are studied with CT if the plain films do not clearly show all the abnormalities or if it is thought that some aspect of the

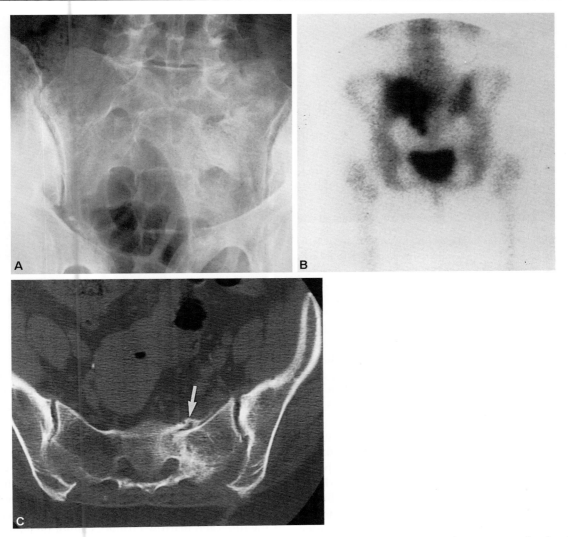

FIGURE 19-7 **Sacral insufficiency fracture.** *A,* Conventional radiograph of the sacrum in an elderly woman demonstrates patchy sclerosis in the left sacral ala. *B,* Posterior view of radionuclide bone scan shows geographic uptake corresponding to the left sacral ala and body. This is a characteristic appearance of a sacral insufficiency fracture on radionuclide bone scan imaging. *C,* Axial CT image demonstrates a fracture *(arrow)* with reactive sclerosis in the ala.

anatomy is not depicted (Figs. 19-10 and 19-11). Re-formations and 3-D reconstruction can depict the extent of the fractures to determine surgical planning. MRI is currently the best way to evaluate the sequelae of glenohumeral dislocation. This modality depicts injury to the soft-tissue structures in addition to the bony injuries. However, if a patient has contraindications for MRI, a CT "double-contrast" study can be performed. The technique begins like a routine shoulder arthrogram, with a needle placed into the glenohumeral joint near the axillary recess. Instead of the standard 10 mL contrast medium placed into the joint, only 1.5 to 2 mL is instilled, together with 0.25 mL 1:10,000 epinephrine and 10 mL air. The epinephrine will delay absorption of the contrast agent to allow for possible delays in completing the CT scan. The needle is removed, and the patient is instructed to move the shoulder through a full range of motion to adequately coat the joint. Plain films are obtained and reviewed to look for leakage of air or contrast medium into the subacromial bursa, which would be diagnostic for a rotator cuff tear. The

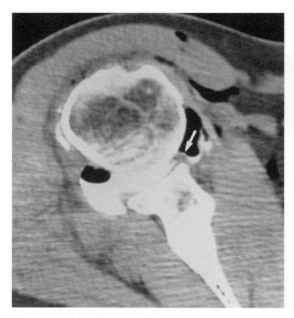

FIGURE 19-12 Normal CT arthrogram of the shoulder. Double-contrast (air and iodinated contrast) axial CT image shows a normal-appearing labrum (arrow).

fication. CT is preferred over MR when assessing myositis ossificans, because the appearance on MRI can mimic a sinister lesion (Figs. 19-17 and 19-18).

☐ CONCLUSION

In summary, CT is a necessary examination in the setting of spinal trauma for evaluation of fractures. The examination can be coupled

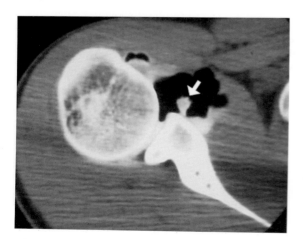

FIGURE 19-13 CT arthrogram of torn labrum. Double-contrast axial CT image shows a labral detachment (arrow) from the underlying glenoid.

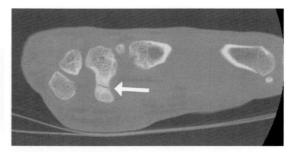

FIGURE 19-14 Fractured hamate bone. Sagittal CT image of the wrist in a patient with wrist pain after falling on an outstretched hand. Fracture of the body of the hamate bone (arrow) is clearly visualized. Conventional films were normal.

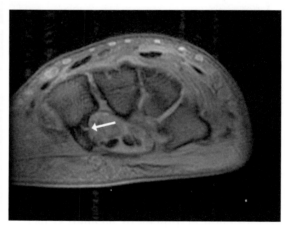

FIGURE 19-15 Magnetic resonance imaging of hamate fracture. T1-weighted axial image shows fracture of the hook of hamate (arrow).

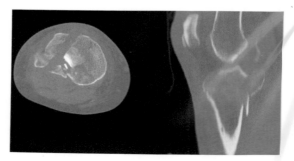

FIGURE 19-16 Tibial plateau fracture. Axial and reformatted sagittal CT images shows a complex fracture of the tibial plateau involving multiple parts and the joint space.

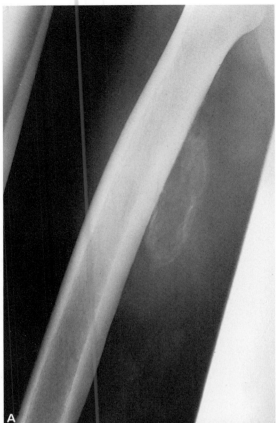

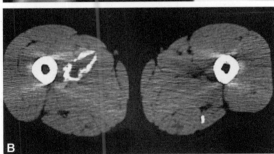

FIGURE 19-17 **Myositis ossificans.** *A,* Conventional film of the thigh in a young patient with pain and swelling shows a calcific mass. The patient could not recall any recent trauma to this area. *B,* CT through the mass shows peripheral, circumferential calcification characteristic of myositis ossificans. Biopsy of myositis ossificans can resemble a sinister diagnosis.

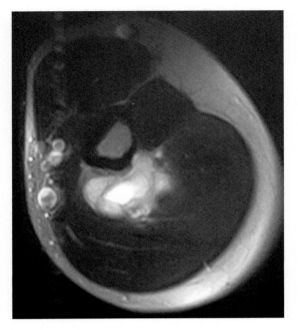

FIGURE 19-18 **Magnetic resonance imaging (MRI) of myositis ossificans.** T2-weighted axial image shows heterogeneous signal intensity. The appearance on MRI is nonspecific for myositis ossificans and can mimic a sarcoma.

with MRI when the patient has neurologic deficits. In evaluation of the shoulder girdle, hip and pelvis, and complex extremity fractures, CT has shown great utility in evaluating the extent of fractures and identifying intra-articular pathology.

SUGGESTED READING

BEARCROFT PW: The use of spiral computed tomography in musculoskeletal radiology of the lower limb: The calcaneus as an example. Eur J Radiol 28:30–38, 1998.

BOHNDORF K, KILCOYNE RF: Traumatic injuries: Imaging of peripheral musculoskeletal injuries. Eur Radiol 12:1605–1616, 2002.

BUCKWALTER KA, RYDBERG J, KOPECKY KK, et al: Musculoskeletal imaging with multislice CT. AJR Am J Roentgenol 176:979–986, 2001.

NEY DR, FISHMAN EK, KAWASHIMA A, et al: Comparison of helical and serial CT with regard to three-dimensional imaging of musculoskeletal anatomy. Radiology 185:865–869, 1992.

PRETORIUS ES, FISHMAN EK: Spiral CT and three-dimensional CT of musculoskeletal pathology. Emergency room applications. Radiol Clin North Am 37:953–974, vi, 1999.

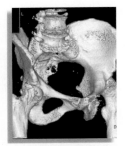

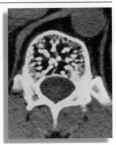

CT in Musculoskeletal Nontrauma

Nancy M. Major, M.D.

20

☐ DISK DISEASE

CT provides the capability of examining in detail not only the disks but also all of the bone and soft-tissue structures in and about the spine, including the facets, the neuroforamen, the thecal sac and nerve roots as they exit the thecal sac, the ligamentum flavum, and the vascular structures. This chapter discusses how CT can be used to diagnose disk disease and spinal stenosis in the lumbar spine. CT essentially has been replaced by magnetic resonance imaging (MRI) for routine evaluation of disk disease and back pain. Multiple studies have shown that MRI is just as good at identifying pathology as CT without the ionizing radiation. CT is useful particularly in the postoperative spine where the imaging artifact from metal can be more problematic on MRI than CT. CT in this setting can evaluate bone fusion mass, as well as residual stenosis. Many centers still perform myelography with CT in patients after surgery. A few studies have been performed comparing the accuracy of diagnosis of plain CT versus myelographic enhanced CT. These show no statistical differences between the two techniques.

CT can be readily performed in a patient who is not MRI compatible who needs evaluation of the spine. In this setting, myelography is

not necessary because pathology is clearly depicted without the myelogram.

Technical Considerations

The proper imaging protocol for a diagnostic lumbar spine study is critical to reduce the chances of missing an abnormality. The patient should be studied in the supine position with the knees flexed over a pillow or other similar object. Anteroposterior and lateral scout films are obtained. The anteroposterior scout film allows the radiologist to determine if transitional vertebrae are present. Recognizing and correctly identifying the levels in the lumbar spine can prevent surgery at the wrong level. The lateral scout view is used to place the cursors over the intended area of scanning. This should include contiguous slices, no thicker than 5 mm from the midbody of L3 to the top of S1. Ten percent of disk protrusions occur at the L3–4 level, and they can clinically mimic protrusions from lower levels; therefore, the L3–4 level must be examined. Some institution's spine protocols perform angled-gantry slices parallel to each vertebral body end plate (Fig. 20-1). This is not advised for two reasons. This leaves spaces or gaps in the central canal that are not imaged that can result in missed free fragments of disk material and

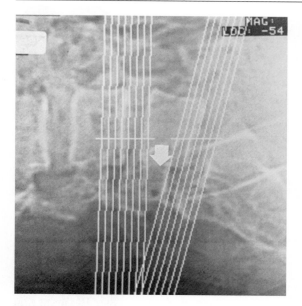

FIGURE 20-1 **Inappropriate scanning protocol.** This lateral scout view has the gantry angled parallel to the L5-S1 end plate with several slices above and below. This is repeated at the L4–5 level. A small but definite space or gap is present between the levels *(arrow)* where a free fragment or spinal stenosis could be missed. In addition, it is mandatory to study the L3–4 level, because up to 10% of disk protrusions occur at this level.

pars defects (spondylolysis), which occur at the midvertebral body level. Second, changing the angle of the gantry will not produce or eliminate disk protrusions with mass effect on the thecal sac. A reasonable protocol is 3-mm-thick slices from the midbody of L3 in a contiguous axial fashion through S1 (Fig. 20-2).

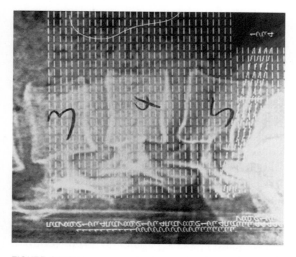

FIGURE 20-2 **Proper scanning protocol.** This lateral scout view has straight axial 3-mm-thick slices from L3 to S1 without gaps. This is an adequate protocol for evaluation of disk disease or spinal stenosis.

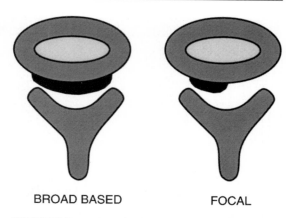

BROAD BASED   FOCAL

FIGURE 20-3 Schematic of focal versus broad-based disk protrusions. A broad-based disk protrusion has a uniform bulge that extends across the entire central canal. A focal protrusion extends only into a portion of the central canal.

Each image should be obtained in bone and soft-tissue windows. It is not accurate to diagnose facet disease or other bony abnormalities from a soft-tissue window image.

Pathology

Terminology is important when evaluating disk disease in the lumbar spine. When a disk bulges or protrudes beyond the end plate, it takes on several names, some of which have more sinister connotations than others. The terms *herniated nucleus pulposus* and *bulging annulus fibrosus* are often mentioned, together with "contained," "extruded," and "sequestered" disks. Terminology is probably not as important as recognizing the pathology and distinguishing a bulge from a sequestered or free fragment (Fig. 20-3). Use terminology that the surgeons at your institution prefer. Disk bulges can be diffuse, broad based, or focal. When disk material migrates from the parent disk, it is termed a *sequestered* or *free fragment.* The surgeon wants to know if disk material of any kind is pressing against neural tissue.

If a disk does impress the thecal sac or a nerve root (Fig. 20-4), it may or may not be symptomatic. Surgeons know it has to be matched with the clinical findings. A large disk protrusion with marked thecal sac impression (Fig. 20-5) is much more likely to be symptomatic.

A large disk protrusion should make one suspicious for a sequestration or free fragment. The largest cause for failure of a percutaneous diskectomy procedure and a not infrequent cause for failed surgical microdiskectomy proce-

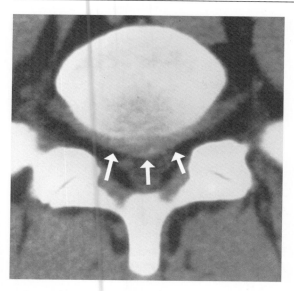

FIGURE 20-4 Small disk protrusion. Axial CT image shows a predominantly broad-based disk protrusion not impressing the thecal sac or nerve roots *(arrows)*. It is therefore a disk protrusion that would not be expected to be symptomatic.

dures is a missed free fragment. A free fragment should be suggested any time disk material is identified in the cut above or below the disk level (Fig. 20-6). If a soft-tissue density is identified above or below the disk space, it should be determined if it is of a similar density as the

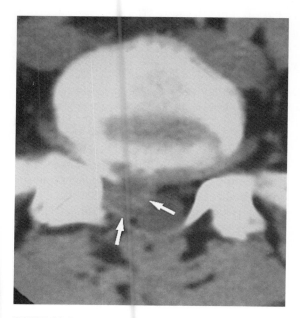

FIGURE 20-5 Disk protrusion with thecal sac impression. Axial CT image shows a focal-based disk protrusion moderately impressing the thecal sac. This disk protrusion may or may not be symptomatic.

thecal sac or if it is of a higher density. If it is clearly a higher density, it is disk material and should be considered a free fragment.

If the soft-tissue density above or below the disk space is isodense to the thecal sac, then it is not a free fragment and is most likely either a Tarlov cyst or a conjoined nerve root. A Tarlov cyst is merely an enlarged nerve root sheath. It is a normal variant and not a cause of any symptoms. It can get quite large and because of persistent pulsations from the cerebrospinal fluid can cause bony erosion (Fig. 20-7). A Tarlov cyst has also been termed a *perineural cyst.*

A conjoined root is a congenital anomaly of two nerve roots exiting the thecal sac together instead of separately (Fig. 20-8). The two roots run in the lateral recess together and appear as a soft-tissue density on CT. A free fragment can have the same appearance but will have an increased density as compared with the thecal sac (Fig. 20-9), whereas a conjoined root will be isodense to the thecal sac. The roots will invariably exit through their appropriate foramen; hence, it is unusual to have an "empty" foramen. Also, the conjoined roots are always associated with a slightly wider lateral recess than the opposite side. Conjoined roots occur in 1% to 3% of all patients and are incidental findings with no reported symptomatology. The reason to recognize them is to not erroneously call these normal variants disk protrusions. Many patients have had neural damage at surgery because of failure to recognize two roots in an area where there is normally only one. Also, many patients have had explorations for "free fragments" when there was a conjoined root mimicking a free fragment. By noting the density differences between the "mass" and the thecal sac, errors can be avoided. Therefore, it is inappropriate to list a differential diagnosis of free fragment, conjoined root, or Tarlov cyst when a soft-tissue mass is found in a lateral recess.

A lateral disk is a disk protrusion that occurs lateral to the neuroforamen (Fig. 20-10). It is one of the more commonly missed disk protrusions simply because it is overlooked. The usual search pattern examines the thecal sac/disk interface and not the area lateral to the foramen. A lateral disk has huge implications for the surgeon. First, a lateral disk will irritate a nerve root that has already exited the neuroforamen and will therefore mimic a disk protrusion at a more cephalad level (Fig. 20-11). For instance,

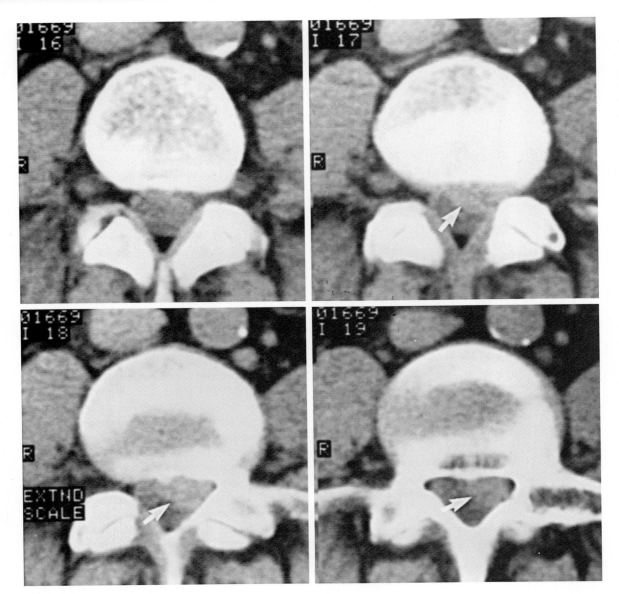

FIGURE 20-6 **Free fragment.** Contiguous axial images show an extremely large, focal, left-sided disk protrusion *(arrows)* that is impressing the left-sided nerve root and thecal sac. This disk also has a broad-based component that is not touching the thecal sac or nerve roots.

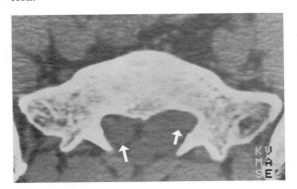

FIGURE 20-7 **Tarlov cyst.** Axial image through the sacrum shows large dilatations of the nerve root sheaths that are causing some erosion into the vertebral body. The cysts are filled with cerebrospinal fluid and are the same density as the thecal sac.

if a disk protrudes posteriorly at the L4–5 level, it will usually press against the L5 root; therefore, if a patient presents with signs and symptoms of an L5 root irritation, the L4–5 level is usually the surgical level because of a disk bulge at that level. However, the L5 root can also be irritated from a lateral disk protrusion at L5-S1. Therefore, if overlooked, it can result in surgery at the wrong level, especially in a patient with disk abnormalities at multiple levels for whom the clinical presentation is relied on to determine which level should be operated on. Another important surgical implication for lateral disks is that a lateral disk does not require a laminectomy because it can be approached from outside the

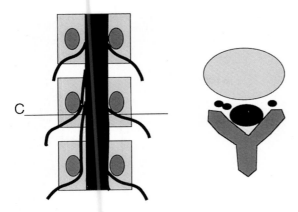

FIGURE 20-8 **Drawing of a conjoined root.** Two nerve roots have arisen from the thecal sac on the right side in an asymmetric manner as compared with the left. When a CT cut is made at the level of the cursor (C), two roots are visualized on the axial cut on the right side, one of which could be confused for a free fragment. They will be lower in density than disk material, however.

bony central canal. The location of a lateral disk is not in an area the surgeon would normally explore. Lateral disks occur in less than 5% of patients but should be searched for in every patient at each disk level.

☐ **SPINAL STENOSIS**

Spinal stenosis has been classically divided into two types: congenital and acquired. Patients who experience congenital stenosis include achondroplastic dwarfs, patients with Morquio's disease, and individuals born with a congenitally small thecal sac who have idiopathic spinal stenosis. Acquired stenosis includes degenerative joint disease with or without degenerative disk disease, post-traumatic stenosis, postsurgical stenosis, Paget's disease, and calcification of the posterior longitudinal ligament. In reality, almost no one ever presents clinically with spinal stenosis unless some component of acquired stenosis is present. Even the most severe form of congenital stenosis, achondroplasia, does not have clinical signs and symptoms until osteoarthritis or degenerative disk disease ensues in early adulthood secondary to an accentuated lordosis (Fig. 20-12).

A preferred classification for spinal stenosis is on an anatomic basis. Stenosis is described as central canal stenosis, neuroforaminal stenosis, and lateral recess stenosis. In each of these areas the most common cause is degenerative joint disease or degenerative disk disease.

Central Canal Stenosis

For decades, radiologists have been asked to measure the central canal to diagnose spinal stenosis. We often encounter patients with bony measurements that are small but have small neural components as well (Fig. 20-13). For stenosis to be clinically manifest, there

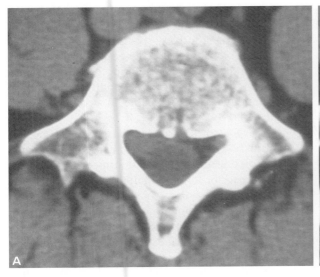
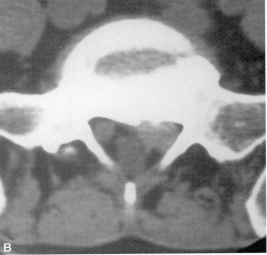

FIGURE 20-9 **Conjoined root and free fragment at different levels in the same patient.** *A,* Axial CT image through the midbody of L4 shows a soft-tissue density in the right lateral recess that is isodense to the thecal sac. This is a conjoined root. *B,* In the same patient, a CT cut through the L5-S1 disk level shows a soft-tissue density in the left lateral recess that is denser than the thecal sac. This is a large free disk fragment.

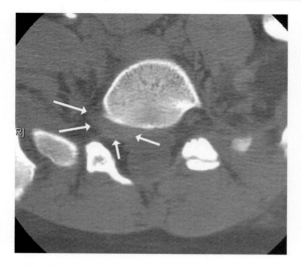

FIGURE 20-10 **Lateral disk.** Axial CT image through L5-S1 level shows a soft-tissue mass on the right side just lateral to the neuroforamen *(arrows).*

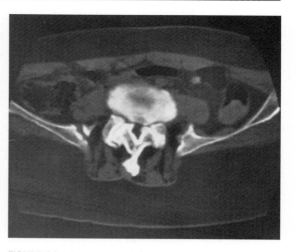

FIGURE 20-12 **Achondroplasia with severe stenosis.** Severe central canal stenosis occurs in patients with achondroplasia because of the congenital stenosis combined with severe degenerative facet disease.

must be a discordance in the size of the bony canal and the thecal sac. Simply measuring the central canal will not address the "fit" of the thecal sac in that canal; hence, measurements are virtually worthless. The only exception to this may be in the cervical spine where a narrow central canal has been correlated to an increased risk for cord injury in football players.

The most useful CT criteria for diagnosing central canal stenosis are obliteration of the epidural fat (Fig. 20-14) and flattening of the thecal sac (Fig. 20-15). Both of these findings can be present without symptoms of spinal stenosis; therefore, stenosis can only be suggested by the radiologist, with clinical correlation required.

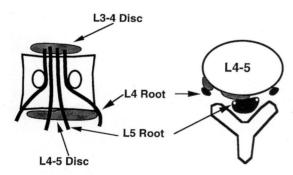

FIGURE 20-11 **Drawing of lateral disk.** This drawing demonstrates how a posterior disk protrusion at L4–5 typically affects the L5 root, yet a lateral disk at the same level affects the L4 root. Because the L4 root is typically affected by a posterior L3–4 disk protrusion, a lateral disk at L4–5 could result in inappropriate surgery at the L3–4 disk space.

The most common cause of central canal stenosis is secondary to facet degenerative disease, which results in hypertrophy of the facets and encroachment of the central canal and the lateral recesses (Fig. 20-16). As mentioned earlier, even patients with the most severe example of congenital spinal stenosis, achondroplasia, rarely present with clinical symptoms until marked facet degenerative disease occurs.

Another common cause of central canal stenosis is hypertrophy of the ligamentum flavum (Fig. 20-17). This is a misnomer because the ligamentum flavum does not actually hypertrophy, but rather buckles inward because of facet slippage and disk space narrowing. Because this is a soft-tissue encroachment, measurements of the size of the bony canal would not reflect this process, which is another reason measurements are not reliable in detecting spinal stenosis.

Paget's disease with enlargement of the vertebral body occasionally can cause central canal stenosis (Fig. 20-18), as can ossification of the posterior longitudinal ligament (Fig. 20-19). It has been reported that up to 25% of patients with diffuse idiopathic skeletal hyperostosis, a common ailment of persons older than 50 years, will have ossification of the posterior longitudinal ligament. Other causes of central canal stenosis include trauma and postoperative changes.

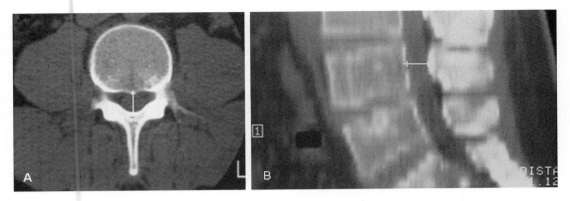

FIGURE 20-13 **Small canal without stenosis.** *A,* The anteroposterior diameter of the canal in this patient measures 11.5 mm, which is extremely small. Note that the thecal sac is not compressed and that the epidural fat is not obliterated. *B,* The anteroposterior measurement taken on a sagittal reformatted image is 11.2 mm. This patient had no clinical findings of spinal stenosis despite a small central canal. The patient has a small thecal sac that is not compressed by the small bony canal. Clinically, the patient did not demonstrate evidence of spinal stenosis.

Neuroforaminal Stenosis

The causes of neuroforaminal stenosis, as in central canal stenosis, can be diverse but are usually caused by degenerative joint disease. Osteophytes emanating from the vertebral body (Fig. 20-20) or from the superior articular facet (Fig. 20-21) are most often the cause, but disk protrusion and postoperative scar can also occur in the foramen.

The nerve root exits the central canal in the superior aspect of the neuroforamen; therefore, encroachment in the inferior aspect, near the disk space, is an infrequent cause of clinical problems. The nerve root is immobile in the neuroforamen, rather than free to move about; hence, even a small amount of stenosis in the superior aspect of the foramen can cause severe clinical symptomatology, whereas severe stenosis of the inferior aspect of the foramen may elicit no symptoms at all. For these reasons, the

FIGURE 20-14 **Obliteration of epidural fat.** Axial image through L2–3 disk space demonstrates central canal stenosis that is compressing the thecal sac. The thecal sac is not visualized because the epidural fat has been obliterated. When the epidural fat is absent, one should suspect spinal stenosis.

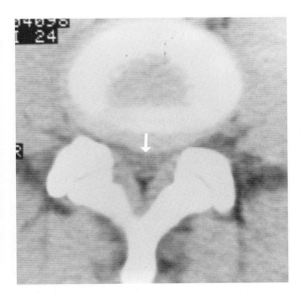

FIGURE 20-15 **Flattening of the thecal sac.** Axial image shows flattening of the thecal sac *(arrow).* This is a good CT sign for central canal stenosis. The patient may not have clinical signs or symptoms of stenosis, but the diagnosis is still suggested.

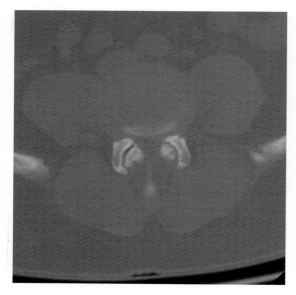

FIGURE 20-16 **Facet hypertrophy.** Axial CT through L4–5 shows a combination of broad-based bulge and facet degenerative disease. The most common cause of spinal stenosis is because of facet degenerative disease with hypertrophy. This is best seen with bone windows because soft-tissue windows can be misleading and make normal facets appear hypertrophied.

amount of narrowing of the neuroforamen often does not correlate clinically.

Although many believe that sagittal re-formations through the neuroforamen are adequate to identify stenosis, axial images are by far more reliable in fully demonstrating the degree of neuroforaminal stenosis and its cause. The

neuroforamen and the nerve root can be seen in its entirety with the axial images, whereas a single sagittal re-formation will show volume rendering of the slice.

A frequent cause of unsuccessful back surgery is failure to preoperatively note neuroforaminal stenosis in a patient undergoing disk surgery resulting in an inadequate procedure being performed. It cannot be stressed enough that disk disease and stenosis, in any of its forms, often occur together and addressing only the disk can result in unsuccessful back surgery.

Lateral Recess Stenosis

The lateral recess is the bony portion of the central canal that is just caudad and cephalad to the neuroforamen. When the neuroforamen ends as one proceeds caudad, the lateral recess begins. It is also called the nerve root canal because the nerve roots, after they leave the thecal sac and before they exit the central canal through the neuroforamen, run in this bony triangular space. In the bony lateral recess, the nerve roots are vulnerable to being impinged by osteophytes, disk fragments, and scar tissue from prior surgery (Fig. 20-22). As with the neuroforamen, the amount of stenosis often does not correlate with the clinical picture; therefore, it is best to just note that the lateral recess is or is not normal in appearance. Any narrowing must be correlated clinically.

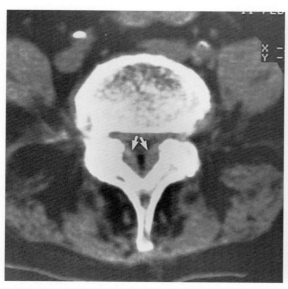
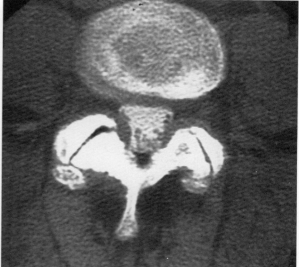

FIGURE 20-17 **Ligamentum flavum hypertrophy.** The ligamentum flavum *(arrows)* is bowing inward and encroaching on the central canal, causing spinal stenosis.

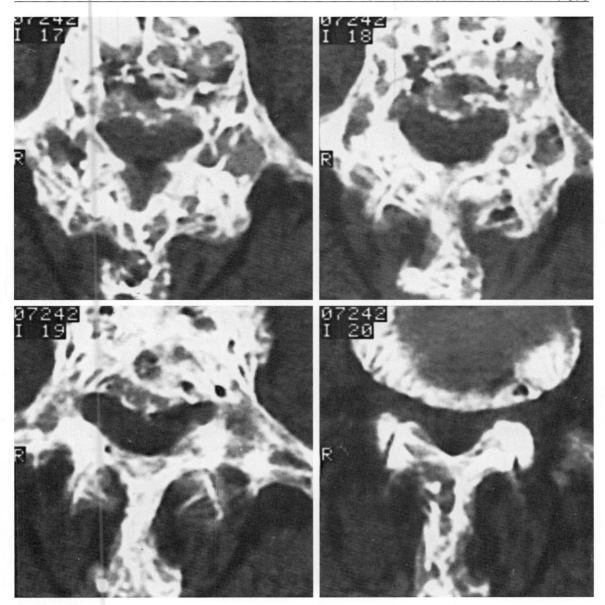

FIGURE 20-18 **Paget's disease.** Contiguous axial images show bony overgrowth secondary to Paget's disease causing central canal stenosis in this patient. This is a typical appearance of Paget's disease in a vertebral body, although it does not always cause stenosis.

□ SPONDYLOLYSIS AND SPONDYLOLISTHESIS

Spondylolysis (pars interarticularis defect) can cause low back pain and sciatica but only occasionally causes spinal stenosis. As discussed in Chapter 19, on rare occasions, a fibrocartilaginous mass builds up around a pars break that can extend into the central canal and impress on the thecal sac or nerve roots (Fig. 20-23). Although this is uncommon, it should be looked for in every patient with a pars break to avoid an unfortunate example of a fusion being performed without removal of the offending soft-tissue mass in the central canal.

Spondylolisthesis is defined as anterior displacement of a cephalad vertebral body with respect to a caudad vertebral body and is graded in severity of slip relative to the lower vertebral body as I (<25%), II (25% to 50%), III (50% to 75%), and IV (75% to 100%). Spondylolisthesis can cause central canal stenosis or neuroforam-

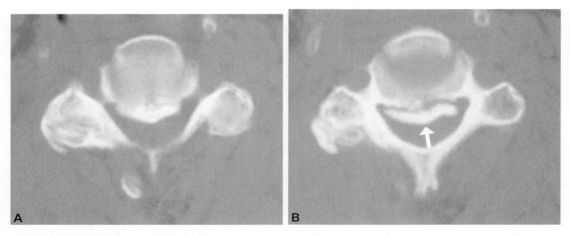

FIGURE 20-19 Ossification of the posterior longitudinal ligament. *A, B,* Axial images through the cervical spine show calcified mass with mass effect on the cord *(arrow).*

inal stenosis. When one vertebral body slides forward on another, the thecal sac can be squeezed at the level of the slip. This rarely occurs with a grade I spondylolisthesis but is not uncommon with the more advanced grades. Occasionally, the broken pars will extend into the neuroforamen and impinge the nerve root (Fig. 20-24). Spondylolisthesis can be caused by either spondylolysis or spondylosis (degenerative disease at the facet joints).

☐ SACROILIAC JOINTS

Plain film examination of the sacroiliac (SI) joints can be extremely difficult to interpret because of the anatomic obliquity of the joints themselves and the thick overlying soft tissues. CT is a more reliable imaging technique than plain radiography and also is more reproducible, more sensitive, and more accurate than plain films and gives the patient less radiation. If the

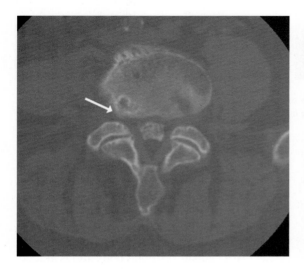

FIGURE 20-20 Neuroforaminal stenosis. An osteophyte arising from the posterior right aspect of the vertebral body is extending into the right neuroforamen causing neuroforaminal stenosis *(arrow).* The left neuroforamen is normal.

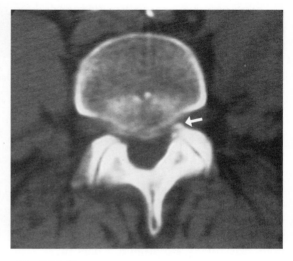

FIGURE 20-21 Neuroforaminal stenosis. An osteophyte from the left superior articular facet is extending into the left neuroforamen causing neuroforaminal stenosis *(arrow).*

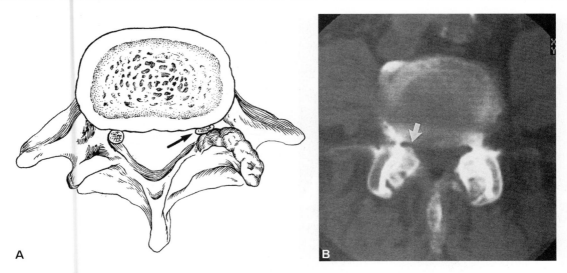

A

B

<u>FIGURE 20-22</u> **Lateral recess stenosis.** *A,* This drawing illustrates how a nerve root *(arrow)* can get impinged in the lateral recess by bony overgrowth. *B,* The right lateral recess *(arrow)* is narrowed from bony overgrowth. The nerve root lies in the lateral recess and may or may not be impinged enough by this process to cause symptoms.

protocol is streamlined, it can be performed rapidly and at a relatively low cost, making it cost effective.

To streamline the protocol and diminish the number of slices necessary to cover the SI joints, the gantry is reversed so that it is at a steep angle parallel to the SI joints (Fig. 20-25). Eight to ten 3-mm-thick slices are obtained that cover the SI joints as seen on the lateral scout film.

SI joint symptoms can occasionally be the cause of back pain. Often, conventional radiographs cannot define SI joint pathology. SI joint abnormalities are part of the symptom complex of many arthritides, especially the spondyloarthropathies.

SI joint sclerosis and erosions can be identified on CT with much more clarity than on plain films (Fig. 20-26). Degenerative joint disease can also cause erosions in the SI joints and can mimic a spondyloarthropathy or an infection (Fig. 20-27). It has been shown that erosions and sclerosis in the SI joints, as shown with CT, increase with aging to the point that patients older than 40 years often have SI joint abnormalities.

Osteitis condensans ilii is diagnosed when triangular-shaped areas of sclerosis are noted in the ilium abutting the SI joint. This is an incidental finding and is not responsible for symptoms.

☐ OSTEITIS PUBIS

Osteitis pubis historically was defined as infection in the pubic symphysis most often identified after bladder surgery. The name would imply an inflammatory change in this joint space. However, the changes are not usually caused by an inflammatory process. Erosions and sclerosis are not infrequently identified at the pubic symphysis and can be a result of degenerative disease or seen as a result of stress changes, particularly when identified in athletes (Fig. 20-28). Coexistent changes or erosions and sclerosis are often seen in the SI joints in these individuals.

☐ COALITION

A frequent use of CT in the ankle is in tarsal coalition. The most common site for coalition is at the calcaneonavicular joint. The next most common locations are at the talonavicular joint and the middle facet of the talocalcaneal joint (Fig. 20-29). It is often difficult to diagnose a coalition if there is a fibrous rather than a bony fusion, but usually there will be enough associated bony abnormalities to allow a diagnosis to be made (Fig. 20-30). There are often coexisting tendon, ligament, and bone edema in patients with

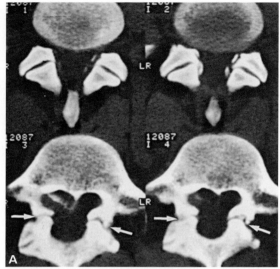

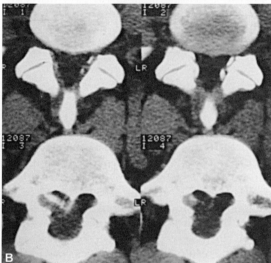

FIGURE 20-23 **Spondylolysis with fibrocartilaginous mass.** *A,* Bone windows through the L4–5 disk and the L5 vertebral body show a pars break *(arrows)* bilaterally. *B,* Soft-tissue windows of the same slices show a large, partially calcified, soft-tissue mass in the right lateral recess *(arrow)* that at surgery was found to arise from the pars break. This has been likened to callus around a fracture that increases when inadequate immobilization occurs.

coalition; therefore, MRI is becoming the study of choice for patients suspected of having a coalition.

☐ TUMORS AND INFECTION

MRI is without question superior to CT in evaluating tumors of the musculoskeletal system. Although it is true that CT is better than MRI at

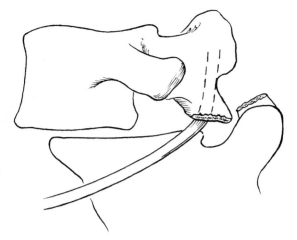

FIGURE 20-24 **Spondylolisthesis.** Drawing indicating how the broken ends of the pars interarticularis can extend into the neuroforamen with spondylolisthesis and impinge a nerve root.

evaluating subtle cortical abnormalities, in reality, it is seldom necessary to improve on the resolution that MRI affords, with the exception, perhaps, of infection, when subtle cortical disruption is key in diagnosing osteomyelitis. MRI is unsurpassed at showing the extent of tumors in the medullary bone and in the soft tissues. There is little role for CT in evaluation of tumors unless

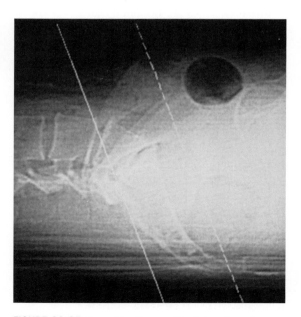

FIGURE 20-25 **Scout film for sacroiliac joints.** Lateral scout view of the sacrum shows cursors are angled parallel to the sacroiliac joints. Eight to ten 3-mm-thick slices are then taken to cover the extent of the joints.

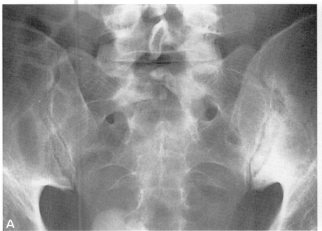

FIGURE 20-26 **CT of the sacroiliac joints in psoriasis.** *A,* An anteroposterior plain film of the pelvis demonstrates left-sided sacroiliac joint sclerosis and erosions. The right sacroiliac joint is possibly involved. *B,* CT shows the left-sided changes nicely and shows that the right joint is definitely not involved.

the internal matrix of a lesion has calcifications requiring resolution of the pattern of internal calcification or if myositis ossificans is a clinical consideration. CT will demonstrate the peripheral nature of the calcifications in that lesion. It is imperative that a biopsy not be performed if myositis ossificans is a consideration because it can resemble a sarcoma to the pathologist and result in unnecessary radical surgery. The plain

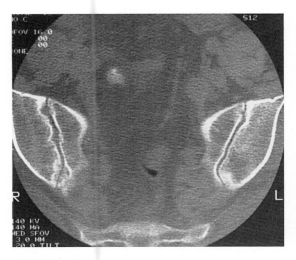

FIGURE 20-27 **CT of the sacroiliac joints in degenerative joint disease.** CT of the sacroiliac joints in this patient shows some minimal sclerosis and definite erosions in the right joint. A small erosion is also present in the left joint. These changes could be caused by any inflammatory arthritis or a spondyloarthropathy, but these were caused by degenerative joint disease. This patient has extensive osteoarthritis in his spine and large joints. This is a typical appearance of degenerative joint disease in the sacroiliac joints.

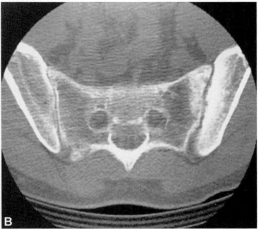

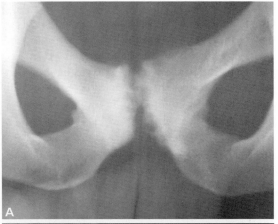

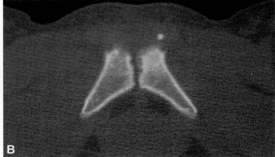

FIGURE 20-28 **Osteitis pubis.** *A,* Conventional radiograph demonstrating erosions along the pubic symphysis. *B,* CT image shows erosions with small bony avulsion. These findings represent stress changes of the pubic symphysis in this long-distance runner.

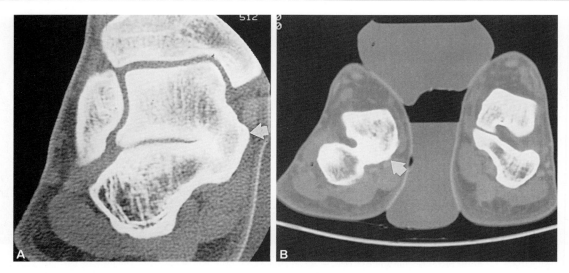

FIGURE 20-29 **Tarsal coalition.** *A*, Coronal CT image shows solid bone fusion of a talocalcaneal coalition *(arrow).* *B*, Normal left ankle for comparison with right talocalcaneal coalition *(arrow).*

film finding that is virtually pathognomonic for myositis ossificans is peripheral calcification (Fig. 20-31). Often, it is difficult to characterize the calcification as either central or peripheral on plain films; CT can help determine the location of the calcification and avert a biopsy in most instances (Fig. 20-32).

CT can be helpful in diagnosing bony involvement of multiple myeloma before plain film findings. CT of the spine will show a "Swiss cheese" pattern of lytic myeloma (Fig.

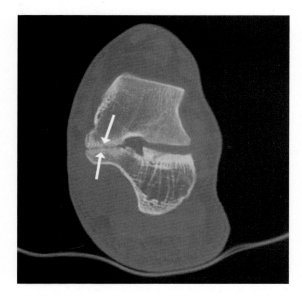

FIGURE 20-30 **Talocalcaneal coalition.** Irregularity along the subtalar joint space is indicative of a fibrous coalition *(arrows).*

20-33). In long-standing myeloma, the pattern is considerably different. The few remaining normal trabeculae undergo compensatory hypertrophy, and the resulting appearance is thick, sclerotic, bony struts with lytic areas in between (Fig. 20-34). This pattern resembles spinal hemangioma (Fig. 20-35) except that the hypertrophied trabecular struts in hemangioma are much more ordered and symmetric.

Another particular lesion that CT is useful for evaluating is an osteoid osteoma. Clinically and radiographically this lesion can be confused with infection. CT can show the location of the nidus that will facilitate its removal by the surgeon. This is especially useful in complex joints such as the hip (Fig. 20-36) or in the spine (Fig. 20-37). Seeing a small lucency surrounded by sclerosis is not pathognomonic for the nidus of an osteoid osteoma. Osteomyelitis with a small abscess can have an identical appearance. The nidus of an osteoid osteoma often partially calcifies and can then resemble a sequestrum in osteomyelitis (Figs. 20-38 and 20-39). CT, plain films, and even MRI can appear identical in both osteoid osteoma and osteomyelitis, with or without a sequestrum; therefore, a differential diagnosis of both entities should be given when a lesion with this appearance is found. Radionuclide bone scan can usually differentiate between osteoid osteoma and osteomyelitis by noting a "double density" sign at the nidus of the osteoid osteoma. This is caused by the increased affinity for the radionuclide by

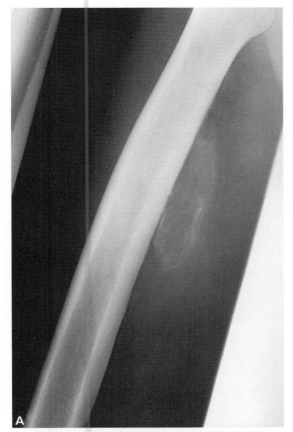

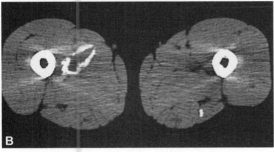

FIGURE 20-31 **Myositis ossificans.** *A,* A plain film of the humerus in this patient with a painful mass shows a faintly calcified mass adjacent to the humerus with some periostitis present. Myositis ossificans and parosteal osteosarcoma were believed to be the main considerations. *B,* CT through the mass shows definite circumferential calcification, which indicates myositis ossificans. No biopsy sample was taken because myositis ossificans can simulate a sarcoma histologically.

the hypervascular nidus. The surrounding reactive new bone takes up the radionuclide to a lesser degree than the nidus. In osteomyelitis a small abscess will be photopenic on radionuclide examination.

CT plays an important role in osteomyelitis by finding sequestrations (Fig. 20-40). The finding of a sequestration has both diagnostic and therapeutic significance. The diagnostic significance is that only a few entities have been described that commonly have a sequestration. These are osteomyelitis, eosinophilic granuloma (Fig. 20-41), and desmoid or malignant fibrous histiocytoma (Fig. 20-42). As mentioned earlier, a partially calcified nidus of an osteoid osteoma can have an identical appearance as osteomyelitis with a sequestrum. All four entities should be considered when a sequestrum is encountered. The therapeutic significance is that the presence of a sequestrum usually requires surgical removal. Antibiotic therapy alone generally does not suffice because the sequestration does not have a blood supply and, therefore, antibiotics cannot reach this location.

☐ MEASUREMENTS

Almost any measurement that is done with plain films, such as scanogram for leg-length discrepancy, can be done more accurately and with considerably less radiation by using CT. The measurements can be easily and accurately obtained with CT by taking an anteroposterior scout film of the extremities and placing cursor points on the bony landmarks for measurement (Fig. 20-43). The computer gives the distance measurements between the chosen points. This technique has been shown to have reproducibility and accuracy, but it suffers from not being able to have the patient bear weight. Most of the time a weight-bearing examination is not necessary; however, if a weight-bearing examination is required, then a CT scanogram cannot replace the conventional scanogram. The radiation dose from the CT scanogram has been estimated at 50 to 100 times less than a conventional scanogram. The cost of a CT scanogram is less than a conventional scanogram because of the low cost of the scout views, which comprise the imaging portion of the examination.

☐ CONCLUSION

CT has utility in evaluating pathology in the lumbar spine. It can demonstrate disk protrusions that are central, lateral, and sequestered. The ability to fully evaluate both the bony and

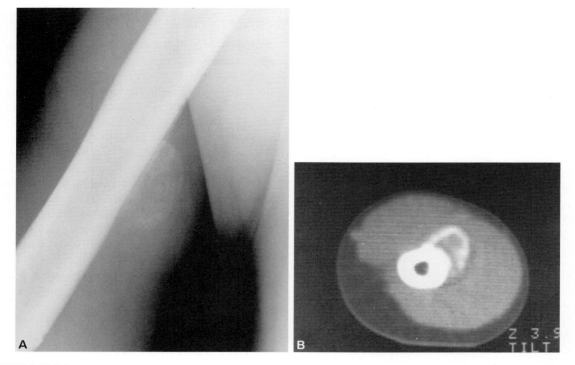

FIGURE 20-32 **Myositis ossificans.** *A,* Conventional radiograph of the humerus shows calcification in a mass adjacent to the right humerus. *B,* Axial CT image through the lesion clearly demonstrates the peripheral nature of the calcification.

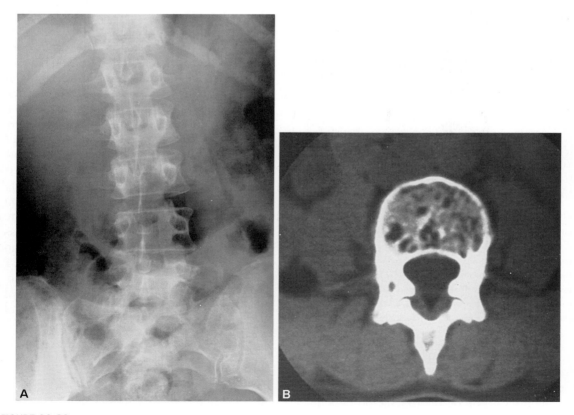

FIGURE 20-33 **Multiple myeloma.** *A,* Anteroposterior view of the lumbar spine in a patient with known myeloma. Except for mild osteopenia, films are normal. *B,* CT through a lumbar vertebral body shows diffuse lytic lesions consistent with multiple myeloma. This is a typical appearance for multiple myeloma in the spine.

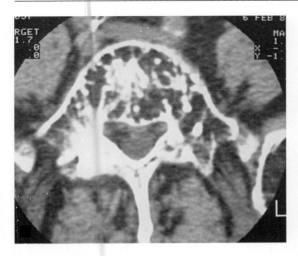

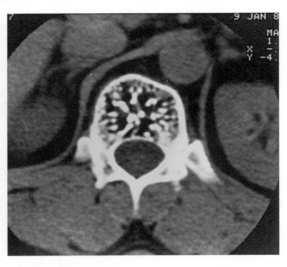

FIGURE 20-34 **Multiple myeloma.** CT scan through L5 shows dense trabecular struts that are hypertrophied. They are separated by multiple cystic areas. This is a characteristic appearance for chronic myeloma with compensatory hypertrophy of the remaining trabeculae. It has a similar appearance to Paget's disease and to hemangioma.

FIGURE 20-35 **Hemangioma.** CT through a vertebral body hemangioma shows strikingly dense, hypertrophied trabeculae that are arranged in a columnar fashion. Note the symmetry of this pattern as compared with that of chronic myeloma.

soft-tissue structures is one of the greatest assets of CT and has helped diminish the incidence of unsuccessful back surgery. Its use in evaluation of sacroiliitis and osteitis pubis is being replaced by MR largely because bone marrow edema is readily appreciated with MRI. However, erosions are more readily appreciated by CT.

CT can readily distinguish an abscess and is used often for evaluation of infection of the appendicular skeleton. MRI is much more efficacious in the evaluation of soft-tissue tumors. MR is also replacing CT in the evaluation of coalition because of its ability to identify bone marrow edema, as well as determining fibrous from

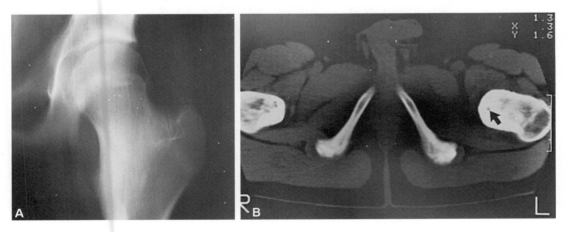

FIGURE 20-36 **Osteoid osteoma.** *A,* A tomogram of the hip in this 20-year-old man with hip pain shows cortical thickening and sclerosis about the medial aspect of the femoral neck *(arrow).* An osteoid osteoma was suspected, but the exact location of the nidus could not be determined. *B,* CT through the femoral neck showed a focal lucency *(arrow)* surrounded by sclerosis. This was removed and found to be the nidus of an osteoid osteoma.

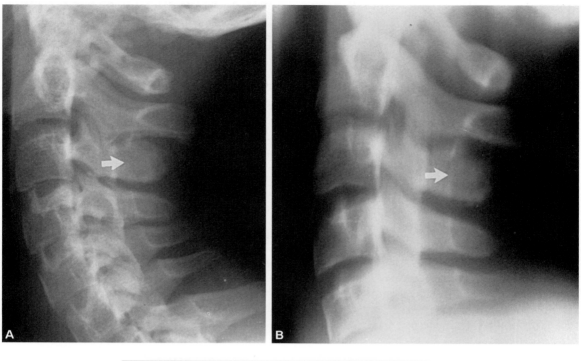

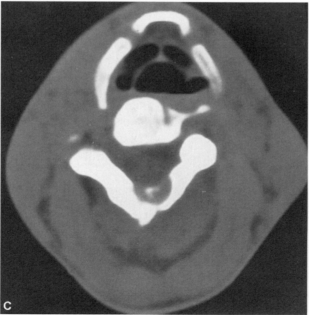

FIGURE 20-37 Osteoid osteoma. *A,* Lateral C-spine view in this young patient with neck pain shows an area of subtle sclerosis with absence of the normal spinolaminar line at C3 *(arrow).* *B,* A conventional tomogram of this area confirms the absent spinolaminar line *(arrow)* but is otherwise noncontributory. *C,* An axial CT through the C3 vertebra shows lucency with a small calcific center that was found at surgery to be the nidus of an osteoid osteoma with partial calcification. Osteomyelitis with a sequestrum could have an identical appearance.

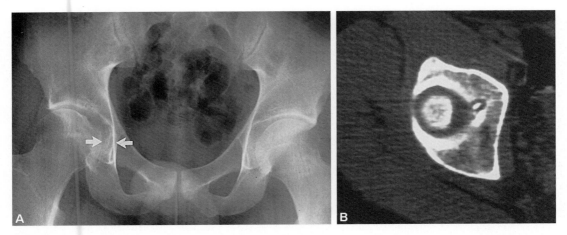

FIGURE 20-38 **Osteoid osteoma with calcified nidus.** *A,* A young patient presented with hip pain and a widened teardrop measurement *(arrows)* on the right as compared with the left. Hip aspiration ruled out an infectious process. *B,* Axial CT of the hip showed an acetabular lucency with a central calcific density consistent with either osteomyelitis with a sequestrum or an osteoid osteoma with a partially calcified nidus. At surgery, this was found to be an osteoid osteoma.

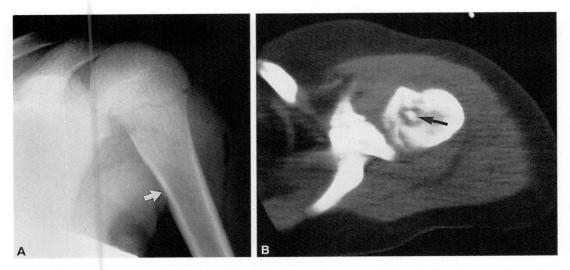

FIGURE 20-39 **Osteomyelitis.** *A,* Anteroposterior plain film of the upper humerus in a child with pain and swelling shows a faint permeative pattern in the bone with periostitis *(arrow).* The differential diagnosis includes osteomyelitis, Ewing's sarcoma, and eosinophilic granuloma. *B,* CT of the humerus shows a lytic lesion with a bony sequestrum *(arrow).* This narrows the diagnosis to osteomyelitis and eosinophilic granuloma, because Ewing's sarcoma will not have a sequestrum. Biopsy showed this to be osteomyelitis.

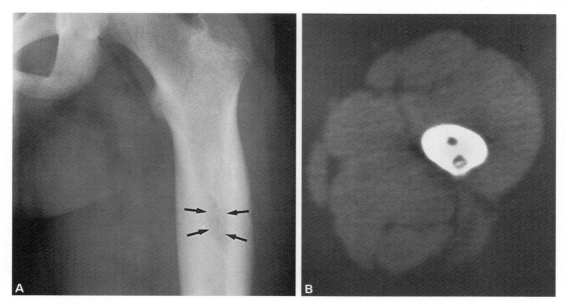

FIGURE 20-40 **Sequestration in osteomyelitis.** *A,* Anteroposterior plain film of the proximal femur in a child with pain shows an area of diffuse sclerosis and cortical thickening with a faint lucency in the intramedullary portion *(arrows)*. *B,* CT of the femur shows lucency with a calcific central portion. Radiographically, this appearance can be seen in osteomyelitis or osteoid osteoma. At biopsy, this was found to be a sequestration in osteomyelitis.

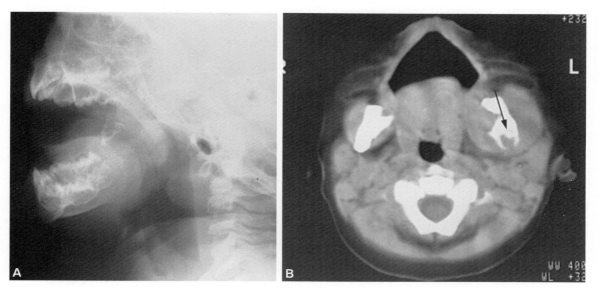

FIGURE 20-41 **Sequestration in eosinophilic granuloma.** *A,* Conventional film of a 2-year-old child who presented with a painful, swollen jaw shows destruction of the mandible near the angle. Infection, Ewing's sarcoma, osteogenic sarcoma, neuroblastoma, and eosinophilic granuloma were diagnostic considerations. *B,* CT showed a destructive lesion that involved much of the mandible. A sequestration *(arrow)* was found that limited the differential diagnosis to osteomyelitis and eosinophilic granuloma. At biopsy, this was found to be eosinophilic granuloma.

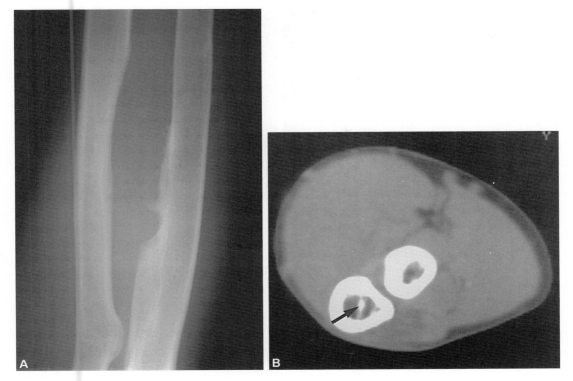

FIGURE 20-42 Sequestration in a desmoid tumor. *A,* A plain film of the forearm shows a destructive lesion of the ulna with some aggressive periostitis. Note the thick benign periostitis as well. *B,* CT through the lesion showed a sequestrum *(arrow),* limiting the differential diagnosis to eosinophilic granuloma, fibrosarcoma, and osteomyelitis. Histologically, this represented a desmoid.

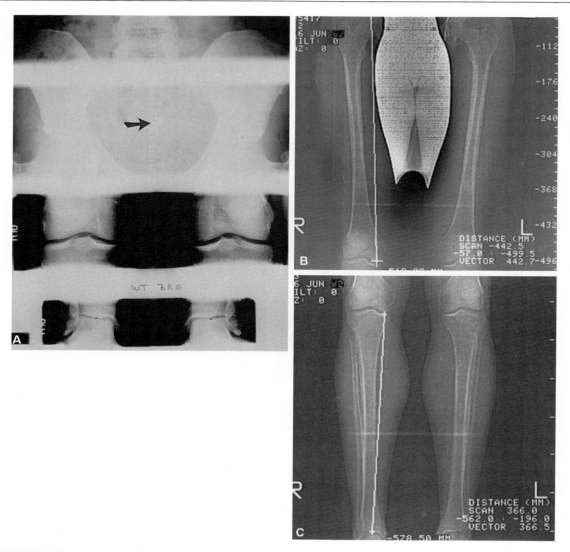

FIGURE 20-43 **CT scanogram.** *A,* This conventional plain film scanogram shows how difficult it can be to visualize the ruler *(arrow)* on all the images. It could not be seen at all on the images of the knees and ankles. *B,* A scout view of the femurs shows the cursor placement at the proximal and distal femur on the right with a distance measurement of 44.2 cm given between the two points. *C,* Scout view of the tibias in the same patient with cursors placed on the medial tibial plateau and on the plafond. The measurement of the distance between the cursors is 36.6 cm. These measurements are repeated on the opposite leg and compared.

cartilage coalition. Scanograms can be performed quickly and effectively in patients who need leg-length measurements.

SUGGESTED READING

GOODMAN RE, VANDER ZR, KAISER GM, et al: Diagnosis of diseases of the lumbar spine: Correlation of computerized tomography with myelography and clinical findings. South Med J 80:855–860, 1987.

HESSELINK JR: Spine imaging: History, achievements, remaining frontiers. AJR Am J Roentgenol 150:1223–1229, 1988.

JACKSON R, BECKER G, JACOBS R, et al: The neuroradiographic diagnosis of lumbar herniated nucleus pulposus: I. A comparison of computed tomography, myelography, CT-myelography, discography, and CT-discography. Spine 14: 1356–1361, 1989.

MODIC MT, MASARYK TJ, ROSS JS, CARTER JR: Imaging of degenerative disk disease. Radiology 168: 177–186, 1988.

PRETORIUS ES, FISHMAN EK: Helical CT of musculo-skeletal infection. Crit Rev Diagn Imaging 42: 259–305, 2001.

RESNICK D, GUERRA J Jr, ROBINSON CA, VINT VC: Association of DISH and calcification and ossification of the posterior longitudinal ligament. AJR Am J Roentgenol 131:1049–1053, 1978.

SARTORIS DJ, RESNICK D: Computed tomography of the spine: An update and review. Crit Rev Diagn Imaging 27:271–296, 1987.

SCHNEBEL B, KINGSTON S, WATKINS R, DILLIN W: Comparison of MRI to contrast CT in the diagnosis of spinal stenosis. Spine 14:332–337, 1989.

WEISHAUPT D, ZANETTI M, BOOS N, HODLER J: MR imaging and CT in osteoarthritis of the lumbar facet joints. Skeletal Radiol 28:215–219, 1999.

21

Incidental Findings

Nancy M. Major, M.D.

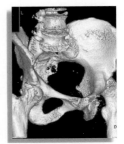

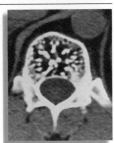

This chapter shows examples of bone pathology encountered during the course of imaging the chest, abdomen, and pelvis for indications other than evaluation of bone pathology. This chapter is not meant to be an atlas of all possible bone lesions, but instead discusses and shows examples of lesions that are commonly encountered or might be potentially confusing during CT examination.

☐ METASTATIC DISEASE/ MULTIPLE MYELOMA

A common indication for CT of the chest, abdomen, or pelvis is the evaluation of possible metastatic disease in a patient who has a known primary cancer. The bones are carefully evaluated for evidence of bony involvement. Bone windows are necessary to accurately characterize the lesion. Conventional radiography is helpful to show the margins of lesions. However, some lesions can be characterized on CT. Not every bone lesion in a patient with a known primary cancer is going to be metastatic disease. A helpful sign of metastatic disease is a permeative appearance in the bone. This would suggest a marrow-based process and an aggressive lesion. This finding can be seen with metastatic

disease, as well as with multiple myeloma (Fig. 21-1). Metastatic lesions can be found in any portion of the body, thus the location of the lesion is not as important as the character of the lesion (Fig. 21-2). Infection, a benign process, can also have a permeative process. One would hope the clinical history might help make the distinction between metastatic disease and infection easier. The presence of a peripheral enhancing fluid collection makes infection much more likely. Magnetic resonance imaging (MRI) is often done in the setting of infection to assess the extent of bone marrow involvement.

Endosteal scalloping or the appearance of the cortex scooped out from the inside of the medullary canal is not a specific diagnosis for metastatic disease or myeloma. This can be seen in many benign entities such as enchondroma, fibrous dysplasia, or nonossifying fibroma (Fig. 21-3). Not all blastic lesions should be considered worrisome for metastatic disease. A bone island, for instance, is a blastic process that is benign. It is essentially a hamartoma of bone. Stellate margins and lack of distortion of bone are useful signs in trying to assess bone island versus metastatic disease (Fig. 21-4).

The presence of a soft-tissue mass around a lytic lesion is also not helpful in distinguishing metastatic disease or multiple myeloma from a

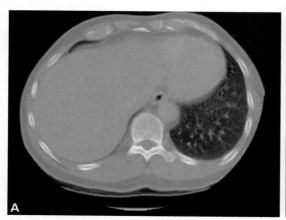

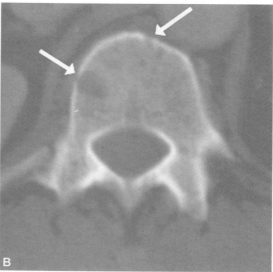

FIGURE 21-1 **Multiple myeloma.** *A,* Axial CT image through the thoracic spine demonstrates "moth-eaten" appearance representing multiple lucencies in vertebral body. *B,* Close up of *A* showing lytic areas of varying sizes in this patient with multiple myeloma *(arrows).*

benign process. There are benign entities that can have an associated soft-tissue mass such as infection, eosinophilic granuloma, and giant-cell tumor (Fig. 21-5), among others.

In the spine, multiple myeloma can have a characteristic appearance. The trabeculae can hypertrophy and become thickened as the bone around these areas is lost due to the disease process. This is a unique appearance for multiple myeloma and plasmacytoma. This characteristic appearance can alleviate the need for biopsy because it is unique to this lesion (Fig. 21-6).

In summary, the greatest concern for a metastatic lesion or myeloma is a permeative process in the bone noted on CT in the correct clinical setting.

☐ HEMANGIOMA

Hemangiomas in the bone can have a variety of appearances. However, in the spine, the trabeculae thicken in an organized fashion unlike myeloma or plasmacytoma (Fig. 21-7). The

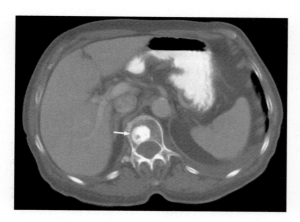

FIGURE 21-2 **Vertebral body metastasis.** Axial CT through the thoracic spine demonstrates a mixed lytic, sclerotic, marrow-based process in the vertebral body *(arrow)* in a patient with known breast cancer.

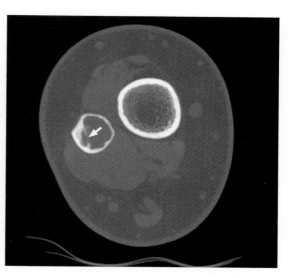

FIGURE 21-3 **Nonossifying fibroma.** Axial image through the fibula shows endosteal scalloping *(arrow)* in this patient with a nonossifying fibroma.

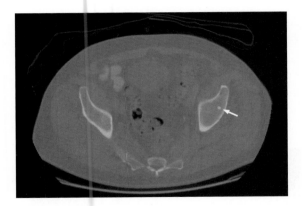

FIGURE 21-4 **Bone island.** Axial image through the ilium demonstrates stellate sclerotic focus *(arrow)*. There is no distortion of surrounding bone. This was an incidental finding.

trabecular thickening is in a vertical fashion, yielding the "corduroy" appearance noted on plain radiograph. Generally, hemangiomas contain some fat within the lesion, and this can be seen with the low density on CT. Sometimes, phleboliths can be seen in association with hemangiomas, and these calcifications can be helpful in making the diagnosis. When the hemangiomas occur in the spine, they are generally well-defined lesions with organized trabecular thickening with fat present within the lesion. They can be located anywhere within the vertebral body and are worth reporting even though they occur so commonly. If the clinician views the study, he or she may be concerned that the hemangioma is something much more sinister. Another reason to note the lesion is if it happens to be located in a pedicle and the patient is being considered for spinal fusion. If the pedicle screw fixation is planned through that area, the surgeon would like to know that he or she may encounter a vascular lesion.

Hemangiomas can also involve the cortex of the bone. When this occurs, it is truly a vascular malformation, and not necessarily a hemangioma. The cortex will demonstrate "holes" within it that are well defined and differ in appearance from the permeative process seen in an aggressive lesion, which is confined to the medullary space. The holes are a result of the vessels tunneling through the cortex.

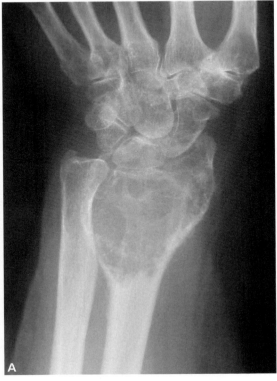

FIGURE 21-5 **Giant-cell tumor.** *A*, conventional AP radiograph demonstrates well-defined expansile lesion without a sclerotic margin, which abuts the articular surface of the distal radius.

Continued

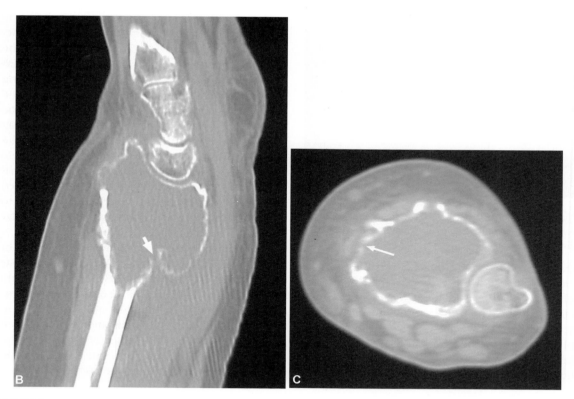

FIGURE 21-5 **Cont'd** *B, C,* sagittal and axial demonstrates the presence of soft tissue density and cortical destruction *(arrow)* in this benign entity. These findings do not imply malignancy.

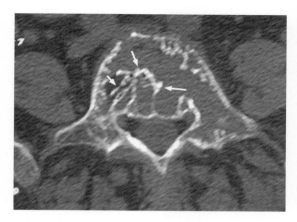

FIGURE 21-6 **Plasmacytoma.** Axial image through lumbar spine demonstrates a fairly characteristic appearance of plasmacytoma on CT. Note the thickening of the trabeculae *(arrows).* This is likely because of the slow-growing nature of this lesion leading to hypertrophy of the remaining trabeculae.

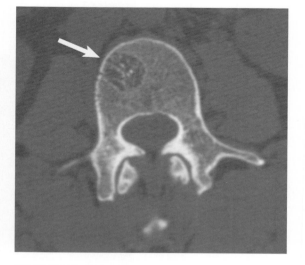

FIGURE 21-7 **Hemangioma.** Axial image through L3 demonstrates a well-defined lytic lesion with organized thickening of trabeculae with intervening fat *(arrow).* This is a characteristic appearance of a hemangioma. This pattern is not seen in multiple myeloma.

SCHMORL'S NODES

Schmorl's nodes are commonly encountered in routine CT imaging. These are not truly nodes but rather herniation of disc material through the end plate of a vertebral body. On CT axial imaging, these lesions occasionally can be difficult to characterize. When trying to determine if the lesion is a Schmorl's node, the end plate must be involved. Associated changes of degenerative disease may also help to determine a Schmorl's node but may not be present. A Schmorl's node can occur in any portion of the vertebral body as long as it involves the end plate, but is most often seen in the center of the vertebral body (Fig. 21-8). It can still be difficult sometimes to determine if the lesion is a Schmorl's node. The lateral scout film may be helpful. If the patient has plain film images of that area, that can be another helpful way to confirm the presence of a Schmorl's node. Schmorl's nodes do not enhance with contrast, because the disk is avascular.

TARLOV CYSTS

Tarlov cysts are nerve sheath dilatations. As mentioned in Chapter 20, usually the density will

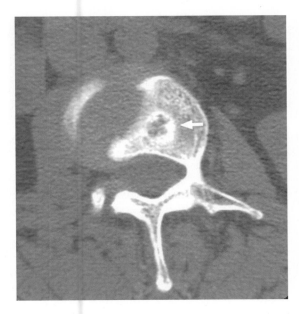

FIGURE 21-8 **Schmorl's node.** Axial image through end plate of lumbar vertebral body (note disk material). A Schmorl's node is noted in the central portion of the vertebral body with a well-defined sclerotic margin *(arrow)*.

allow adequate distinction of a Tarlov cyst from disc fragment. However, if a Tarlov cyst becomes large enough, and particularly when located in the sacrum, it can lead to bone erosion from the pressure effect of this process (Fig. 21-9). Recognition of this abnormality is important to avoid a biopsy. The margins are well defined, and the density of the lesion immediately adjacent to the excavated bone is that of cerebrospinal fluid. A soft-tissue mass causing bone erosion would have a higher density than cerebrospinal fluid. Generally, the findings are straightforward. However, in the confusing case, MRI is strongly indicated before an attempt to perform a biopsy. The MRI will show the fluid nature of the lesion. There is no bone marrow edema associated with Tarlov cysts on MRI. A pelvic mass or sacral tumor eroding into the bone may have an associated finding on MRI of bone marrow edema.

PAGET'S DISEASE

Paget's disease is a not infrequently encountered abnormality on CT. Paget's disease can affect any bone in the body and has three different appearances: it can be purely lytic, in which case it has a well-defined leading edge; it can be purely sclerotic; and it can be mixed lytic and sclerotic. Paget's disease will have associated findings of bone overgrowth, cortical thickening, and trabecular thickening (Fig. 21-10). The trabecular thickening is not organized as in a hemangioma, thus it can be distinguished from this entity. Paget's disease can be distinguished from multiple myeloma by the cortical thickening and

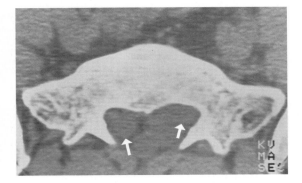

FIGURE 21-9 **Tarlov cyst.** Axial CT image through the sacrum demonstrates dilated nerve root sheaths *(arrows)* with density similar to cerebrospinal fluid. Note the bone erosion from long-standing pressure effect.

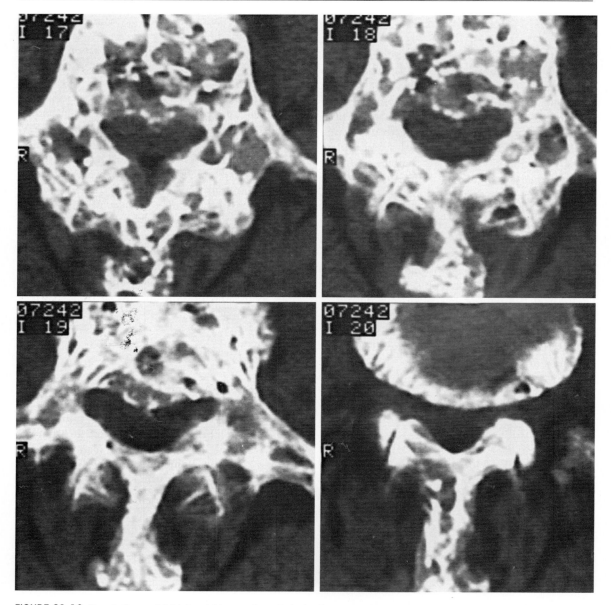

FIGURE 21-10 **Paget's disease.** Multiple axial images through the lumbar spine show marked trabecular thickening and overgrowth of bone. Overgrowth of vertebral body, posterior elements, or both can lead to stenosis.

bone overgrowth. These processes are not a part of myeloma. Paget's disease generally begins at one end of the bone at the articular surface and will migrate to the other end in long bones. In the pelvis (a commonly encountered location for Paget's disease), there may be thickening of iliopectineal and or ilioischial lines, but this is not always the case. It seems that the most confusion comes when imaging a patient for prostate carcinoma and a blastic process is encountered in the pelvis. Remember to look for the additional findings to suggest Paget's disease.

Prostate cancer will not be associated with bone overgrowth, cortical thickening, or hypertrophied trabeculae.

☐ FIBROUS DYSPLASIA

Fibrous dysplasia is a congenital disorder of bone leading to the presence of fibrous tissue, chondral tissue, and even cysts within the bone. Because of these different tissue types, it can have a wide variety of appearances on CT. In

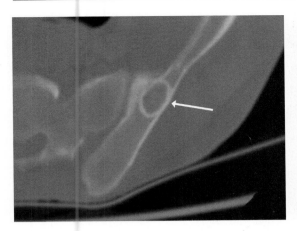

FIGURE 21-11 **Fibrous dysplasia.** Axial image through the left ilium shows a well-defined lesion with a "hazy" matrix and sclerotic margin *(arrow)*. Note the cortical thickening of the ilium adjacent to the sacroiliac joint.

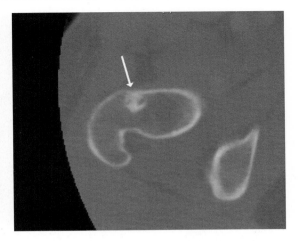

FIGURE 21-12 **Fibrous dysplasia.** Axial image through right femoral neck showing sclerotic focus *(arrow)* and characteristic appearance of fibrous dysplasia in this location.

general, fibrous dysplasia will be asymptomatic and, therefore, an incidental finding. It is a well-defined lesion that can occasionally be seen to have thickened cortices, but will not demonstrate the trabecular thickening of Paget's disease or the bone overgrowth (Fig. 21-11). Calcifications may be seen within this lesion caused by the chondroid elements that are reported in about 10% to 30% of lesions of fibrous dysplasia. There can be associated endosteal scalloping because this is a medullary-based process. There may be a sclerotic border particularly if it occurs in the intertrochanteric region (Fig. 21-12). In summary, fibrous dysplasia can look like many things on CT, but it will not look aggressive. There will be no associated soft-tissue mass or periosteal reaction (unless a pathologic fracture is present). If a soft-tissue mass is encountered or periosteal reaction is present (without the identification of a fracture) in association with a bone lesion, fibrous dysplasia is not the diagnosis.

In general, for bony lesions that are encountered during CT that cannot be diagnosed clearly, conventional radiography can be useful for further evaluation. When evaluating primary lesions of the bone, a conventional radiograph is the way to determine benign versus aggressive processes. CT should be used only to evaluate matrix. Thus, when the CT is performed before the conventional radiograph, check the patient's jacket for films of the area. If none have been performed, perform them and compare your CT findings with that of the plain films.

☐ CONCLUSION

In summary, although all possible lesions cannot be reviewed in this chapter, some helpful tips with commonly encountered examples have been provided. Remember that all bone lesions are best characterized on a conventional radiograph, and when faced with difficulty determining the causative factor of the lesion and proper diagnosis, start with a conventional radiograph. This will save a lot of headaches and unnecessary biopsies. CT is useful when evaluating lesions in the pelvis because plain films in this area are often difficult to interpret because of overlying bowel gas.

▪ SUGGESTED READING

MATAMEDI K, ILASLAN H, SEEGER LL: Imaging of the lumbar spine neoplasms. Semin Ultrasound CT MR 25(6):474–489, 2004.

RESNICK D: Diagnosis of Bone and Joint Disorders. 4th ed. Vol. 3. Philadelphia: W.B. Saunders. 2203–2205, 2718–2721, 2002.

WHITEHOUSE RW: Paget's disease of bone. Semin Musculoskelet Radiol 6(4):313–322, 2002.

Index

Page numbers in *italics* refer to illustrations; page numbers followed by t refer to tables